Advance Praise for
Interpretive Phenomenology in Health Care Research

"This collection takes us far along the path to wholeness in nursing science by articulating important and meaningful stories that are often overlooked in the quest for generalization and normalization. Anyone who thinks science is alienating and disconnected from human life will appreciate the recontextualized picture this book offers. And those who think rational empiricism has the whole story will have their eyes opened to what is missing."

–LISA DAY, PHD, RN, CNS
CLINICAL NURSE SPECIALIST
NEUROSCIENCE AND CRITICAL CARE
UNIVERSITY OF CALIFORNIA,
SAN FRANCISCO MEDICAL CENTER

"Bravo! A much needed cutting-edge phenomenological exploration of care-giving in the contemporary moment. Flying in the face of managerial demands for cool efficiency, these remarkable nurses instead propose full engagement with patients as situated and embodied persons. An invaluable guide to grasping the world as experienced, reclaiming health-caring across specialties."

–ADELE E. CLARKE, PHD
PROFESSOR OF SOCIOLOGY
UNIVERSITY OF CALIFORNIA, SAN FRANCISCO
CO-EDITOR, *BIOSOCIETIES*

"No one has done more to enhance our understanding of caring practices than Patricia Benner, whose groundbreaking work and its influence is richly presented in *Interpretive Phenomenology in Health Care Research*. It represents the fruits of an intellectual community at work, pushing our understanding of caring and patient and family lifeworlds into new, enriched dimensions. The volume's solid presentation of interpretive phenomenology, together with empirical case studies, extends its relevance far beyond nursing to the many other disciplines conducting research in health care.

–DEBORAH R. GORDON, PHD
DEPARTMENT OF ANTHROPOLOGY, HISTORY, AND SOCIAL MEDICINE
UNIVERISTY OF CALIFORNIA, SAN FRANCISCO
CO-EDITOR, *BIOMEDICINE EXAMINED*

INTERPRETIVE PHENOMENOLOGY
IN HEALTH CARE RESEARCH

GARRETT K. CHAN, PhD, RN, FAEN, FPCN
KAREN A. BRYKCZYNSKI, DNSc, RN, FAANP, FAAN
RUTH E. MALONE, PhD, RN, FAAN
PATRICIA BENNER, PhD, RN, FAAN

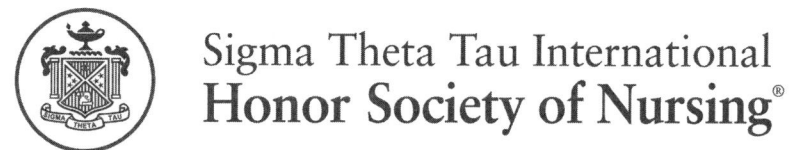

Sigma Theta Tau International
Honor Society of Nursing®

Sigma Theta Tau International

Copyright © 2010 by Sigma Theta Tau International

All rights reserved. This book is protected by copyright. No part of it may be reproduced, stored in a retrieval system, or transmitted in any form or by any means, electronic, mechanical, photocopying, recording, or otherwise, without written permission from the publisher.

Any trademarks, service marks, design rights, or similar rights that are mentioned, used, or cited in this book are the property of their respective owners. Their use here does not imply that you may use them for similar or any other purpose.

Sigma Theta Tau International
550 West North Street
Indianapolis, IN 46202

To order additional books, buy in bulk, or order for corporate use, contact Nursing Knowledge International at 888.NKI.4YOU (888.654.4968/US and Canada) or +1.317.634.8171 (outside US and Canada).

To request a review copy for course adoption, e-mail solutions@nursingknowledge.org or call 888.NKI.4YOU (888.654.4968/US and Canada) or +1.317.917.4983 (outside US and Canada).

To request author information, or for speaker or other media requests, contact Rachael McLaughlin of the Honor Society of Nursing, Sigma Theta Tau International at 888.634.7575 (US and Canada) or +1.317.634.8171 (outside US and Canada).

ISBN-13: 978-1-930538-88-7

Library of Congress Cataloging-in-Publication Data
Interpretive phenomenology for health care researchers : studying social practice, lifeworlds, and embodiment / Garrett Chan ... [et al.].
    p. ; cm.
  Includes bibliographical references and index.
  ISBN 978-1-930538-88-7 (alk. paper)
 1. Nursing--Research. 2. Experiential research. 3. Phenomenology. 4. Medical care--Research. I. Chan, Garrett, 1970- II. Sigma Theta Tau International.
  [DNLM: 1. Nursing Care--methods. 2. Nursing Methodology Research--methods. 3. Nurse-Patient Relations. 4. Nursing Care--psychology. 5. Philosophy, Nursing. 6. Qualitative Research. WY 20.5 I6194 2010]
  RT81.5.I584 2010
  610.73072--dc22
                                                    2010001970

First Printing, 2010

Publisher: Renee Wilmeth
Acquisitions Editor: Cynthia Saver, RN, MS
Editorial Coordinator: Paula Jeffers
Cover Designer: Gary Adair
Interior Design and Page Composition: Rebecca Batchelor

Principal Editor: Carla Hall
Development Editor: Teresa Artman
Proofreader: Linda Seifert
Indexer: Johnna VanHoose Dinse

DEDICATIONS

To Patricia Benner for her pioneering work and body of scholarship that created a new way to understand nursing and caring practices.

To all past, present, and future interpretive phenomenologists who open up possibilities by articulating lifeworlds.

And, to my partner, Russ McLaren, for being a tremendous support during my journeys.

—GARRETT K. CHAN

To Herbert L. Dreyfus a phenomenal teacher and philosopher par excellence.

To my teacher, Patricia Benner, whose work has inspired me and guided my research trajectory.

To my father, Casimir H. Brykczynski, whose steadfastness I have admired and tried to emulate.

To my dear mother, Emma, whose smile and consistent positive outlook have enabled me to persevere during many challenging times.

—KAREN A. BRYKCZYNSKI

To all my teachers in nursing, beginning with my mother and including my students from whom I learn so much.

—RUTH E. MALONE

This book is dedicated to the outstanding doctoral and post-doctoral students with whom I have had the privilege of working over the past 30 years. You remain a source of inspiration and truly colleagues in a wonderful scholarly community!

—PATRICIA BENNER

ABOUT THE AUTHORS

Michael Acree, PhD—Chapter 16

Michael Acree, PhD, is director of the Biostatistics Core at the Osher Center and research specialist in the Department of Medicine at the University of California, San Francisco. He obtained his doctorate from Clark University in psychology, and he has worked primarily in research and teaching as a methodologist and biostatistician. He has taught both graduate statistics and qualitative research methods for 13 years and is completing a book on the history and philosophy of statistical inference. Acree is also developing methodologies for the study of alternative and complementary medicine.

Patricia Benner, RN, PhD, FAAN, FRCN—Introduction and Chapter 7

Patricia Benner, RN, PhD, FAAN, FRCN is professor emerita from the University of California, San Francisco. She is currently a visiting professor at the University of Pennsylvania, School of Nursing, for the 2009 fall semester. Benner received her bachelor's degree in nursing from Pasadena College (now Point Loma Nazarene University), her master's degree in medical surgical nursing from the University of California, San Francisco, and her PhD from the University of California, Berkeley, in stress and coping and health, under the direction of Hubert Dreyfus and Richard Lazarus.

Benner is a noted nursing educator and has just completed the first national nursing education study in 30 years under the auspices of the Carnegie Foundation for the Advancement of Teaching. She is involved in a large collaborative research study with The Tri-Service Military Nursing Research, with Captain Maggie Richards, on the new knowledge developed and experiential learning in the Iraq and Afghanistan Wars. Her work has had wide influence on nursing, both in the United States and internationally. She is a Fellow of the American Academy of Nursing, and she was elected an honorary fellow of the Royal College of Nursing. Her work has influence beyond nursing in the areas of clinical practice, clergy education, and clinical ethics. She has received two honorary doctorates. She is the author of *From Novice to Expert* and 12 other notable books. Her latest book, *Educating Nurses: A Call for Radical Transformation*, co-authored with Molly Sutphen, Victoria Leonard, and Lisa Day, was published by the Carnegie Foundation for the Advancement of Teaching and Learning and Jossey-Bass Publishing Company.

Karen A. Brykczynski, RN, DNSc, FNP, FAANP, FAAN—Chapters 7 and 8

Karen A. Brykczynski, RN, DNSc, FNP, FAANP, FAAN, is professor at the University of Texas Medical Branch (UTMB) School of Nursing in Galveston, Texas. She teaches in the Master's Advanced Practice Nursing Program. The findings from her interpretive phenomenological study of the clinical practice of nurse practitioners served as the underlying framework for the National Organization of Nurse Practitioner Faculties curriculum guidelines and were applied by the American Association of Colleges of Nursing in developing The Master's Essentials. Her current research investigating how nurse practitioner faculty incorporate the holistic dimensions of nursing practice into nurse practitioner education was sponsored by an educational research grant from the National League for Nursing. Her current faculty practice consists of providing primary health care to underserved individuals at a free nursing clinic established by the UTMB School of Nursing. She received her Bachelor of Science in Nursing and Master of Science in Nursing from Adelphi University School of Nursing in New York and her Doctor of Nursing Science in Family Health Care Nursing from the University of California, San Francisco, School of Nursing. Her post-masters Family Nurse Practitioner preparation was from the University of Colorado Health Sciences Center's School of Nursing in Denver, Colorado, which she completed as a Robert Wood Johnson Nurse Faculty Fellow in Primary Care.

Garrett K. Chan, APRN, PhD, FAEN, FPCN—Introduction and Chapter 6

Garrett K. Chan, APRN, PhD, FAEN, FPCN is an assistant clinical professor at the University of California, San Francisco, lead advanced practice nurse and associate medical director in the Emergency Department Observation Unit, and relief clinical nurse specialist in the Palliative Care Service at Stanford Hospital & Clinics. His program of research and clinical practice focuses on palliative care in the emergency department (ED). He uses interpretive phenomenology and quantitative methodologies to investigate his phenomena of interest. His current research will investigate the symptom management and genomics of acute dyspnea in the ED. Chan received his Bachelor of Science in Nursing from San José State University and his master's and PhD from the University of California, San Francisco. He is a Fellow in the Academy of Emergency Nursing and in the Hospice and Palliative Nurses Association.

Catherine A. Chesla, RN, DNSc, FAAN—Chapter 1

Catherine A. Chesla, RN, DNSc, FAAN, is professor and Thelma Shobe Endowed Chair in Ethics and Spirituality at the School of Nursing at the University of California, San Francisco (UCSF), where she teaches in the master's and doctoral nursing program and conducts research. Teaching foci include family theory and research and interpretive phenomenological research approaches. Her research focuses on family caring practices in those living with chronic illness in ethnically diverse families. Her current National Institutes of Health-funded research is a community based participatory research project that establishes a partnership between UCSF with two Chinatown service agencies to adapt and test a family-focused cognitive behavioral intervention for Chinese immigrants with type 2 diabetes.

Susan Folkman, PhD—Chapter 16

Susan Folkman, PhD, is the director of the Osher Center for Integrative Medicine and the Osher Foundation Distinguished Professor of Integrative Medicine at the University of California, San Francisco (UCSF). She has also been professor of medicine at UCSF since 1990, and from 1994 until 2001 she was co-director of the UCSF Center for AIDS Prevention Studies (CAPS). Folkman received her PhD from the University of California at Berkeley. She is internationally recognized for her theoretical and empirical contributions to the field of psychological stress and coping. Her work since 1988 has focused on stress and coping in the context of HIV disease and other chronic illness, especially on issues having to do with caregiving and bereavement.

Steffanie Goodman, MPH—Chapter 16

Steffanie Goodman, MPH, is clinical research manager at the Osher Center for Integrative Medicine where she has worked in program development and research for 5 years. She graduated magna cum laude from the University of Vermont and earned a master's in public health from Columbia University's Mailman School of Public Health. Goodman's academic experience includes the development and instruction of university and graduate level curriculum in eco-psychology and integrative medicine. Her professional experience includes coordination and implementation of multiple research studies, serving as liaison for the Osher Center research department and development and implementation of health education programs.

Annemarie Kesselring, RN, PhD—Chapter 1

Annemarie Kesselring, RN, PhD, did her nursing training in Switzerland and received her Bachelor of Science in Nursing, Master of Science, and PhD at the University of California, San Francisco. She used qualitative research methods in her program of research that focused on embodied experiences of women living with breast cancer and families' decisions surrounding organ donation of a brain-dead family member. She is an associate professor emerita at the University of Basel, Switzerland, where she was one of the two professors responsible for opening the first university program for nursing science.

Christine Kinavey, RN, PhD, CNS—Chapter 12

Christine Kinavey, RN, PhD, CNS, is an assistant adjunct professor in the Department of Family Health Care Nursing and the Department of Social and Behavioral Sciences at the University of California, San Francisco, and a clinical nurse specialist in the Regional Spina Bifida Program, Kaiser Oakland Medical Center, Department of Genetics, Oakland, California.

Vickie Leonard, RN, PhD, FNP—Chapter 1

Vickie Leonard, RN, PhD, FNP, currently works at the California Childcare Health Program, a community-based program of the University of California, San Francisco (UCSF) School of Nursing that is funded by the California Department of Education to improve health and safety practices and the well-being of children in child care in California. She is a clinical nurse specialist in maternal and child health and a nurse practitioner who has also worked with children in both primary care and subspecialty clinic settings. She was a research associate for the Carnegie Foundation for the Advancement of Teaching's national study of nursing education, *Educating Nurses: A Call for Radical Transformation*, directed by Patricia Benner. She earned her Master of Science in Nursing and PhD from the University of California, San Francisco.

Richard MacIntyre, RN, PhD, FAAN—Chapter 13

Richard MacIntyre, RN, PhD, FAAN, teaches courses in community health, research, and health policy, and is working with a team of Robert Wood Johnson (RWJ) fellows on diffusion of innovation in clinical nursing education. He served as associate dean for nursing at Samuel Merritt University from 2005-2007 with responsibility for the school's second degree programs and learning centers in San Francisco, San Mateo, and Sacramento. Previously MacIntyre served as the division chair for Health Professions at Mercy College, New York. During that time, he was elected secretary and then president of the Council of Deans of Nursing, Senior Colleges, and Universities in New York State and was a member of the American Association of Colleges of Nursing (AACN) Task Force on the Nursing Faculty Shortage, the National Leadership Council of the Association of Nurses in AIDS Care (ANAC), and served on the editorial board of the Journal of the Association of Nurses in AIDS Care. MacIntyre was a member of the original group that developed the ANAC standards for treating anemia in patients with HIV/AIDS and is a frequent national and international lecturer on complementary and alternative medicine and HIV/AIDS. His publications include a book on asymptomatic HIV written while a Fulbright professor at the University of Tromsø, Norway, and subsequently published by Rutgers University Press. MacIntyre was the founding chair of the American Association of Colleges of Nursing Organizational Leadership Network and is a Fellow of the American Academy of Nursing.

Ruth E. Malone, RN, PhD, FAAN—Chapter 3

Ruth E. Malone, RN, PhD, FAAN, is professor and vice chair, Department of Social & Behavioral Sciences, School of Nursing, University of California, San Francisco. Her current research focuses on tobacco control and the activities of the multinational tobacco companies. She has utilized interpretive research approaches in secondary theoretical analyses and in analyzing archival documents, interview and focus group data in multiple studies funded by the National Institutes of Health and the California Tobacco-Related Disease Research Program. Her theoretical interests center on how corporate entities and other institutions structure public health and health care practices.

Susan McNiesh, RNC-OB, PhD—Chapter 2

Susan McNiesh, RNC-OB, PhD, is an assistant professor in the School of Nursing at San Jose State University where she teaches in the baccalaureate, RN- BSN, and masters degree programs. Her specialty area is maternal-child nursing. She received her PhD from the University of California, San Francisco, and her doctoral work used interpretive phenomenological methods towards an understanding of how students in an accelerated nursing program took up the practice of nursing. Her research interests continue to focus on experiential nursing with a current focus on RN- BSN transitions and the role of simulation in experiential learning.

Karen Plager, RN, DNSc, FNP-BC—Chapter 10

Karen Plager, RN, DNSc, FNP-BC, is a professor at Northern Arizona University School of Nursing. She is a family nurse practitioner (FNP), teaches primarily graduate course work in family nursing, family primary care, and advanced health assessment, and coordinates the Family Nurse Practitioner track. She received her FNP (1989) and DNSc (1995) from the University of California San Francisco, where she studied family nursing, primary care, and hermeneutic phenomenology. She is involved in international nursing education through work in Madagascar (since 2005). She is also involved in developing study abroad opportunities for nursing and other health professional students, including helping develop a public and environmental health field study course in Kenya. She has also done qualitative research and published on outcomes assessment of master's nursing graduates.

Bonnie Raingruber, RN, PhD—Chapter 9

Bonnie Raingruber, RN, PhD, is a nurse reseacher and associate professor of Internal Medicine at the University of California, Davis. She is a professor of nursing and director of the Center for Health and Human Services at California State University, Sacramento. Raingruber teaches clinical reasoning, cooperative education, and mental health nursing. She serves on the American Nurses Credentialing Center's content expert panel in child adolescent mental health. Raingruber has written more than 75 publications and is the author of *Using Your Head To Land On Your Feet: Developing Critical Thinking and Clinical Reasoning Skills as a Beginning Practitioner.* Her program of research focuses on workforce development, obesity prevention, and alternative and complementary interventions for cancer patients. She received both her doctorate and master's degree from the University of California, San Francisco, where she was awarded dissertation of the year in 1998. Her bachelor's degree in nursing was from California State University, Chico.

Carol Robinson, RN, MPA, CNAA, FAAN—Chapter 9

Carol Robinson, RN, MPA, CNAA, FAAN, is the Chief Patient Care Services Officer/Director of Nursing for the University of California Davis Health System, located in Sacramento, California. Robinson received her Bachelor of Science in Nursing from the University of Virginia, Charlottesville, in 1973 and her Master in Public Administration from the University of San Francisco, San Francisco, California, in 1986. Carol became a fellow in the Johnson & Johnson/Wharton Fellows Program in Management for Nurse Executives in 1996 and a Fellow in the American Academy of Nursing in 2002. She has served as the director of Nursing and associate director of Hospital and Clinics at the University of California, Davis Medical Center (UCDMC) since 1991. Her accomplishments during the course of her career include leading the team to achieve designation as a Magnet Hospital, developing the UCDMC Level I Trauma Center Program, and chairing the committee on the development of the Davis Tower Building devoted to patient care.

Lee SmithBattle, RN, DNSc—Chapter 11

Lee SmithBattle, RN, DNSc, is a professor of Nursing at the School of Nursing at Saint Louis University in St. Louis, Missouri. She has conducted studies on teenage childbearing and the development of public health nursing expertise. She has also introduced and studied innovative approaches in nursing undergraduate education. Her studies have been funded by the National Institutes of Health, the American Nurses Foundation, and Sigma Theta Tau International. She has interviewed one sample of teen mothers and their families every four years for 16 years and has published more than 30 articles in nursing and interdisciplinary journals. She teaches doctoral courses on knowledge development from a philosophical perspective and qualitative research methods. She also teaches an undergraduate elective on teenage sexuality that has incorporated team-based learning and the development of dramatic performances based on students' interviews with teens.

Elisabeth Spichiger, RN, PhD—Chapter 15

Elisabeth Spichiger, RN, PhD, is a research associate and lecturer at the Institute of Nursing Science at the University of Basel, Switzerland, where she teaches in the bachelor's and master's nursing programs and conducts research. She is also a scientific collaborator at the Inselspital Bern University Hospital, Switzerland, where she is responsible for promoting practice development and nursing research. Her teaching focuses on qualitative research. Using an interpretive phenomenological approach, she explored patients' and families' experiences with hospital end-of-life care. Her current research focus is on symptom management in patients with cancer.

Cynthia Stuhlmiller RN, MS, DNSc—Chapter 5

Cynthia Stuhlmiller RN, MS, DNSc, is adjunct nursing faculty at Daemen College, Buffalo, New York, and affiliate graduate faculty in public health at the University of Hawaii (UH) where she previously held collaborative professorial appointments between the Department of Human Services and UH School of Social Work (2008-2009), the UH Mental Health

Services Research Evaluation Training Program and UH Department of Public Health (2007-2008), and the Hawaii Department of Health, Mental Health Division and UH School of Nursing (2004-2007). She was professor and foundation chair of mental health nursing at Flinders University South Australia (2000-2005), and University of Technology, Sydney Australia (1997-2000). Stuhlmiller was a Fulbright Senior Scholar in Tromsø, Norway (1993), and has been faculty in Norway, New Zealand, and the United States. Her clinical background in mental health includes work with a variety of populations. She is a pioneer in the treatment of post traumatic stress disorder (PTSD), having helped found the first National Center for PTSD in Menlo Park, California (1981-1993). She is known for her work with emergency workers, disaster survivors, action-based therapies, experiential learning, and most recently computer-aided cognitive behavioral therapy.

Helena Sunvisson, RN, PhD—Chapter 4

Helena Sunvisson, RN, PhD, works as a senior lecturer in the nursing program in the School of Health and Medical Sciences at Örebro University in Sweden. She holds courses for patients with Parkinson's disease and their families in the Neurology Department in the Örebro University Hospital. Her research, using mainly qualitative research methods, focuses on patients' and carers' experiences of neurological diseases and palliative care. Current research concerns include understanding cultural meanings of dementia in Sweden and Iran from the viewpoint of the patient, the informal carer, and nurses using interpretive phenomenological approaches. She is also interested in understanding how creative dancing twice weekly influences adolescent girls' wellbeing using a randomized controlled trial intervention.

Sara Manny Weiss, RN, PhD—Chapter 14

Sara Manny Weiss, RN, PhD, is a staff nurse on the Inpatient Behavioral Health Unit at Marin General Hospital, Marin County, California. She was an assistant professor of Nursing at Sacramento State University and the project director for the San Francisco Adult Day Services Outcomes Study, funded by eight private foundations, prior to her current appointment. She received her Bachelor of Science in Nursing, her Master of Science in Adult Psychiatric Nursing, and her PhD from the University of California, San Francisco.

Judith Wrubel, PhD—Chapter 16

Judith Wrubel, PhD, is research specialist at the Osher Center for Integrative Medicine at the University of California, San Francisco (UCSF). She received her PhD in Human Development and Aging at UCSF. She has worked for 30 years as a qualitative analyst specializing in interpretive phenomenology and has served as co-investigator and lead qualitative analyst on numerous studies, including longitudinal studies of caregivers of people newly diagnosed with HIV, and of people with serious and terminal illnesses. Her book, *The Primacy of Caring: Stress and Coping in Health and Illness*, which she co-authored with Patricia Benner, is a groundbreaking work that examines the lived experience of illness. The book, a winner of the American Journal of Nursing Book of the Year Award in two categories, has been translated into four languages and is used as a basis for curricula in nursing schools and as a text for anthropology and medicine courses.

TABLE OF CONTENTS

About the Authors IV
Foreword XV
Introduction XVII

Part 1 Interpretive Phenomenology: Theory and Practice   **1**

1 Why Study Caring Practices? 3

2 A Fusion of Horizons: Meaning and Understanding in Becoming a Nurse 23

3 Distal Nursing 41

4 Research and Ontology: Neurology and Parkinson's Disease Sufferers' Lived Experiences of Embodiment and Dwelling in Lifeworlds 59

5 Health, Disorder, and the Psychiatric Enterprise: Reclaiming Lost Connections 75

6 Understanding End-of-Life Caring Practices in the Emergency Department 91

7 The Living Tradition of Interpretive Phenomenology 113

Part 2 Interpretive Phenomenological Studies   **143**

8 Articulating, Preserving, and Promoting Holistic Aspects of Nurse Practitioner Practice 145

9   Sustaining Purpose and Motivation: Weaving Caring and Self-Care Together in Nursing Practice 169

10 Sustaining Family Life and Health Through Rituals, Routines, and Practices in Well Families with School-Age Children 195

11 Listening with Care to Teen Mothers and Their Families 217

12 Life-Course Considerations for Adolescents Born with Spina Bifida: Toward Authentic Care and Transparency of the Other 243

13 Our Patients: Heretics, Believers, Agnostics, and Ecumenists. 259

14 Dwelling in the World: Realms of Meaningful Involvement in Late Life. 287

15 Patients' and Family Members' Experiences of Hospital End-of-Life Care 313

16 End of Living: Maintaining a Lifeworld During Terminal Illness 337

    Index. 359

FOREWORD

Any volume with Patricia Benner as an author or editor is noteworthy. She has expanded the thinking of the nursing profession for decades, beginning with her 1984 book, *From Novice to Expert*. This book describes how nurses, because they belong to a practice profession, grow from novice to expert with experience. Before that work, the simplistic perception within and around the profession was that new graduates should be able to begin their careers fully formed. Publication of *From Novice to Expert* brought about a renewed appreciation for the complexity of becoming a nursing professional. Only by fully understanding the intricacies of career development could the profession begin to envision new ways of facilitating that advancement.

In opening nurses' minds to the generative powers of understanding those intricacies, Benner helped lead a worldwide movement that questioned decontextualization—a focus on main effects, even if the basics do not hold for every population or situation—in favor of a view that values interaction effects and looks at individuals embedded in their family, social, cultural, ethnic, and work environments. This focus on the similarities and differences that constitute the "lived experience" has led to all sorts of new insights, not the least of which is an appreciation for the complexities shaping women's health (McBride & McBride, 1981). When one gives up expecting to find only one pattern and stops trying to fit every patient into that mold, creativity is more likely to be unleashed, and the likelihood of finding an appropriate intervention is increased.

In 1994, Benner edited the first volume of readings in interpretive phenomenology, which provided an assortment of examples of how rich clinical understandings become when one takes people's lived experiences seriously. And now, thankfully, *Interpretive Phenomenology in Health Care Research* embraces the complexities of caring—balancing the tensions all nurses feel between task and relationship, between continuity and change, between efficiency and effectiveness, and between standardization and customization. Benner's work, as a whole, criticizes the commoditization of caring by reminding us to examine the meaning that patients make of their experiences for new insights into how to achieve quality care. The various narratives that constitute this volume prove the richness of this strategy and bear witness to the therapeutic value that patients and professionals alike find in that meaning.

Interpretive Phenomenology in Health Care Research is also important because it was first developed as a Festschrift to celebrate Benner's work upon her retirement from the University of California, San Francisco. In other fields, a *Festschrift* has long been the highest honor that one's students and colleagues can pay a pioneering thinker, because it is a book-length tribute to the person's work. Typically, such a book reflects on the person's contributions, discusses work undertaken in the spirit of the contributions, extends the ideas to discuss new situations, and often includes comments by the honoree. *Festschrifts* have been rare in the nursing profession. Only one comes to mind—a book published by Sigma Theta Tau International that celebrates the work of Virginia Henderson (Herman, 1998). *Interpretive Phenomenology in Health Care Research*, then, is a hopeful sign of how much progress the profession has made in recent decades to have nurses with a body of scholarship substantial enough to merit such reflection and extension.

This book comes at a good time, because the nursing world is catching up to Benner and her colleagues in appreciating the value of complexity (Lindberg, Nash, & Lindberg, 2008). There is renewed appreciation for the idea that mechanical thinking is not effective in meeting today's challenges. The world of nursing—hospitals and other clinical and community agencies, universities, and businesses—is complex, interconnected, interdependent, and diverse. Thus, the approach taken by Benner and colleagues—with its emphasis on respect, connection, sense-making, information exchange, and empowerment—is more important in the 21st century than it was when Benner began her nursing career in the 20th century.

–ANGELA BARRON MCBRIDE, PHD, RN, FAAN
DISTINGUISHED PROFESSOR AND UNIVERSITY DEAN EMERITA
INDIANA UNIVERSITY SCHOOL OF NURSING
PAST PRESIDENT, SIGMA THETA TAU INTERNATIONAL (1987-89)

References

Benner, P. (1984). *From novice to expert: Excellence and power in clinical nursing practice*. Menlo Park: Addison-Wesley.

Benner, P. (Ed.). (1994). *Interpretive phenomenology: Embodiment, caring, and ethics in health and illness*. Thousand Oaks, CA: Sage.

Herman, E. K. (Ed.). (1998). *Virginia Avenel Henderson: Signature for nursing*. Indianapolis, IN: Sigma Theta Tau International.

Lindberg, C., Nash, S., & Lindberg, C. (Eds.). (2008). *On the edge: Nursing in the age of complexity*. Bordentown, NJ: Plexus Press.

McBride, A. B., & McBride, W. L. (1981). *Theoretical underpinnings for women's health*. Women and Health, 6(1/2), 37-55.

INTRODUCTION

PATRICIA BENNER AND GARRETT K. CHAN

Taken collectively, this book of interpretive phenomenology (IP) studies reveals in intimate, descriptive, and interpretive accounts what it means to be human and what is common to human lives. Human beings are curious about ourselves and the world we live in. These curiosities about the phenomena that constitute and are constituted by our being in the world have led scientists to ask questions to understand our world. Scientists in the qualitative research community have developed many methodologies, or, "how do we know the world or gain knowledge of it" (Denzin & Lincoln, 2000, p. 19) to understand and interpret the world. The type of research questions and lines of inquiry drive qualitative research methodology. In many forms of rational-technical research, the goal is to make generalizations through decontextualizing particular events and phenomena, take a historical view of their occurrence, break them down to their most elemental or atomistic level, and then create a theoretical system to tie them back together again. This is a powerful and useful strategy, but it necessarily overlooks the person *in* the situation, the context, the intents, particular content and meanings, and relational intertwining of events and persons.

While qualitative research methodologies have roots in both the positivist and interpretive traditions (e.g., History, Dilthey, Law, and Hermeneutic studies of sacred texts), phenomenologists have turned away from an epistemological approach to personhood because of their built-in Cartesian interpretation of what it is to be a human being. Descartes believed that answering the epistemological question of how a person knew things, the ontological question of how a person was or existed, could be answered or rendered irrelevant (Benner & Wrubel, 1989). Phenomenologists have turned toward ontological questions of understanding the human embodied, lived experience and the background concerns, habits, practices, relational qualities, and skills in actual situations that make up human being and human worlds (Benner, 1994; Dreyfus, 1991; Heidegger, 1927/1962; Merleau-Ponty, 1945/2001).

Heidegger's (1927/1962) phenomenological view on the nature of being a person proposes that humans are self-interpreting beings. When we are born into this world, we come into a pre-existing world that has meaningful contexts and practices. Social identity and membership constitutes the person prior to any individual identity and private subjective existence. Over the course of living a life in a world with meaningful contexts and practices, humans are constituted as they come into an already formed lifeworld (i.e., culture, language, family, community, society, and so on) (Benner & Wrubel, 1989). These pervasive taken-for-granted skills, practices, and meanings go largely unnoticed by human beings because they both constitute the person and make the world intelligible to persons creating possibilities and conditions for actions (Leonard, 1994). Heidegger asserts that a person has an effortless, nonreflective understanding of self in the world because the person is always situated in a meaningful context and because the person "grasp[s] meaning directly" through being born into and formed by a pre-existing world (Benner & Wrubel, 1989, p. 41). In contrast, in the goal of abstract or conceptual thinking, the person purposefully stands outside of the situation. This is an epistemological stance highly valued in Western society. Human beings, however, are always situated (in a culture, a historical time, and lodged in particular social relationships), and most of a person's being occurs in this engaged activity. Interpretive phenomenology (IP) is interested in illuminating the kind of knowing that occurs when one is involved in a particular world and social situation rather than standing outside of it as an onlooker (Benner & Wrubel, 1989).

Traditional rationalist inquiry attempts to uncover a world that is constituted by formal abstractions with an underlying structure governed by rules, axioms, and principles to guide action in everyday life (Packer & Addison, 1989). The model of the person, both the researcher and the one being researched, is that of a disengaged knower standing over against an objective world. The researcher is detached and abstracts a theory from the phenomenon and shared understandings, practices, and meanings. The context is stripped away from the phenomenon as it is considered irrelevant and possibly obscuring the important underlying structures. This clearing of the context distorts the phenomenon (Taylor, 1985) and, in particular, denies access to praxis. "The practical activity is intrinsically linked to its context and has a complex temporal organization" (Packer & Addison, 1989, p. 19).

Classical empiricism holds that the world is constituted by independent entities that possess absolute, measurable, and context-free properties independent of human concerns and practices (Packer & Addison, 1989). Empiricist inquiry attempts to measure the entity's properties and discover the laws that cause interaction between entities. A de-contextualized, rational, and atomistic view of the world does not allow for a full understanding of lifeworlds where humans are members and participants in a historical, cultural, and familial world and engaged in particular relationships and activities guided by meanings and concerns of the actors (Benner & Wrubel, 1989; Leonard, 1994). Rational-empirical methods remove human emotions, senses, and nuances from the research as they are deemed irrelevant and possibly over-shadowing important underlying objective structures or the outside, context-free reality (Packer & Addison, 1989).

Because of human concerns, actions, and the complexity of a human life, qualitative distinctions and the lived experience of the phenomenon cannot be fully captured or described by fragmented, objective, elemental empirical science (Benner & Wrubel, 1989; van Manen, 1990). Importantly, knowledge of our life world is not well articulated or understood if we engage only in elemental rational empirical science (Fjelland & Gjengedal, 1994). Interpretive phenomenology fills gaps in understanding that are left by rational-empirical science research approaches and offers us plausible insights that bring us in more direct contact with the lived world, engaged activities, concerns, and embodied know-how and understanding (Plager, 1994; van Manen, 1990). Understanding context-bound and situated lifeworlds and lived experiences of human beings are the goals of interpretive projects (Packer & Addison, 1989).

Imaginative responses can be developed by nurses from reading these first-person accounts of the lived experiences of birthing, learning, parenting, skillful capacities within a social practice, and social dwelling within a lifeworld. This second book of readings on IP comes 16 years after the first edited book of readings on interpretive phenomenology (*Interpretive Phenomenology: Embodiment, Caring, and Ethics in Health and Illness*, Benner, 1994). Both books reveal the social lifeworld that is excluded in a "clinical" model of diagnosing pathology or finding "coping deficits": that is, focusing on the alteration or absence of normal, healthy coping, a stance called "normalizing" Foucault (1973/1974). Collectively, the readings in this book affirm that until one knows what the person's coping concern is—what the stakes and limitations are—one cannot judge coping efficacy nor understand situated cognition and interpersonal concerns.

Normalizing discourses—that is, identifying deficits related to a norm or standard (Foucault, 1973/1994)—makes understanding the human experience of illness difficult. Numerous nursing-care implications become evident as a result of understanding what persons with illness, disabilities, or a sense of stigma confront in their lived experience of recovery and coping with illness or disability. Nurses can find ways to connect with the human experience of illness as shaped by the concerns and coping issues of a person living with a disability, a chronic or acute illness, or an injury in a particular lifeworld. Each chapter in this book can create an enriched clinical imagination for all caregivers, both formal and informal. Careful articulation and understanding of the lived experience of aging, illness, and disability open new strategies for patient's and nurse's situated possibilities, caregiving, coaching, and patient education (Benner & Wrubel, 1989).

The goal of putting together this group of readings, apart from presenting theories and research findings that have much to offer in guiding nursing practice, is to demonstrate the positive project of IP which is to make the person *in context*: that is, persons engaged in skillful activity, relationships, practices, and habits all within a particular social lifeworld, making it more accessible and visible.

This book is testimony to a lively connected group of concerned scholars who formed both a virtual and face-to-face scholarly community and tradition. All were interested in how ontological structures of concerns and care set up human lifeworlds where things stood out as more or less important, and also shaped meanings of illness, disability, finitude, and the situated possibilities of human responses to illness. Inherently, this body of work focuses on what gets passed over in the highly successful project of Cartesian Medicine to study disease at the cellular, tissue, organ, genomic, and biochemical levels. This work does not take an oppositional stance against medical achievements, elevating one and devaluing the other. Indeed, the stories within this work show that nurses participate fully in medical care historically and daily. The larger goal of this work is an attempt to enlarge the scholarly discourse about rationality; embodiment; lifeworld, with a beginning assumption that all are intertwined with the human experience of illness; embodied vulnerabilities; development; growth; finitude; possibility; and despair.

In addition to deliberative, thoughtful intentionality, human beings are endowed with embodied intentionality and tacit intentionality and even a nonagential social intentionality that stems from social communities, rituals, and practices, and taken-for-granted background meanings that come into play in practical situations of skilled know-how and skilled dwelling in meaningful human worlds. For example, an aged person with failing memory can be sustained by a community who shares many of the person's life experiences. These social aspects of our common humanity are accessible and intelligible only when we enter people's lifeworlds and study those persons as they are engaged in meaningful projects and contexts.

Part I: Interpretive Phenomenology: Theory and Practice

Chapters in Part I will explore additional theoretical and philosophical discourses and debates within interpretive phenomenology that began with Benner's work in *Interpretive Phenomenology: Embodiment, Caring, and Ethics in Health and Illness* (1994). Additionally, these chapters offer guidance when considering interpretive phenomenology as an interpretive approach focused on studying and articulating human phenomena particularly within health and health care. All chapters in Parts I and II underwent a process similar to a topic-specific journal such as *The Clinics of North America* and *Advances in Nursing Science*. Chapters were peer-reviewed by at least two editors, and comments were shared with the authors. The authors revised and resubmitted their manuscripts prior to acceptance for inclusion in the book.

Chapter 1: Why Study Caring Practices?

Kesselring, Chesla, and Leonard open the book with a clear articulation of the self-defining and formative aspects of socially embedded caring practices. Human beings are not formed by beliefs, mental representations, and deliberative thought alone. A lifeworld beckons the person and gives social birth. Belonging and being nurtured in an infant/parent relationship sets up the conditions of possibility to exist, and to dwell in the world through connection and relationship. Physical birth is accompanied by social birthing and formation that never ends for the healthy, connected human being. Sharing common taken-for-granted meanings as a result of being a member-participant in a social world can easily be misunderstood in a culture of competitive individualism, or even expressive individualism (Taylor, 1985; 1991). From a stance of expressive individualism, it can seem that "holding common taken for granted meanings" means or refers to *sameness* and conformity of persons holding background meanings in common. However, this is a misinterpretation born of expressive individualism that imagines a self of possession and powers of self-creation apart from social context (Taylor, 1989). Likewise, atomistic individualism and a Cartesian understanding of the person as a private subject who stands alone and over against the world and others (the monological observer) overlook our essential social birthing and our essentially social existence. Instead, participating in taken-for-granted, shared, commonly held meanings is the essential condition for intelligible disagreement and differences within a language and culture, and is also the starting place for meeting the other from a different culture and language group (Gadamer, 1960/1975). Kesselring, Chesla, and Leonard point to ways to bring caring practices from the margins in bureaucratic institutions where the focal practices of caring have been rendered less visible because of the ascendency of a "device paradigm" that, for these authors, includes technical biomedicine (Borgmann, 1984).

Despite the marginality of caring practice, Kesselring, Chesla, and Leonard show that caring practices form the very conditions of possibility for health care. Bureaucracies and managerial practices find it difficult to disclose and acknowledge the role of caring practices in health care because caring practices exist in the skills and dispositions of the persons skilled at caring practices and are less amenable to command and control managerial practices. As Joseph Dunne (1997) points out

> A practice is not just a surface on which one can display instant virtuosity. It grounds one in a tradition that has been formed through an elaborate development and that exists at any juncture only in the dispositions (slowly and perhaps painfully acquired) of its recognized practitioners. (p. 378-380)

Chapter 2: A Fusion of Horizons: Meaning and Understanding in Becoming a Nurse

It is fitting in this collection of research that Susan McNeish gives a careful interpretive, thick description (Geertz, 1987) of how second-degree students take up the practice of nursing: how they are formed by moving from a lay person to gain an insider's perspective on *being* a practitioner. The student in maternal child care, particularly labor and delivery, learns that the human passage of birth can be ignored or passed over by a technological environment. Students must learn to dwell in the technological world while fostering and supporting the meaningful focal practices of giving birth as a human passage. This is possible at first through their own primordial understanding of what it means to dwell in a meaningful world. They grasp first-hand how significant it is in this culture to acknowledge the birth as an advent, a new beginning of a human life; and experientially learn how many ways this human passage and its significance can be usurped by excessive concern about technical interventions. McNeish gives us a glimpse of the formation of clinical imagination in nursing students. Both technology and human caring have a role, but the technology must somehow be tamed to allow for the human passage, and the focal practices of birthing a baby show up in the context of a medicalized hospital setting.

Chapter 3: Distal Nursing

Malone attacks the same problem that nurses encounter in preserving their nursing practice in a highly technical and efficiency-oriented health care delivery system. "Distal nursing" becomes central, and care of the body and relational work in nursing are marginalized as "niceties" that nurses can no longer do in order to be more efficient. Malone argues against the cult of efficiency and reclaims care of the embodied person in her articulation of central, focal nursing practices.

To understand practitioners and caring practices, one has to be able to study the person *in* a social context and also engaged in carrying out the practice. This is amply illustrated throughout this work. Caring practices form the identity, character, and skills of the practitioner, just as the beginning nurse, or parent, or teacher takes up caring, nurturing practices in their halting ways at first, with the intent of supporting and nurturing the one cared for. Because caring practices are ubiquitous, even in their most unnoticed and marginalized state in institutions of health care, they require informed interpretive methods that begin where a self-interpreting being must begin: with their own understanding of a story. Then through dialog, examining parts and whole, and reflecting upon what one is projecting onto the story, much like understanding a literary text, the researcher/reader begins to understand the story in its own terms.

Chapter 4: Research and Ontology: Neurology and Parkinson's Disease Sufferers' Lived Experiences of Embodiment and Dwelling in Lifeworlds

Sunvisson begins to bridge the divide that exists between the pathological description of movement and the understanding of embodied "dwelling in the world" in persons with Parkinson's disease (PD). Sunvisson draws upon the work of Merleau-Ponty (1945/2001) to describe how the environment or situations call the body to move in particular ways. Movement, or motor intention, is more fluid the less the person has to consciously guide movements through single-sequence commands, especially in times of stress or feeling uncertain. However, when persons with PD feel optimistic, happy, amused, or engaged and involved in situations, tremors and sudden immobility are minimized. Healing, then, comes when caregivers pay attention to coping with the environment and situations in addition to the medical treatment for PD. This work offers a breakthrough rough correlation between the lived body experiences of PD and the diagnostic accounts of specific mechanisms of pathology.

Chapter 5: Health, Disorder, and the Psychiatric Enterprise: Reclaiming Lost Connections

Stuhlmiller describes the consequences of ignoring the lifeworld and environment of persons with a mental illness when reducing the person to a set of psychological alterations. She creates a dialog between the psychologizing work of Post-Traumatic Stress Disorder and the everyday understandings and coping of rescue workers in the Loma Prieta (California) earthquake I-880 freeway collapse. The common difficulties of all persons engaged in disasters and war environments is that the trauma itself can be internalized, and boundaries can blur so that the rescuer also becomes a victim of the sights and sounds of the disaster. Unlike war, rescuers at the I-880 freeway collapse were not engulfed in the disaster and danger in the same way that soldiers in a combat zone are. As civilians, rescuers can effectively use their everyday meanings and sayings to help them deal with the tragedies that they observe. They can return to an intact home and family situation unlike soldiers who must stay in a combat zone. Stuhlmiller raises the provocative challenge of how "overly identifying" helping with danger of a disease, such as Post-Traumatic Stress Disorder disrupts the lifeworld resources embedded in meanings and the coping of helping others during a tragedy. She also notes the dangers of creating an unwitting epidemic of Seasonal Affective Disorder (SAD) that disrupts cultural practices and meanings developed to dwell in the darktime of winter in northern areas. Not everyone suffers to the same extent by lack of sunlight during the winter time.

However, the diagnosis itself, can override the protective effects of extra socializing, use of candlelight, exercise, and rituals to celebrate the season of rest and await the reawakening of spring.

Stuhlmiller's point is that a diagnostic psychologizing culture can disrupt the usual coping resources of the local cultural practices embedded in a shared lifeworld. Stuhlmiller's work illustrates the possibility of critique, and deconstruction through better understanding human and lifeworld possibilities outside the usual normalizing discourses.

Chapter 6: Understanding End-of-Life Caring Practices in the Emergency Department: Developing Merleau-Ponty's Notions of Intentional Arc and Maximum Grip through Praxis and Phronesis

Chan's interpretive ethnography in an Emergency Department opens an understanding of *optimal grasp* of clinicians and how that perceptual grasp may differ from the understanding of the patient's family. Professional caregivers come to dwell in different perceptual worlds in part because of their experiences of caring for patients near the end of life and must learn to translate and understand the worlds of patients and families. Chan explores how the clinical situation of a patient who is approaching death calls the health professionals to employ different care techniques, such as initiating cardiopulmonary resuscitation to a patient who suddenly experiences a cardiac arrest, or sitting with family members and guiding them through the expected phases of imminent death.

Chapter 7: The Living Tradition of Interpretive Phenomenology

Brykczynski and Benner conclude Part I by examining the critique and dialogs created by IP in nursing. Often, critics of this tradition of IP misunderstand the work as opposing rational-empirical science. Brykczynski and Benner point out that the IP scholarly community does not uphold nor support a single or unified paradigm of science, but rather advocates for scientific pluralism. The critical dialog offers a rich opportunity to clarify and better articulate the methodological rigor and demands of IP with the goal of expanding the current view of rationality beyond a narrow, technical rationality. Studying the person *in* the situation is required in nursing practice because nurses coach patients through their illness, injury, or birthing, or when facing death. An objectified, detached view of practice covers *over* the patient and nurse as well as the relational caring practices that allow the nurse to coach, accompany, bear witness, and empower patients and their families.

The critiques in the dialog with IP studies and philosophy primarily focus on the method of IP rather than on the intent and content of the studies. Most often, these critiques have been done from a rational-empirical, single paradigm science with little or no recognition of the nature of the questions asked nor the intent of the studies that govern the selection and use of IP.

Part II: Interpretive Phenomenological Studies

Part II represents a collection of research studies that demonstrate a range of interpretive investigations. These studies explore a wide variety of topics of inquiry, and the reader will note that there are many ways to present the data and findings. The goal of presenting these studies is to allow readers to see the "family resemblances" in the method across studies while examining the variations created by the phenomena being studied.

Chapter 8: Articulating, Preserving, and Promoting Holistic Aspects of Nurse Practitioner Practice

Brykczynski's work articulates how the caring practices of nursing are transported and translated into the work of nurse practitioners. She expands the dialog about the nature of advanced nursing practice. Her articulation of the Domains of Skill and Practice of Nurse Practitioners became a developmental force for nurse practitioners when they were adopted as the descriptive and assessment rubric for national guidelines for nurse practitioner curricula and assisted with describing distinctions between physicians, physician assistants, and nurse practitioners. Her descriptive articulation encouraged further development of the caring practices of nurse practitioners as they expanded their roles to include diagnosis and prescription of treatments.

Chapter 9: Sustaining Purpose and Motivation: Weaving Caring and Self-Care Together in Nursing Practice

Raingruber and Robinson retrieve healing practices and self-care from the margins of nurses sustaining themselves in their demanding practice of nursing. They affirm the essential truth that "self-care is not selfish." Rather, self-care creates its own clearing in the same way that caring for others opens up new possibilities for those cared for. In this clearing of self-care, nurses find a renewed sense of motivation and purpose, which enriches their caregiving practice. Raingruber and Robinson demonstrate this generative function of self-care through teaching nurses alternative strategies for self-care in the midst of caring for others. Learning self-care and modes of relaxation and healing strengthened the community of practice for these nurses, in addition to renewing their energy and sense of connection to their caregiving work. Raingruber and Robinson describe concrete strategies for promoting self-care and a sense of balance and well-being for caregivers at a retreat designed for enhancing self-care of nurse caregivers. Institutions intent on improving caring practices are well advised to consider this kind of exemplary approach to improving the self-care of nurse caregivers.

Chapter 10: Sustaining Family Life and Health through Rituals, Routines, and Practices in Well Families with School-Age Children

Plager identifies three kinds of family rituals and practices in her research on health promotion in families:

- Gathering practices
- Play practices
- Protection practices

In her work, she articulates how families form health promotion, risk prevention, and prevention of illness practices. In this chapter, she focuses on the focal caring practice of the evening meal. These three areas of the social formation of families open up new perspectives on the formative health promotion and protective practices of families. Her attention to the family meal as a ritual and focal practice of forming the family as a social space is contrasted with current threats to this practice.

Plager's work opens the revelatory nature of focal practices within any social group to create a place of social formation and place where people are gathered together focusing on a focal activity. In a culture of extreme individualism, social focal practices tend to be marginalized even as they provide a continuity: for example, in a family legacy of gathering practices.

Chapter 11: Listening with Care to Teen Mothers and Their Families

SmithBattle draws on Plager's articulation of family legacies in studying family and teen mothers' multigenerational caregiving practices. SmithBattle found that teen mothering was often aided by mothers and grandmothers, and that the birth of a child sometimes became a source of challenge and inspiration for constructing a better life for both the mother and child. When SmithBattle began her 16-year longitudinal study of teenage mothers, the literature was replete with normalizing discourses, such as Klein's (1978) label of teenage pregnancy as a "syndrome," which includes multiple sources of failures. SmithBattle rightly pointed out that this "failure discourse"—often framed as children raising children—created policies and public programs that further stigmatized teenage mothers and failed to understand the variation in the experience and life course of teenage mothers that she had observed in her own public health nursing practice, and now has documented with a careful, 16-year longitudinal study. By its absence of normalizing and pathologizing discourses, SmithBattle's work demonstrates the wisdom and insight that can be gained by studying variation and not just grouped generalizations. Clinical public health nursing, in the end, has gained new clinical imagination and sense of possibilities for teenage mothers.

SmithBattle's work demonstrates and articulates the narrative structure of living a particular life over time. It also illustrates the power of uncovering and articulating social legacies as well as ritual practices in order to study social life, particularly like the social life of a family. In presenting her work to public health nurses, SmithBattle encountered public health nurses who stated that they wished they had teenagers like those in SmithBattle's study. Of course, they actually do, but their normalizing discourse focusing on deficits rather than possibilities, aspirations, and challenges that mobilize many teenage mothers remain hidden to their disciplinary frameworks for encountering and perceiving the teenage mothers in their caseload first as damaged adolescents. Smith-Battle's work demonstrates that mothering cannot be studied apart from its social context and family legacies. Her work reaffirms that the work of mothering "requires a coherent social world and relationships that foster a sense of self and future." The formative and constitutive work of social birthing and development that is common to all human beings is amply illustrated in SmithBattle's work.

Chapter 12: Life Course Considerations for Adolescents Born with Spina Bifida: Toward Authentic Care and Transparency of the Other

Kinavey's chapter articulates the challenges created by physical and social environments for adolescents and young adults with spina bifida. Her participants describe the impact of social marginalization and multiple "normalizing" cultural practices and discourses that persons with spina bifida encounter from their earliest childhood. Her study participants describe the experience of difference, stigma, marginalization, and what for the adolescent can be a totalizing social identity of stigma and social rejection. Nurses who can acknowledge this systematic marginalization and stigma with their patients with spina bifida can open new understanding for children, adolescents, and young adults with spina bifida.

Chapter 13: Our Patients: Heretics, Believers, Agnostics, and Ecumenists

MacIntyre examines possible stances in relation to modern medicine in the context of the AIDS epidemic. He notes that to defy the authority of medicine in today's context is as difficult as it was for the person in the Middle Ages to deny the Church and the existence of God. He articulates and illustrates the following stances in relation to the authority of the medical establishment: heretics, believers, agnostics, and ecumenists. His work as a whole provides a profound insider's account of the lived experience of getting the HIV test and having one's T cells counted in the 1980s within the San Francisco Bay Area. MacIntyre's work recovers the sense of ambiguity and doom during the early period of the discovery of AIDS. Initially in the community, many were dying, and there were no effective treatments except for management of infections and symptom management. It was a time of crisis in faith in medical power even though medical science had made the virus visible as the cause. Medicine had not yet produced a cure, or even drugs capable of limiting the reproduction of the virus and the assault on the immune system. People wrestled with a sense of doom and fatalism even as they were told that they needed to elaborate their positive emotions in order to strengthen their immune system. The usual medical moral absolution of the discovery of the virus, the scientific cause, did not remove doubt about the person's sense of complicity with the development of the epidemic within the gay community.

MacIntyre is right in his interpretation of the different stances of heretics, believers, agnostics, and ecumenists in relation to healing and cure that exist with most people. Health care providers cannot ignore the range of endorsement and rejection of modern medicine even in the clinic visit or hospitalization. MacIntyre does not ignore nor deny the dominance and power of the medical model in the current context, but his work is a harbinger of the beginning erosion of Cartesian dominance as people confront what is left out of purely physical accounts of the human experience of health promotion, well-being, and recovery, which fall outside the separation of the physical from the social and sentient embodied person.

Chapter 14: Dwelling in the World: Realms of Meaningful Involvement in Late Life

In Weiss' work (Chapter 14), the reader is confronted or *returned* to an acknowledgement of our common humanity in old age. Social discontinuities will be experienced, in some form, by all who advance in age by losing family and friends through death, relocation; and losing bodily capacities, such as the appearance of fragilities of the aging body. However, as Weiss points out, losses are experienced differently by persons with different lifeworlds, concerns, alterations in bodily capacities, and experiences of possibility and despair. A normalizing discourse that would consider the aged as "wholly other" (Levinas, 1989) can be rejected after the universal aspects of our common humanity are articulated in the lives of two of her participants, Ann and David. Clinicians can imagine what will be experienced as helpful to Ann and David as well as other persons with different experiences, concerns, social place, and bodily capacities associated with aging. The existential skills of dwelling in a particular lifeworld are enhanced and constrained by embodied continuities, discontinuities and skills, social-relational connections, and dwelling in an altered temporality of a foreshortened future. All human beings experience some measure of loss associated with finitude and the loss of openness in one's life horizons. All the participants whose lived experiences of illness and disability are articulated and exemplified can help nurse readers develop an enriched clinical imagination that can open new possibilities in caregiving and coaching patients.

Chapter 15: Patients' and Family Members' Experiences of Hospital End-of-Life Care

Spichiger's careful articulation of what is perceived as attuned care demonstrates that both technical skilled know-how and *phronesis*, or attuned clinical judgment, are required for compassionate and effective end-of-life care. Spichiger's articulation demonstrates that not all symptoms can be managed completely: that sometimes the most that can be offered is assistance with symptom management as well as assisting patients and families living through the exigencies of approaching death with its existential as well as physical suffering. Spichiger's work shows how important it is to the family that care is given expertly, with imagination and understanding of the patient in ways that preserve as much personal identity and continuity for the dying person and family as possible.

Chapter 16: End of Living: Maintaining a Lifeworld During Terminal Illness

We appropriately end this book with a selected publication from the writings of Judith Wrubel and her colleagues at the Osher Center for Integrative Medicine at UCSF. Wrubel, a long-time colleague of Patricia Benner, is a central member of this group of researchers developing an IP tradition in nursing research. Her dissertation (Wrubel, 1985) has long been considered as exemplary in illustrating excellent IP research, and so is read as an exemplary dissertation by most IP students.

In Chapter 16, Wrubel, Acree, Goodman, and Folkman demonstrate how quantitative and qualitative data can be used to inform and enrich each other within the same study. This chapter is a fitting ending to this selection of IP work to demonstrate the usefulness of the notion of dwelling in a lifeworld to understand lived experience. This chapter highlights persons who have extreme disruptions to their experience of dwelling in their lifeworld at the end of their life because of relocation, cognitive impairment, commitment to no longer tenable goals, and/or ongoing substance abuse.

Wrubel and her colleagues articulate how it is possible to dwell in one's familiar habitus and lifeworld through substituting and finding new more realistic goals, engaging in one's spiritual practices, and continued engagement with one's close others so that a sense of social participation and belonging are not lost. Focusing on the situated possibilities with a person's familiar lifeworld and facilitating the existential skills of dwelling can enlarge clinical imagination for how to facilitate sustaining meaningful engagement in life even as death is close at hand. Social death does not always have to precede physical death. This chapter, like those preceding it, demonstrates how to develop a more equal dialog between the biomedical discourse and the lived socially embedded experiences common to all human beings dwelling in lifeworlds.

Summary

All the members of the scholarly community of IP researchers focus on socially constituted caring practices, practical knowledge, the existential skills of dwelling, and skilled know-how. These researchers seek to articulate what these practices look like, how they are disclosed, and what makes them possible. The goal is to increase the insight and wisdom of caring practices by all caregivers—nurses, teachers, parents, friends, families, and so on—so that caregivers respond to the meanings and concerns disrupted by the particular vulnerabilities that a person might experience. It is only through the experience of common humanity—embodiment, vulnerability, finitude, temporality, engaging in the common human experience of dwelling in lifeworld—that social space and the capacity to meet others with understanding and compassion can occur. By their nature, all caring practices are culturally embedded and also dependent upon the experience of a common humanity.

We could revolutionize caregiving and medical care if caregivers could use *both* scientific understandings of disease, and imaginative responses to lived disruptions caused by disease, injuries, and disabilities. On the surface, this seems obvious. However, the general grip of the biological and medical discourse is dominant in that it is considered the "true," "objective," or more definitive discourse than what is excluded from the dominant model. This work calls for a dialog between the Cartesian biomedical discourse and what Merleau-Ponty (1945/2001) calls the "middle terms" of lived experience of health and illness, dwelling in a lifeworld, embodied intentionality, and so on. Both the pathophysiological understandings of biomedicine *and* accounts and understandings of lived experience, lifeworld, interpersonal concerns, and so on are needed for attuned and imaginative caregiving.

Rational empiricism, with its attendant epistemology, aims for generalization and generates theories about biological and social structures, functions, processes, and causal mechanisms. The method of generalization in rational empiricism is based upon decontextualization of events and phenomena, making them a-temporal and a-historical (Dreyfus, 1991). Categorization through generalization abstracts objectified features and elements that can be considered essentially the same (generalizability) across situations after they have been stripped of the influences of maturation, change over time and contextual shaping or particularities of the "abstracted features of members," thus formed into general categories. This is a valid and powerful strategy that enables research to see patterns and notice new relationships between variables.

Like all human science, though, a theoretical screen is embedded in the method: The method is finite and limits what can be found, noticed, and analyzed by rational empirical generalizations. IP augments this picture, studying knowledge embedded in social practice; in engaged skilled actions; and in cultural practices, rituals, and concrete ways how people cope with everyday life events, such as illness, injury, birth, suffering, and dying. IP researchers augment the stories that can be told by rational empirical research studies of human beings—and, more importantly, can create a dialog of communication and mutual influence on health, disease, and the lived experience of illness.

IP studies presented here and published by other authors create new understanding and insights that can contribute to the development and evaluation of health policy. Health policy draws upon many different disciplines, such as ethics, public health, management, and the decision sciences. However, getting a deeper understanding of how programs affect peoples' lives can influence policy. Also, IP studies can help design programs for the teenage mother, the adolescent with spina bifida, and persons who are HIV-positive; as well as palliative care programs; long-term care programs; and so on. IP studies identify key issues and factors that drive or restrain change, articulate the effective and ineffective processes, and illuminate possibilities for future directions to health or clinical policies.

IP researchers do not seek a unified or single science method to study the lives of self-interpreting human beings engaged in lifeworlds of concern, culture, projects, habits, practices, and so on. In addition to theoretical grids about the nature of the "mind-brain" and "body" they seek, as noted earlier, to add what Merleau-Ponty (1945/2001) considers the middle terms of the lived social sentient body believing that social sentient human embodied intelligence and action in the world are best understood by studying the person in context, engaged in acting in a social lifeworld.

IP researchers maintain that articulating the lived experiences of a person looks for singular universals, such as the universals of finitude, historical thrownness, social constitution, relational social birthing, existence, and vulnerability are common in human beings and can be articulated by single lives lived in particular contexts. Commonalities and distinctions among persons, concerns, culture, habits, and practices (these "middle terms" of the social sentient embodied person [Merleau-Ponty, 1945/2001]) are amply demonstrated in accessible ways in this collection of studies and the earlier collection (Benner, 1994; Dreyfus, 1991). Such work accesses and articulates lived experiences of healthy, ill, injured, developing, and suffering persons in their lifeworlds in order to assist caregivers to understand what is needed for attuned and wise coaching and caregiving. High-end, embodied, skilled know-how and coping, such as expertise and excellent human performance, can also be studied and understood using IP. From such studies, clinical imagination and enlightened health care policies can be developed.

A Note About This Book

Chapters in this book underwent a process similar to that used by topic-specific journals such as *The Clinics of North America* and *Advances in Nursing Science*. At least two editors peer-reviewed the chapters and provided feedback to authors. The authors revised and then resubmitted their peer-reviewed manuscripts for approval to be included in the book. When possible, citations note the original year of publication, followed by the year of the source that was used. Also, figures and tables provide illustration when feasible. Emphasis that has been added by an author is indicated in *italic* unless otherwise noted. Finally, and most importantly, narrative and dialog passages from patients, nurses, clients, and study participants are highlighted in sidebars, to add their collective voices to the rich tapestry of life experience that embodies the sentiment and importance of interpretive phenomenology in the world of nursing and health care.

References

Benner, P. & Wrubel, J. (1989). *The primacy of caring: Stress and coping in health and illness*. Menlo Park, CA: Addison-Wesley.

Benner, P. (1994). The tradition and skill of interpretive phenomenology in studying health, illness, and caring practices. In P. Benner (Ed.), *Interpretive phenomenology: Embodiment, caring, and ethics in health and illness* (pp. 99-126). Thousand Oaks, CA: Sage.

Borgmann, A. (1984). *Technology and the character of contemporary life: A philosophical inquiry*. Chicago: University of Chicago Press.

Denzin, N. K. & Lincoln, Y. S. (2000). Introduction: The discipline and practice of qualitative research. In N. K. Denzin & Y. S. Lincoln (Eds.), *Handbook of Qualitative Research* (pp. 1-28). Newbury Park: Sage.

Dreyfus, H. L. (1991). *Being-in-the-world: A commentary on Heidegger's being and time* (Division 1). Cambridge, MA: The MIT Press.

Dunne, J. (1997). *Back to the rough ground: Practical judgment and the lure of technique.* Notre Dame, IN: University of Notre Dame Press.

Fjelland, R. & Gjengedal, E. (1994). A theoretical foundation for nursing as a science. In P. E. Benner (Ed.), *Interpretive phenomenology: Embodiment, caring, and ethics in health and illness* (pp. 3-26). Thousand Oaks, CA: Sage.

Foucault, M. (1994). *The birth of the clinic: An archaeology of medical perception*. (Tavistock Publications, Trans.). New York: Vintage Books. (Original work published 1973).

Gadamer, H. J. (1975). *Truth and method*. (G. Barden & J. Cumming, Eds., Trans.). London: Sheed and Ward. (Original work published 1960).

Geertz, C. (1987). Deep play: Notes on the Balinese cockfight. In P. Rabinow & W. Sullivan (Eds.), *Interpretive social science: A second look* (pp. 195-240). Berkeley, CA: University of California Press.

Heidegger, M. (1927/1962). *Being and Time* (J. M. E. Robinson, Trans.). New York: Harper & Row.

Klein, L. (1978). Antecedents of teenage pregnancy. *Clinical Obstetrics and Gynecology, 21,* 1151-1159.

Leonard, V. W. (1994). A Heideggerian phenomenological perspective on the concept of Person. In P. E. Benner (Ed.), *Interpretive phenomenology: Embodiment, caring, and ethics in health and illness* (pp. 43-63). Thousand Oaks, CA: Sage.

Levinas, E. (1989). Time and the other. In S. Hand (Ed.), *The Levinas reader* (pp. 37-58). Oxford, UK: Basil Blackwell.

Merleau-Ponty, M. (2001). *Phenomenology of perception*. (C. Smith, Trans.). London: Routledge. (Original work published 1945).

Packer, M. J., & Addison, R. B. (1989). Introduction. In R. B. Addison (Ed.), *Entering the circle: Hermeneutic investigation in psychology*. Albany, NY: SUNY Press.

Plager, K. A. (1994). Hermeneutic phenomenology: A methodology for family health and health promotion study in nursing. In P. E. Benner (Ed.), *Interpretive phenomenology: Embodiment, caring, and ethics in health and illness* (pp. 65-84). Thousand Oaks, CA: Sage.

Taylor, C. (1985). Theories of meaning. In *Human agency and language, philosophical papers I* (pp. 248-292). Cambridge, UK: Cambridge University Press.

——— (1989). *Sources of the self: The making of modern identity*. Cambridge, MA: Harvard University Press.

——— (1991). *Ethics of authenticity*. Cambridge, MA: Harvard University Press.

——— (1995). Comparison, history and truth. In C. Taylor *Philosophical arguments* (pp. 146-164). Cambridge, MA: Harvard University Press.

van Manen, M. (1990). *Researching lived experience*. Albany, NY: SUNY Press.

Wrubel, J. C. (1985). *Personal meanings and coping processes: A hermeneutic study of personal background meanings and interpersonal concerns and their relation to stress appraisals and coping.* Unpublished dissertation, Berkeley, CA: University of California.

PART I
Interpretive Phenomenology: Theory and Practice

1 Why Study Caring Practices?............3

2 A Fusion of Horizons: Meaning and Understanding in Becoming a Nurse ...23

3 Distal Nursing 41

4 Research and Ontology: Neurology and Parkinson's Disease Sufferers' Lived Experiences of Embodiment and Dwelling in Lifeworlds 59

5 Health, Disorder, and the Psychiatric Enterprise: Reclaiming Lost Connections....................75

6 Understanding End-of-Life Caring Practices in the Emergency Department 91

7 The Living Tradition of Interpretive Phenomenology 113

CHAPTER 1

Why Study Caring Practices?

**ANNEMARIE KESSELRING,
CATHERINE CHESLA, AND
VICTORIA LEONARD**

One of Patricia Benner's most important contributions to the nursing profession has been her ability to radically redirect our attention away from the study of discrete objects and behaviors, and their causal mechanisms, to the study of practices and the cultivation of narrative understandings of patients, their illness experiences and lifeworlds, and the ways in which nurses care for them. She has created a body of work (1984, 1994, 2000; Benner, Hooper-Kyriakidis, & Stannard, 1999; Benner & Sutphen, 2007; Benner, Tanner, & Chesla, 1996, 2009; Benner & Wrubel, 1989) that broke new ground by applying the philosophical arguments of hermeneutic philosophy found in the writings of Bourdieu, Dreyfus, Foucault, Heidegger, Kierkegaard, Levinas (1947/1987), MacIntyre, and Taylor to nursing's work. (For specific references, see text.) Through the study of narrative accounts of practice, Benner and her students have opened new understandings of important focal practices (such as nursing, mothering, and familial care) and helped preserve the goods (i.e., the well-being of patients, children, and families) that are central to those caring practices.

In this chapter, we articulate the notion of a practice, as well as the goods that help constitute a practice, from a hermeneutic perspective. Then we discuss ways in which aspects of modern life and culture undermine and marginalize caring practices. Finally, we examine how the study of practices through interpretive phenomenology both opens our understanding of human experiences (such as illness, mothering, and nursing) but also helps to preserve and extend those very practices, and the goods they exist to protect, by making them visible and pulling them in from the margins where they often languish, eclipsed by our cultural obsession with the empirical study of causal relationships between objective variables that have been extracted from the flux of human experience.

THE NOTION OF A PRACTICE

The Oxford English Dictionary (Oxford University Press, 2009) defines "practice" to mean

1. Perform an activity or exercise (a skill) repeatedly in order to improve or maintain proficiency in it.

2. Carry out or perform an activity or custom habitually or regularly.

3. Be engaged in a particular profession.

4. Observe the teaching and rules of a religion.

All four definitions point to activities that are repeatedly performed over time. Undoubtedly, activities, skills, crafts, routines, behaviors, habits, and duties are components of any practice. However, none of these notions addresses the ways in which practices have a constituting social power and a profound generative influence on the self-understanding of those who practice them, and on the relationship of those who practice them to the specific world in which they practice. Practices are so transparent and taken for granted that they typically escape scrutiny or are mistaken for an assemblage of discrete skills that bear no relation to the situations in which they are enacted. In fact, though, practices powerfully constitute us as human beings, and "focal" practices (Borgmann, 1984), in particular, serve to protect and preserve those goods in the culture that make life worth living.

> It is certainly the purpose of a practice to guard in its undiminished depth and identity the thing that is central to the practice, to shield it against the technological diremption into means and end. Like values, rules and practices are recollections, anticipations, and, we can now say, guardians of the concrete things and events that finally matter. Practices protect focal things not only from technological subversion but also against human frailty. (p. 209)

The teleological nature of practices derives from the ontological fact, according to Heidegger (1926/1962), that as human beings, we care: Things matter. We exist and act in the world because of those things that matter to us because of what Heidegger calls the "for the sake of which." In a practice, these things that matter—these "goods"—set up the possibility for excellence and expertise in a world redolent with significance. Care provides the ground from which practice is possible. It is interpretive phenomenology that can best help us to understand these practices. As a research approach, interpretive phenomenology both reveals practices in their depth and also, importantly, helps to preserve and shape the ethos of a practice.

Practices as we define them are rooted in the social structures of the world into which a person is born and, in Bourdieu's (1980/1990) words, are acquired as an embodied "habitus" (italic in the original). The habitus

> tends to generate all the "reasonable," "common-sense" behaviors (and only these) which are possible within the limits of [. . .] regularities, and which are likely to be positively sanctioned because they are objectively adjusted to the logic characteristic of a particular field, whose objective future they anticipate. (p. 55-56)

It is first and foremost the embodied habitus—not the mind—that generates the vast majority of those human activities that constitute practices and everyday living, and which, per se, are sensible and "meaning-full" within the boundaries of the situation at hand and its inherent, yet subliminally anticipated, future. The concept of habitus ought not to be understood as a bridge between the social world and a person, but rather as the generation of an individual gifted with a culturally and socially sentient body: endowed with an embodied understanding and capacity for action and discernment through the very practices of the world she or he has been born into, and is part of.

Bourdieu (1972/1977) argues that "it is necessary to abandon all theories which explicitly or implicitly treat practice as a mechanical reaction" structured by external rules. He additionally acknowledges that theories that reduce human action to "conscious and deliberate intentions" (p. 73) also miss the mark. Rather, he notes that practical action contains within itself the possibility for responsive adaptation to the situational context: that humans demonstrate situated freedom and agency.

"Practical sense," in Bourdieu's thinking, is rooted in the social world through the habitus, and simultaneously in "a quasi-bodily involvement in the world which presupposes no (mental) representation either of the body or of the world, still less of their relationship (1980/1990, p. 66)." For Bourdieu, practical belief, "is not a 'state of mind' . . . but rather a state of the body" (p. 68). All practices are embodied. "What is learned by body is not something that one has, like knowledge that can be brandished, but something that one is" (p. 73). And embodied practices—such as skillfully sitting or standing in relation to others, speaking and relating to older or younger people, playing games as a girl or a boy—create, re-create, and perpetuate the very social and cultural self-understandings that practices carry from generation to generation, albeit in ways that also respond to changing cultural contexts and meanings. Practices are "something extremely vague and general: more or less any stable configuration of shared activity, whose shape is defined by a certain pattern of dos and don'ts"

(Taylor, 1989, p. 204). Practices connect us to others. Through practices we share with others, we understand who we and who our fellow contemporaries are. That is, we learn to eat certain foods with a fork, with chop sticks, or by hand; are able to judge what feels (is) good or bad, easy or difficult, engaging or boring; and so on.

Yet, eating practices encompass more than just using specific utensils. The quality of foods and drinks to be prepared, the meanings associated with them, the art of cooking and serving, how to behave at the table, the company of others, table talk, festive and dietary meals are all part of eating practices (see also Elias, 1969, 1982; Plager, 1994). Eating practices convey who we are—hence, the proverb: Tell me what and how you eat, and I shall tell you who you are. Therefore, for an individual, major changes in eating practices may indicate that he or she is ill or in a foreign culture, and previously taken-for-granted issues linked to his or her eating identity rise to awareness. This state of "breakdown" is, in fact, one of the few ways in which taken-for-granted practices gain full attention and become visible.

In his ontological account of what it is to be a human being, Heidegger (1962) argued that human beings are "thrown" into a world of practices, meanings, and traditions, yet we are not mere pawns in a world already and permanently defined. According to Dreyfus (2004), there is the possibility for agency and a kind of freedom to redefine one's local world by recognizing

> one's current style as a style [that] enables one to collect now-marginal practices from the past which in turn allows one to engage in a loosely ordered multiplicity of activities that give life meaning or beauty, while at the same time contributing to slowly changing the totalizing background practices that endanger human freedom. (para. 107)

Both the vagueness and flow of practices allow for variations in how specific activities are enacted, and thus promote some changes in practices over time. Possibilities of doing things differently within a specific practice—for example, bringing up children with more or less freedom to move about in the community—are not idiosyncratic, but an integral and largely taken-for-granted part of what it means to bring up children as a parent with a particular history who is engaged in the practice of parenting in a particular familial and cultural context. It is part of the definition of a practice that excellence matters, and extending and refining what excellence means is always a defining good aspired to by the practitioner. Although the practice of bringing up children is an inherent part of every culture, and in most cultures goes largely unexamined, the ways of bringing up children—for example, to what extent children are allowed to be with, speak, or play in the presence of adults—differ. Variations in the practice attract attention, mainly from those who are unfamiliar with the variations. These variations in the practice get judged as good or less good, and may be adopted by others—and hence, generate more or less subtle transformations of both the practice and its integral self-understanding.

Practices are learned. Some, like eating, are learned very early and without integration of formal knowledge. Others—for example, professional practices, such as nursing or doctoring—are built upon a foundation of biopsychosocial theories, empirical knowledge, and practical experience. Beginners in a practice profession learn to use and adapt rules and theoretical knowledge in concrete situations. With time, they analyze and, to a certain extent, predict the development of familiar situations. Their mode of thinking is mainly analytic; they tend to be preoccupied with solving the tasks at hand, follow prescribed procedures, and their performance is normative and mostly safe. Engaged, expert professional practitioners, however, experience a quantum leap. After years of experience with a large number of patients and families, they no longer analyze the situation at hand but grasp it whole, and respond adequately and fluently to its salient human and medical features. Expert practitioners are able to successfully master complex and quickly changing situations. Because they respond adequately, quickly, and fluidly to the immediate demands of the situation and act (often creatively) in anticipation of its development, they may not always adhere to institutional rules and procedures. In places where their expertise is not recognized by superiors and colleagues, nonadherence to protocols makes them vulnerable to institutional sanctions (Benner, 1984; Benner, Tanner, & Chesla, 1996; Dreyfus & Dreyfus, 1986).

In his discussion of practice, MacIntyre (1984) distinguished goods external and internal to a practice. He defines practice as any

> coherent and complex form of socially established cooperative human activity through which goods internal to that form of activity are realized in the course of trying to achieve those standards of excellence which are appropriate to, and partially definitive of, that activity, with the result that healing powers to achieve excellence, and human conceptions of the ends and goods involved, are systematically extended. (p. 187)

External goods are associated, primarily by outsiders, with a certain practice and include status, fame, or money. Caring practices such as nursing, child rearing, or family care of the chronically ill are endowed with less status, power, and money than for instance, doctoring. External goods are reasons for ranking and rewarding (Foucault, 1975/1979, p. 181) as well as "objects of competition with winners and losers" (Spichiger, Wallhagen, & Benner, 2005).

Institutional systems that focus primarily on rewarding practice with external goods risk undermining those goods *internal* to the practice and ultimately, the practice itself. For example

> *When health insurance plans rewarded physicians for authorizing fewer specialty referrals for their patients, physicians frequently practiced for the sake of the external good of financial reward rather than for the good of their patients. Patients and the practice of medicine were both hurt by this institutional practice. (Sainford, Karsh, Booske, & Smith, 2001)*

Benner's work has made nursing's work visible and helped to rescue often-marginal caring practices from being extinguished in health care institutions that have commodified care and collapsed means and ends in their drive toward efficiency. This collapse of means and ends is exemplified, for instance, by substituting fetal monitoring machines for the art of labor coaching. This change ignored the constituting power of the relational practice of coaching a woman through a difficult labor as well as the ways in which these practices allow the nurse to know the patient and follow her childbirth trajectory, her coping, or her labor progress; and to identify those subtle cues that signal impending danger or emotional breakdown. It is these practices that allow nurses to treat patients as the "for the sake of which" in their practice—as the moral horizon of their action—as opposed to objects to be processed in a service agenda.

Although the technical skills required for nursing must be performed in a competent manner, what nurses find meaningful about their practice is the opportunity to provide care in its totality, not merely as a technical fix. But, the relational skills that are the heart of nursing practice are often invisible in the cultures of commodifying institutions; and nursing is defined, instead, as a set of technical skills, easily parsed and delegated. It is no wonder, then, that in a 2001 study (Aiken et al., 2001) more than 40% of nurses working in hospitals reported being dissatisfied with their jobs. The study indicated that one out of every three hospital nurses under the age of 30 planned to leave their current job in the next year.

> *"What nurses find meaningful about their practice is the opportunity to provide care in its totality, not merely as a technical fix."*

Goods internal to a practice, implicit notions of the "for the sake of which" (Heidegger, 1926/1962), can be experienced and attained only by being involved in and enacting that very practice. This contributes to nursing work's invisibility.

For the experienced nurse who cares for a family of a child who is being treated with chemotherapy at home, an internal good might be to work with the distraught parents until they regain some confidence in their ability to care for the ill child without neglecting the needs of their other children. The nurse might have an order to make a home visit to teach infusion skills, but recognizes that the ultimate good of the child's recovery is best served by talking to the parents about their fears and concerns around home infusion of chemotherapy rather than about the technical skill of how to use a pump.

THE VULNERABILITY OF CARING PRACTICES IN INSTITUTIONS

Many practices are practiced with the support of institutions: for example, in nursing's case, hospitals and nursing homes (MacIntyre, 1984). Institutions are not themselves practices yet may enhance and sustain the development of expertise in practices by financing them or by providing the space and climate for them to be enacted and recognized. Institutions may also curtail or thwart the development of excellence in practices when practical wisdom and know-how in dealing successfully and ethically with particular situations—what Aristotle named "phronesis"—is judged as insignificant and is largely substituted with "techne," or theoretically deduced knowing-that (Dreyfus & Dreyfus, 1986; Malone, 2003; Weiss, Malone, Merighi, & Benner, 2002).

Quality assurance and threats of malpractice litigation enhance institutional zeal for providing safe medical and nursing care at reasonable cost. Thus, institutions increasingly demand that personnel base interventions upon protocols derived from "scientific evidence," "universal principles," or other theoretical frameworks. And institutions, which rely strongly on hierarchical rankings of professions, increasingly demand "normalizing judgments" and discipline from their employees (Foucault, 1975/1979, p. 177) in observing rules and protocols.

The problem with unwavering adherence to standardized procedures is that not all protocols are adequate to fit specific, complex situations. Practitioners may therefore overlook situational features that do not show up in the protocol or the theory they use, potentially missing relational imperatives in the situation. Thus, instead of deciding on a course of action based upon situational cues, they pseudo-decide based upon an algorithm's general rules (Gordon, 1984).

High-quality care and the development of patient- and family-centered practices are also truncated by impersonal, top-down hierarchical management; division of labor; and unclear delegation of responsibility to amorphous teams (Aiken et al., 2002; Blegen et al., 2004; Clarke & Aiken 2003, 2006; Eisenberg, Bowman, & Foster 2001; Lundstrom et al., 2002; Sainfort et al., 2001). Guillemin and Gillam (2006) documented nurses' moral distress when in a maze of unclear responsibilities, hierarchical thinking, and general lack of respect toward a patient who decided to forgo further treatment, they were unable to commit to and advocate for the patient.

The immediately aforementioned studies and scholarly papers point alarmingly to real and looming losses of quality of care in hospitals and contribute to the burnout of discouraged professionals. The lack of recognition of, or even loss of, expert practice in institutions disheartens practitioners and enhances emotional and moral disengagement and the spread of "ethical blindness" (Rubin, 1996, p. 171) toward patients' and families' needs and suffering.

In the institutional effort to contain or reduce costs for services, individualized person-care may become a luxury as attention is instead focused upon defined and discrete tasks and measurable outcomes in the production of health care. Caring practices are threatened with marginalization and depleted of their core meaning and internal good: namely, easing the suffering of patients and their families and relating to their plight. As individual "person-care" is replaced by anonymous "health-care," the very sick and the chronically ill are discharged sicker and quicker to their homes (Weiss et al., 2002). And, interventions and high-tech treatments (such as medication titration, mechanical ventilation, or intravenous chemotherapy) are delegated to families—or, if systems are in place, to professional practitioners in the community.

Both the looming loss of core practice values in institutions and the increasingly complex requirements of care for very sick and dependent chronically ill patients in the community change the professional focus of nursing. Where care was formerly predominantly focused on individuals while they were hospitalized or institutionalized, attention now needs to be focused on families who care for an ill member in their home, as well as on the many elderly who live alone. However, the relational work that is central to such care is often considered peripheral—or worse, invisible and unnecessary—and, therefore, nonreimbursable. Nurses are again faced with the demoralizing choice of reducing care to technical procedures, contributing to job dissatisfaction (Aiken et al., 2001) and increased personal vulnerability (Borgmann, 1984), or sacrificing themselves in order to do the relational work that is central to their practice and a constituting good.

Most nurses who deviate from technically oriented orders do so because they recognize that the patient is best served by more relational work, and they are forced to either provide relational care in the guise of procedural care or to provide the care on their own time. However, in these attempts to serve the ultimate good of their practice, nurses work to pull in these focal caring practices from the margins and preserve them. Another way that these focal practices are preserved is by studying them and thereby making them visible. Nurses have looked to Benner's work for direction on how to develop the skills and understanding to take up practices in research work without obscuring or violating them, or disaggregating them into meaningless "factors."

> *"Most nurses who deviate from technically oriented orders do so because they recognize that the patient is best served by more relational work."*

PRACTICE AND SCIENCE

"Practice has a logic which is not that of the logician" (Bourdieu, 1980/1990, p. 86). In his critique of theoretical reason, Bourdieu warned scientists not to err into "the antinomy between the time of science and time of action, which tends to destroy practice by imposing on it the intemporal time of science" (p. 81). Conventional, atemporal, decontextualizing scientific methods ask for objectification and distinctive definitions: separation of the parts from the whole as well as theoretical hypothesizing of possible logical relationships among the parts. Their data are snapshots of fragmented points in time. Such hyperrational approaches defy the flow of practice's logic: They are incommensurable with its intricate fabric and, hence, their results both distort and hide the fundamental nature of practice.

Notions of the goods internal to practice are often vague, nonexplicit, non-(self)-reflexive, and nonintellectual. They, too, are founded in the "paradoxical logic of all practical sense":

> The idea of practical logic, "logic in itself," without conscious reflexion on logical control, is a contradiction in terms, which defies logical logic. This paradoxical logic is that of all practice, or rather of all practical sense. Caught up in 'the matter in hand,' totally present in the present and in the practical functions that it finds there in the form of objective potentialities, practice excludes attention to itself (that is, to the past). It is unaware of the principles that govern it and the possibilities they contain; it can only discover them by enacting them, unfolding them in time. (Bourdieu, 1980/1990, p. 92)

Self-reflection and intellectual, reflexive attention to distinct actions or features indicate that the flow of practice is interrupted; typically, this may occur when there is a need for systematic problem solving. Once the problem is taken care of, the fluidity of work again resumes, and concern for what is salient in the situation guides the practitioner's activities and subliminal awareness. The in-practice, engaged state allows for a self- and world-forgetting concentration on the task at hand.

> In contrast to logic, a mode of thought that works by making explicit the work of thought, practice excludes all formal concerns. Reflexive attention to action itself, when it occurs (almost invariably only when the automatisms have broken down), remains subordinate to the pursuit of the result and to the search (not necessarily perceived in this way) for maximum effectiveness of the effort expended. So it has nothing in common with the aim of explaining how the result has been achieved, still less of seeking to understand (for understandings' sake) the logic of practice, which flouts logical logic. (Bourdieu, 1980/1990, p. 91)

Understanding that "practice excludes attention to itself" is central to Bourdieu's critique of studying practices by imposing rational thinking upon the practitioner. Research questions that demand self-reflection and logical reasoning of practitioners, such as explicating their decision making or defining the goals they aspire to, catapult them out of practice's flow; and the answers harvested are likely to be distorted or false post hoc constructions of what they *thought* they did or reasoned (Schutz, 1962). The practitioner's lived, real concerns and embodied practical sense, however, escape analytic scrutiny. Paradoxically, practices are fundamental to a society's survival, but their being taken for granted and escaping rational analytic exploration make them vulnerable to political and institutional devaluation, and difficult to study well.

"Analysis requires a deep commitment to the data, to uncovering the logic of the practice that the narratives reveal."

The study of practices requires deftness in drawing narratives forth from participants and the ability to stay curious about what seems obvious to the participant and pursue it. Analysis requires a deep commitment to the data, to uncovering the logic of the practice that the narratives reveal. It is a process that contrary to rational empirical science, is best done in concert with others who can validate findings, challenge assumptions, and point out possibilities in the data not yet seen. And it is time-consuming work that can challenge one's own sense of adequacy when facing down daunting layers of data that must be distilled into an essential narrative that can be shared with others as evidence for the interpretive case being made.

One must be creative with strategies that allow the researcher to preserve the worldhood of a participant and present it to outsiders in a convincing way. Relative to the analysis of quantitative data, it is a messy and underdetermined process.

> *"One must be creative with strategies that allow the researcher to preserve the worldhood of a participant and present it to outsiders in a convincing way."*

Why Study Caring Practices?

Descriptions that adequately capture the constituting goods of nursing practice while at the same time avoiding sentimental or trivializing accounts require sensibility to that practice and skill in articulation. By studying practices in their full depth, research makes the work of focal caring practices visible, thereby helping to preserve and protect them. Research on practices also amplifies the drive toward excellence as it gradually articulates examples of both excellent and poor practice, and the situational and personal aspects that facilitate each.

As health care changes and as patients increasingly move out of hospitals for care, nurses must acquire the formal knowledge, practical know-how, and understanding required to provide care for families and individual community dwellers. Formal knowledge is made available through scientific, deductive methods. However, understanding the illness experiences of others to be able to care for them well in their homes can come only from studying patients' experiences—through eliciting stories and other accounts of what is experientially important (Benner, 1984; Benner & Wrubel, 1989).

Narrative accounts elucidate what caring for ill people and families is all about. Research that brings forth stories and allows the articulation of exemplary caring situations does not "objectify the most fundamental presuppositions of practical logic, [but] seeks to understand, in and for itself, and not to improve it or reform it" (Bourdieu, 1980/1990, p. 91).

Taylor (1985) differentiated two ways of formulating a problem using words. In the first, hypotheses to be tested are defined by using words for objects or facts that can be neatly defined—those with what Taylor called "clear contours": that is, those objects or facts that are not difficult to find words for, and agreement as to meaning is easily achieved. The second way of formulating a problem involves the more demanding task of articulating in words those "objects lacking definite contours," such as feelings or meanings, and the self-understandings inherent in practices that we "do not quite know what to focus on in focusing on them." It is through formulating that the words or objects come into clearer view, and we are able to articulate and understand them. Through "genuine formulation . . . we only know afterwards what we are trying to identify" and to bring to our "explicit awareness what we formerly had only an implicit sense of" (Taylor, 1985, p. 256). When research focuses on the first, easily achieved, notion of formulation, it often passes over those hard-to-articulate and often-hidden aspects of the problem that are often central to its resolution or treatment.

Studying caring practices aims exactly at providing words for and bringing to explicit awareness what families and practitioners know but are unable to express. Through stories told and interpreted by the use of qualitative methods, professional and lay caring–practitioners gain in-depth understanding of their situation and of self. And learners at all levels of practice experience may become aware of how *being with* a patient or family "dictates the ethics, craft, and tact of caregiving" (Benner, 2000, p. 303; italic by the authors).

How to Study Caring Practices?

Here, we offer guidance from our experiences in using interpretive phenomenology to study the practices of patients and families, particularly those who live with cancer or other life-threatening conditions (Kesselring), those engaged in mothering and childcare (Leonard), and families accommodating chronic illness (Chesla). We offer practical observations and guidelines from our work. We are deeply committed to bringing practices to light, particularly those that gather local participants into communities, thereby helping to preserve them. We are not naïve to the fact that study practices is a fragile art, one that can hide or distort that which is studied, as easily as illuminate it. Still, our commitment is to remain open to the everyday world of those we engage in our studies, and do the best we can to encounter their worlds and share their understandings (Dreyfus, 2004).

Studying practices requires creating a context in which participants can demonstrate, in their words or actions, their everyday ways of being meaningfully involved in their worlds. Frequently, this means creating a research project that enables narration of the everyday such that participants' background understandings, which arise from local (cultural) worlds, become visible to the interpreter. We are required to configure the research such that participants' concerns in action can be appreciated. Practically, this means doing participant observation in meaningful contexts, and/or conducting interviews in various forms and formats, but there are important qualitative distinctions in how these observations and interview opportunities are structured.

> "Our commitment is to remain open to the everyday world of those we engage in our studies, and do the best we can to encounter their worlds and share their understandings."

The need to attend carefully to the basic design of an interpretive phenomenological study is frequently underappreciated. Studying the lifeworld of participants regarding any aspect of their everyday world requires careful attention to getting "into the hermeneutic circle" in the right way. Benner (2000) emphasized the need to create disclosive spaces in which participants recognize the concerns of the researcher and can begin to move toward addressing the questions of the project. Researchers work to create understanding by positioning themselves and framing their questions such that the lived concerns of the participant are elicited. We believe that significant time and thought are required to frame the research in a way that allows access to the practices of the community of concern.

The contemporary scientific context in which we design our research is, as Bourdieu has eloquently argued, so thoroughly structured by particular kinds of logic that it takes creativity and risk to formulate questions in terms of the logic of practice. And questions must be carefully drafted to illuminate craft. Our initial intuitions may be misdirected because of theoretical overdrive. When thinking about issues we wish to study, it is easy to fall into theoretically habitual ways of thinking. For example, questions about how social support or family cohesiveness affects family health come readily to mind. Although these questions are important, and certainly should be appreciated as background theoretical context for framing family research, they don't travel far enough down the road toward families' practical experiences.

> *"Observing meaningful practices involves careful, solicitous observation in the settings and situations where such practices unfold."*

In framing research, we need an appreciation of the theoretical constructs that frame the phenomenon of interest and the empirical findings regarding this phenomenon; but, finally, we need to be willing to engage with the problematic of everyday life to frame questions that will elicit participants' experiences, skills, and practices in a more holistic, less reductionist way:

> *A study of family care practices might be framed as a question: How do parents of children with severe disabilities create and re-create their relationships with their children as they grow and develop? What are the varieties of ways that parents engage with their children with severe disabilities?*

A second problem that prevails in structuring interpretive phenomenological research projects is standing outside the hermeneutic circle of the phenomena of interest and simply proposing to "understand lived meanings." It is insufficient to simply point to current rational empirical science, and suggest that it misses much of the lived meaning of those who have been studied. For almost any patient or family issue, that is probably true. However, justifying a project requires specifying a significant problematic in living to be articulated, or a significant practice that needs expression, to change contemporary understanding or change health care practices. The researcher's stance on the problem can help with this articulation: Her clinical or experiential grasp of the phenomenon to be studied can serve as a starting point, along with thorough theoretical and empirical grounding, for framing the project. Next, we describe qualitatively distinct ways to structure a research project that increase opportunities for discerning practices.

Disclosing Practices Through Observation

The best, and perhaps only, way to study the temporal unfolding of practices is to observe practices in action. Observing meaningful practices involves careful, solicitous observation in the settings and situations where such practices unfold. For example:

> *Observation in families' homes allows the ineffable movements of families solving problems together and living their lives to be seen by the researcher. Observing in hospitals or community practice settings allows the ineffable yet skillful practices of nurses to be observed with the press of the situation intact. The contextual features of situations that draw forth practices are present for observation if the researcher has the appropriate sensibility to perceive them.*

> *Observation, while providing openings on unfolding practices that other forms of research engagement simply can't provide, remains a complex endeavor. The problem of how to position oneself as an observer, when to show up, how long to stay, and what to watch are all problems that must be thought through in advance, and require experience and mentoring to do well. The key is to structure observations in such a way as to increase the likelihood of having practices show up: When trying to study parents' care of chronically ill children, it makes sense to observe bedtimes, mealtimes, treatments, and periods of transition between caregivers. Selecting these times will increase the likelihood of observing any problematic care as well as the creative or habitual responses by parents. However, selecting these times also creates the risk of missing significant events, such as the capacity of families to make use of down-time for play or joy.*

For example, in a study of the capabilities of patients with Alzheimer's disease and family caring practices surrounding those patients, Phinney observed quiet and active times in family home life. Her work demonstrates the insight that is possible in well-structured observation. She described how patients with Alzheimer's disease disclosed worlds as memory failed. For example, threads of practices remained regarding helping prepare a meal, but were fragmented. As practices, they were held together only by family members who surrounded and supported the person with Alzheimer's. Family members were necessary to fill in the gaps in patients' understanding or engagement with the practice (Phinney, 2006; Phinney & Chesla, 2003).

Although less ideal than studying participants in the flow of their everyday lives, interactions in varied interview and action contexts also provide insight into participants' practices. Gathering multiple members of a family for an interview and providing unstructured time for narrating family life experiences creates a disclosive space for enacting their ways of relating to one another. Similarly, gathering participants who share a significant life experience for group interviews creates the possibility for them to disclose both narratives about their shared experiences as well as reflections upon those experiences.

In addition, background practices can be elicited in participants' direct interactions with one other, as the following example shows:

> *In group interviews with Chinese immigrants about family care of type 2 diabetes, one wife told of an argument she had with her husband about his capacity to work. He believed that his diabetes prevented him from holding down a job. Her story elicited from other group members culturally shaped responses: They chided her to "believe him" and to "support him" fully in his belief that he could not work. Another wife noted that diabetes medicines made her husband feel tired and weak as well. In their responses, the group coached the wife to enact a culturally nuanced practice to be a good Chinese wife and support her husband in all things. The first wife responded to coaching with silence, but in subsequent 1-on-1 interviews, continued to question the truth of her husband's claim.*

Creating varied contexts in which researchers can interact with participants as they narrate their everyday practices allows the researcher better access to those practices.

Disclosing Practices Through Interviews

Interviews are a familiar form of exchange in contemporary life. Most participants in North America are familiar with the cadence and structure of a fact-based, survey interview. Participants experience quick, disengaged forms of interviews in many areas of their lives, including when they seek health care. Less familiar is the tempo, tone, and emotional structure of a narrative interview that invites disclosure of practices. Several factors contribute to the success of generating such a disclosive space. These include the attitude, or philosophical positioning, of the interviewer to the field of the everyday; the interpersonal comfort of the researcher in asking about significance-filled events and people; maintaining a stance of curiosity and openness to unanticipated answers from the participant; and listening with a sensibility for significance and probing further in that direction.

> "Appreciating that interviews comprise access to disclosive spaces, as opposed to opportunities to interrogate participants, helps position the researcher for understanding."

Successful movement in the unstructured moments of an interpretive phenomenological interview is enhanced by a researcher's appreciation of how humans live in the world. Does one need to study Heidegger or Foucault to conduct a good interpretive phenomenological interview? No, but it helps. Appreciating that interviews comprise access to disclosive spaces, as opposed to opportunities to interrogate participants, helps position the researcher for understanding. Appreciating that humans are world disclosers (Dreyfus & Spinosa, 2003; Spinoza, Flores & Dreyfus, 1997) in the everyday as well as in the interview, both participant and researcher are simply setting about the task of disclosing a common world, creating a rich possibility for meeting. And, entering the interview with an appreciation that the important story lies *in the practices*—rather than in the reflections on those practices, the causes or results of those practices, or in some deep self-understanding that has to be unearthed—throws the researcher into the encounter in an affirmative way.

Skill in eliciting, and comfort with hearing, significant accounts greatly enhance the possibility of uncovering practices. In everyday encounters, humans can be numbed to living lives of significance. Many present-day encounters invite or require distance, disengagement, and emotional blunting. Researchers are responsible for establishing the research encounter as a place in which the participants are invited to describe involvements that matter to them. Researchers can establish this space by demonstrating a seriousness of purpose; by remaining nondirective but curious about the participant's experience, particularly early in the interview; by directly naming some core issues that may arise in the participant's situation; and by responding to every utterance with respect.

For example, when exploring issues of diabetes care in group interpretive interviews with Black women, Chesla (a Caucasian researcher) worked with Jones (a Black research assistant) to put the issue of race on the table early in the interviews. They spoke frankly about their interest in learning about family practices—positive, meaningful, satisfying, and unsatisfying—for caring for type 2 diabetes within Black families. They acknowledged their interest in presenting the range of experiences in Black families; their concern to create balanced, rather than pejorative, representations of Black family experiences; and their efforts to confront race as Black and Caucasian researchers working together. Naming what was significant, acknowledging historical misrepresentation of Blacks in previous research, and pointing to the difficulties in working across race, created a starting place for serious discussions of habits and practices within the participant's lives.

Uncovering Practices in Text Interpretation

Practices are best apprehended in texts of observations and in narratives of direct concrete experiences that are obtained from participants within interviews. While we attend carefully to the whole/parts review of the text, we have found that special attention to narrative portions of the whole text yields the most essential insights into participants' practices. Because narratives embody participants' concerns (or what matters to them) but seldom express these concerns directly, thoughtful dwelling with narratives—gathered via interviews or through observations—is imperative. We have found that interpreting a participant's concerns within each narrative is the best way to understand everyday practices. This aspect of analysis is the most interpretive and requires the greatest risk in articulating our understanding of their verbal expressions or action, but is also the most productive. Thus, for each narrative, the following questions deserve attention:

- What matters to the participant here?
- Why is the participant telling this story and why now?
- How does this narrative align with or discriminate the concerns of this participant with other narratives in the whole text?
- How does it fit with the whole of her expressions (both narrative and reflexive)?
- How/who is the participant in this story?
- How does the participant show up in this story?
- Within what kind of world does this story make the best sense?

Interpreting the concerns of a participant within a whole case also enables the articulation of the generative force of practices in a participant's life. The accretion of understanding across the narratives within a case, as well as the capacity of the participant to review past experiences within a lengthy interview, allows participants to review and researchers to understand transformative practices.

For example, Chesla interviewed Alzheimer's disease family caregivers four times over an 18-month period of care:

> *One wife traced her transformation in caring for her husband. Shortly after the diagnosis, the wife attended Alzheimer's support groups; after listening to the group discussion, she started feeling sorry for herself for having to provide demanding, detailed daily physical care for her husband. However, after a period of time, she reached a turning point in which she recognized, "Wait a minute. This is ridiculous. This man cared for me all my life, and I love him. It's no big deal that I have to help him get dressed in the morning. It's the least I can do." With this realization, the woman stopped going to the support meetings, got back in synch with her own concerns, and acknowledged the good she experienced in her life by caring for her husband. Caring for her spouse constituted her life in a new way, and created a positive possibility for absorbing her husband's decline into her life and habits.*

The study and elucidation of practice is not just a research activity. Clinical work can also create a disclosive space for understanding and extending practices. For instance, in working with childcare providers who regarded their work as a series of tasks, Leonard helped them to see that their work was not just a series of tasks but a practice that had as its overarching good the formation of children. Simple caring practices—such as having a conversation structured by affection and curiosity rather than simple commands, and feeding as an activity that embodied care and concern about choices rather than simply placing food on the table—were reframed as important activities grounded in an ethical concern and issuing in important, life-changing formative experiences for young children.

We have merely touched upon the profound ways that studying practices can help to deepen and extend understanding in nursing. Others in this book provide wonderful examples of what this work looks like, and any understanding of how or why to study practices should move from a theoretical description such as we have provided here, to examples of the work itself. We have additionally highlighted how particular orientations to the conduct of interpretive phenomenological research can increase the likelihood that practices will be laid bare.

In a world moving at an ever more frenetic pace, creating a disclosive space for really *seeing* practices is a world-preserving act that helps us see that we act for the sake of something that really matters. As Kierkegaard (1848/1962) would argue, it is a way to outwit a leveled world and revive qualitative distinctions and world-defining commitments to that which matters. If there were ever a time in human history that required world-preserving action, it is now. We have Patricia Benner to thank for nursing's access to this world-preserving work.

References

Aiken, L. H., Clarke, S. P., Sloane, D. M., Sochalski, J. A., Busse, R., Clarke, H., et al. (2001). Nurses' reports of hospital quality of care and working conditions in five countries. *Health Affairs, 20,* 43-53.

Aiken, L. H., Clarke, S. P., Sloane, D. M., Sochalski, J.A., & Silber, H. (2002). Hospital nurse staffing and patient mortality, nurse burnout, and job dissatisfaction. *Journal of the American Medical Association, 288,* 1987-93.

Benner, P. (1984). *From novice to expert. Excellence and power in clinical nursing.* Menlo Park, CA: Addison-Wesley.

Benner, P. (1994). *Interpretive phenomenology: Embodiment, caring, and ethics in health and illness.* Thousand Oaks, CA: Sage.

Benner, P. (2000). The quest for control and the possibilities of care. In Wrathall, M. & Malpas, J. (Eds). *Heidegger, coping, and cognitive science: Essays in honor of Hubert L. Dreyfus,* (Vol. 2, pp. 293-309). Cambridge, MA: The MIT Press.

Benner, P., Hooper-Kyriakidis, P., & Stannard, D. (1999). *Clinical wisdom and intervention in critical care: A thinking-in-action approach.* Philadelphia: Saunders.

Benner, P., & Sutphen, M. (2007). Learning across the professions: The clergy, a case in point. *Journal of Nursing Education, 46*(3), 103-108.

Benner, P., Tanner, C., & Chesla, C. (1996). *Expertise and nursing practice: Caring, clinical judgment, and ethics.* New York: Springer.

Benner, P., Tanner, C., & Chesla, C. (2009). *Expertise and nursing practice: Caring, clinical judgment, and ethics* (2nd ed.). New York: Springer.

Benner, P., & Wrubel, J. (1989). *The primacy of caring: Stress and coping in health and illness.* Menlo Park, CA: Addison-Wesley.

Blegen, M. A., Vaughn, T., Pepper, G. Vojir, C., Stratton, K. Boyd, M., et al. (2004). Patient and staff safety: Voluntary reporting. *American Journal of Medical Quality, 19*(2), 67-74.

Borgmann, A. (1984). *Technology and the character of contemporary life.* Chicago: University of Chicago Press.

Bourdieu, P. (1977). *Outline of a theory of practice.* (R. Nice, Trans.). Cambridge, UK: Cambridge University Press. (Original work published 1972).

Bourdieu, P. (1990). *The logic of practice.* (R. Nice, Trans.). Stanford, CA: Stanford University Press. (Original work published 1980).

Clarke, S. P., & Aiken, L. H. (2003). Failure to rescue: Measuring nurses' contributions to hospital performance. *American Journal of Nursing, 103,* 42-47.

Clarke, S. P., & Aiken, L. H. (2006). More nursing, fewer deaths. *Quality and Safety in Health Care, 15*(1), 2-3.

Dreyfus, H. L. (2004). Heidegger and Foucault on the subject, agency and practices. Retrieved 31 August 2007 from http://socrates.berkeley.edu/~hdreyfus/html/paper_heidandfoucault.html

Dreyfus, H. L., & Dreyfus, S. E. (1986). *Mind over machine: The power of human intuition and expertise in the era of the computer.* New York: Free Press.

Dreyfus, H. L., & Spinosa, C. (2003). Further reflections on Heidegger, technology and the everyday. *Bulletin of Science, Technology & Society, 23*(5), 339-349.

Eisenberg, J. M., Bowman, C. C., & Foster, N. E. (2001). Does a healthy health care workplace produce higher-quality care? *Journal on Quality Improvement, 27*(7), 444-454.

Elias, N. (1969) *The Civilizing Process Vol. 1 The History of Manners*. Oxford: Blackwell). (Original work published 1939).

Elias, N. (1982). *The Civilizing Process Vol. II State Formation and Civilization*. Oxford: Blackwell. (Original work published 1939).

Foucault, M. (1979). *Discipline and punish*. (A. Sheridan, Trans.). New York: Vintage Books. (Original work published 1975).

Gordon, D. R. (1984). Identifying the use and misuse of formal models in nursing practice. In Benner, P., *From novice to expert. Excellence and power in clinical nursing* (pp. 225-243). Menlo Park, CA: Addison-Wesley.

Guillemin, M., & Gillam, L. (2006). *Telling moments: Everyday ethics in health care*. Melbourne, Australia: IP Communications.

Heidegger, M. (1962). *Being and time*. (J. Macquarrie & E. Robinson, Trans.). New York: Harper & Row. (Original work published 1926).

Kierkegaard, S. (1962). *The present age*. (A. Dru, Trans.). New York: Harper & Row. (Original work published 1848).

Levinas, E. (1987) *Time and the other*. (R. A. Cohen, Trans.). Pittsburgh: Duquesne University Press. (Original work published 1947).

Lundstrom T., Pugliese, G., Bartley, J., Cox, J., & Guither, C. (2002). Organizational and environmental factors that affect worker health and safety and patient outcomes. *American Journal of Infection Control, 30*(2), 93-106.

MacIntyre, A. (1984). *After virtue* (2nd ed.). Notre Dame: University of Notre Dame Press.

Malone, R. E. (2003). Distal nursing. *Social Science and Medicine, 56*, 2317-2326.

Oxford University Press, retrieved March 2009 from http://www.askoxford.com

Phinney, A. (2006). Family strategies for supporting involvement in meaningful activity by persons with dementia. Journal of Family Nursing, 12(1), 80-101.

Phinney, A., & Chesla, C. A. (2003).The lived body in dementia. *Journal of Aging Studies, 17*, 283-299.

Plager, K. A. (1994). Hermeneutic phenomenology: A methodology for family health and health promotion study in nursing. In Benner, P. (Ed.), *Interpretive phenomenology: Embodiment, caring, and ethics in health and illness* (pp. 65-83). Thousand Oaks, CA: Sage.

Rubin, J. (1996). Impediments to the development of clinical knowledge and ethical judgment in critical care nursing. In P. Benner, C. Tanner, & C. Chesla, *Expertise and nursing practice: Caring, clinical judgment, and ethics* (pp. 170-192). New York: Springer.

Sainfort, F., Karsh, B. Z., Booske, B. C., & Smith, M. J. (2001). Applying quality improvement principles to achieve healthy work organizations. *Journal on Quality Improvement, 27*(9), 469-483.

Schutz, A. (1962). Common-sense and scientific interpretation of human action. In *The problem of social reality. Collected papers Vol. 1*. The Hague, Netherlands: Marinus Nijhoff.

Spichiger, E., Wallhagen, M. I., & Benner, P. (2005). Nursing as a caring practice from a phenomenological perspective. *Scandinavian Journal of Caring Sciences, 19*, 3003-3009.

Spinosa, C., Flores, F., & Dreyfus, H. L. (1997). *Disclosing new worlds: Entrepreneurship, democratic action, and the cultivation of solidarity*. Cambridge, MA: The MIT Press.

Taylor, C. (1985). *Human agency and language. Philosophical papers 1*. Cambridge, UK: Cambridge University Press.

Taylor, C. (1989). *Sources of the self: The making of the modern identity*. Cambridge, MA: Harvard University Press.

Weiss, S. M., Malone, R. E., Merighi, J. R., & Benner, P. (2002). Economism, efficiency, and the moral ecology of good nursing practice. *Canadian Journal of Nursing Research, 34*(2), 95-119.

CHAPTER 2

A Fusion of Horizons: Meaning and Understanding in Becoming a Nurse

SUSAN MCNIESH

Taking up the practice of nursing occurs in a situated context that is rarely explicitly articulated and often taken for granted. Entering the clinical setting, nursing students encounter the juxtaposition of two worlds: one the medical and technological; and the other located in the local, meaningful, and particularly situated world of the patient and family. For example, in the context of labor and delivery, nurses often administer highly technical interventions that require careful monitoring and management of dual patient (mother and fetus) responses. While the nurse must be concerned with the potential risks for both mother and infant, she must also attend to the birth as a significant life passage for the patient, infant, and family.

In part, learning the practice of nursing in a medical and technological world requires a "fusion of horizons" (Gadamer, 1975/2004) as the lifeworld of student nurse intersects with the lifeworld and focal practices of patients and families. But it is not only these two horizons that are present: The technical understandings and practices related to medicalized birth (as practiced in a hospital setting within the United States), as well as the structural aspects of a bureaucratic institution also shape the experiences of medical and nursing personnel, the student, and the patient and family members.

Gadamer (1975/2004) described our gaining understanding as the fusion of horizons. Gadamer's horizon speaks to the limits of what can be seen from a particular vantage point. In an analogous form, one can picture a flooded rice field that visually appears as green stems poking up in clusters or clearings. Because of our background understandings of how the field would look if it weren't flooded, we know that what appears as distinct clusters or clearings of green would be seen as a whole phenomenal field if the water were drained. In the same way, there are shared background understandings of whatever phenomenon one is engaged with that provide a relational context. The phenomenon is foreground, but it arises from the context of a background that infuses it with meaning. Horizon is the limit of what one can see from one historical standpoint, but as one exposes and interprets more background meaning, the horizon changes and becomes clearer.

In a comparable way, the intersecting worlds of students, patients, and Westernized medicine can be viewed as sharing the same phenomenal field of background meanings, shaped by a common historical time and cultural epoch. A human science, such as research on nursing education, is concerned with the embodied practices and concerns of students, patients, families, nurses, faculty, researchers, doctors, and other medical personnel. Traditional science is inappropriate for human sciences, which require an understanding of participants' meanings and interpretations as situated and engaged (Dreyfus, 1991; Heidegger, 1927/1962). In traditional science, the researcher attempts to be an uninvolved scientist contemplating distinct objects separated from one's own existence. Rational empiricism assumes the researcher can achieve an outside perspective that is objective and value-free—what might be termed a God's-eye view or a "view from nowhere" (Nagel, 1986). In this view, phenomena are decontextualized: broken down into atomistic, isolable units; abstracted; and made ahistorical. Instead, using an interpretive account, practical behavior occurs within our involvement in the world. The interpretive phenomenology method strives to uncover and articulate the taken-for-granted and shared meanings that constitute these skills and practices, and their interconnectedness within the practice of nursing.

> "The intersecting worlds of students, patients, and Westernized medicine can be viewed as sharing the same phenomenal field of background meanings, shaped by a common historical time and cultural epoch."

My purpose in this chapter is to articulate the background meaning of taking up the practice of nursing in an experiential setting: that is, during clinical practica in pre-licensure nursing. Exemplar cases used to enhance this articulation of taking up the practice of nursing were collected while I was the faculty of record for clinical practica in maternal/child nursing. Clinical journals were written and collected as part of background coursework for the clinical experience, and students met in a postconference setting and were encouraged to provide narratives of their clinical day. Written permission from the students was gathered at that time to contact them in the future for consent to use the clinical journals in potential research. Subsequent human subjects review was obtained, students were re-contacted, and formal written consents were obtained to use the students' narratives.

MEANINGS AND UNDERSTANDING

Because human beings are born into a pre-existing world, certain background meanings are both shared and tacit (Heidegger, 1927/1962). For Heidegger, each experience is understood based upon our individual "thrownness"—that is, our lived experience of being born into an existing culture. One's being is always situated in a particular community at a particular historical time (Dreyfus, 1994). Understanding is lived and "is itself a kind of practical experience in and of the world that, in part, constitutes the kinds of persons that we are in the world" (Schwandt, 2000, p. 196).

Being born into an existing human world means that from the beginning, humans are immersed in interpretive webs of practices that themselves contain interpretations about the human world. To be human is to interpret and to understand or encounter meaning (Gadamer, 1975/2004). Persons cannot stand outside the hermeneutic circle of their preunderstandings (nor would the individual want to) to gain a more objective view. Background meanings condition our understandings and interpretations. In this way, learning is about taking up new interpretations, new meanings, and new ways of perceiving and acting as students encounter ruptures in their ordinary smooth flow of everyday being-in-the-world-as-student. Whatever is encountered in interpretation is encountered from within our background understandings, so it is always partial and temporary.

> *"Clinical concrete cases are always more complex, uncertain, and ambiguous than can be captured in theory, although theory can act as a guide, especially for the novice."*

Meanings of Practice

Becoming a nurse involves the taking up of a practice. A practice is not mere activity, but rather is a cluster of patterned and interrelated ways of being that relies upon socially embedded practical knowledge (Dunne, 1997). The individual student as practitioner takes the best action in a particular situation of inescapable uncertainty based upon prior experiences and background cultural meanings. Nursing education tends to emphasize the formal and explicit knowledge, leaving the embodied, taken-for-granted skills and knowledge of bedside nursing unattended or undescribed (Benner, Tanner, & Chesla, 1996).

As with all practice knowledge, in nursing education, there is a limit to formal theory that must be extended and contextualized through experience. Clinical concrete cases are always more complex, uncertain, and ambiguous than can be captured in theory, although theory can act as a guide, especially for the novice. Knowledge gained through experience broadens, extends, and refines existing knowledge and allows the fledgling practitioner to begin to recognize what is important in situations and also compare situational similarities with prior experiences. Practices develop in response to "problematic situations of uncertainty, complexity, instability, uniqueness, and value conflict" (Schon, 1983, p. 117) but also in response to meanings and goals. Thus, indeterminism and the ways that taken-for-granted background meanings cannot be made completely explicit limit the ability to formalize social practices (Benner & Wrubel, 1989; Dreyfus, 1999; Dunne, 1997), and knowledge gained through practical experience fills in the gaps.

One notices coherency and fluidity to the expert practitioner's use of shared goals, skills, knowledge, and equipment (Benner, 1997). For example, when an experienced nurse enters a patient's room, she will notice—in an embodied and a nonreflective manner—salient aspects of the situation. For example, the nurse will observe the patient's color, body posture and movement, level of consciousness, and a host of other patient cues, all within the time it takes to walk to the patient's bed. In addition, the nurse will be scanning the room for equipment placement and functioning as well as other situational features that tacitly cue the nurse toward further action. This is an example of taken-for-granted meanings and skillful practices forming an embodied intentionality (Merleau-Ponty, 1945/2006). The nurse learns to dwell in a world that is salient for providing good nursing care.

> *"Techniques or tasks completed without engaging in caring relationships with particular patients with particular sets of needs and concerns do not constitute a practice."*
> *–Patricia Benner*

Practices are also situated "for the sake of" something else that is of concern to our *being* (Heidegger, 1927/1962). Practices as socially embedded human actions are defined by MacIntyre (1984) as any

> *coherent and complex form of socially established cooperative human activity through which goods internal to that form of activity are realized in the course of trying to achieve those standards of excellence which are appropriate to, and partially definitive of, that form of activity, with the result that human powers to achieve excellence, and human conceptions of the ends and goods involved, are systematically extended. (p. 187)*

According to MacIntyre, "internal goods" refer to social goods within the practice itself, and "external goods" refer to ulterior motives toward gains to practitioners outside the practice.

Human beings dwell in the world as concerned about, and caring for, people as well as objects (Heidegger, 1927/1962). According to Benner (1997), care ethics are embedded within the social community of nursing practice. Care ethics are situated, or based in, communally defined notions of the good and are attentive to the needs, desires, and possibilities of the parties involved—in particular, the patient and family members. Benner distinguishes the taking up of the *practice* of nursing from merely accomplishing tasks: "Techniques or tasks completed without engaging in caring relationships with particular patients with particular sets of needs and concerns do not constitute a practice" (p. 50).

Communities of Practice

Taking up a practice such as nursing occurs within a community of practice. Learning is situated and relational, and meanings are negotiated (Lave & Wenger, 2006). There is no discrete set of content that stands alone and apart from the practice setting. In the integrative learning of a social practice, notions of the good are also taken up in the formation of an everyday ethical comportment (Benner, 1997). For example, within a labor and delivery unit, nursing students learn to take cues from the particular patient regarding the meaning of modesty and the level of body exposure that is comfortable for the patient during labor, delivery, and the post-partum period. As with any hospitalized patient, the student meets the patient in a vulnerable and exposed state of undress, and the nurse and patient together constitute, typically in an unspoken manner, an understanding of what is meant by modesty.

For the nursing student, such learning is transformative in that the new understanding or skill literally changes the individual's embodied ways of perceiving and orienting to the situation, as well as his or her anticipation toward how to respond. Learning shifts from a focus on the individual to participation within a social world (Lave & Wenger, 2006). For the nursing student, world-transforming identity changes as well as taking up practical skills and knowledge occur by engagement within the everyday world of a community of practice and in encountering and caring for patients and families.

The Nursing Student and the Phenomenon of Care

Lived experience itself is interpretive. The meaning of our being and presence in the world is continually reinterpreted through our practical engagements with other people, things (such as equipment), and events that are of concern. According to Heidegger (1927/1962), caring in its broadest sense as "things mattering" is essential to an understanding of human being. It is embedded in our every day involvements *in order to* and *for the sake of*. As a being who "belongs to involvements," the individual shares with others "a primordial familiarity with world" (p. 119), in which each is involved in the same, concernful way.

To care about something or someone sets us up to act in certain ways toward certain possibilities. We are drawn to act based upon what we have already experienced. Growing up in a particular culture affords the nursing student access to an understanding of connection and involvement with the Other. The Other is always already there in the world in which we are born and raised. Heidegger (1927/1962) described the meaning of Others in this way:

> By 'Others' we do not mean everyone else but me—those over against whom the "I" stands put. They are rather those from whom, for the most part, one does not distinguish oneself—those among whom one is too . . . the "too" means a sameness of Being as circumspectively concernful Being-in-the-world . . . Being-in is Being-With Others. (p. 154-155)

As social beings, we are always already in a world with others and therefore have an existential readiness to deal with people as they go about their Being-in-the-World; Being-With is already there. We inhabit the world as a "we." Nursing students learn to understand the Other through the concrete experiences of Being-With and caring-for the Other, a type of care that Heidegger referred to as *solicitude*. Solicitude in the everyday world often shows up in a deficit mode as being without, being against or for, or passing by, but we come to know the Other in our concernful solicitude toward them. The Being-With of solicitude is understood as a shared space of "we" rather than "you and I." The Other is always there referentially, so that even in its absence, it remains although in the background of understanding as students encounter patients and their families in the clinical setting.

A Postmodern/Technological Age

A cultural epoch, according to Heidegger (1952/1977), comprises any number of styles of understanding being, but typically one style becomes dominant and thus defines the age. Heidegger argued that, "Metaphysics grounds an age, in that through a specific interpretation of what is and through a specific comprehension of truth it gives to that age the basis upon which it is essentially formed" (p. 115). This specific truth claim becomes the system of explaining the world. According to Heidegger, a culture's epochal style is so pervasive that it is invisible to its members. That is, the styles of a culture exist in practices, habits, equipment, skills, and social relationships. The style of a culture determines what shows up as important for its inhabitants. The notion of understanding *being* as human then fades into the background as a taken-for-granted way of being in the world is taken up, and takes over self-understanding. Therefore, taking up the practice of nursing in any historical time will reflect the style of that age, and the style of the age influences what shows up as important to the nursing student as well as the faculty.

Beginning in 1950, later writing by Heidegger suggested that Western civilization had entered a new epoch: the technological understanding of being (Dreyfus & Spinosa, 2004). This new postmodern period is the age of possibilities. Everything, including human beings, is optimized. In television ads, the U.S. Army encourages potential young enlistees to "Be all that you can be." Even children's lives are filled with sports, Scouting, art and music lessons, and tutoring so they, too, can make the most of their possibilities. Adult individuals can "reinvent" themselves or create or extend their identities via the Web. The understanding of being has changed from an instrumental view to an informational view, or as suggested by Dreyfus and Spinosa, "the postmodern human being is not interested in collecting but is constituted by connecting" (p. 7). Now what matters is maximum flexibility or adaptability.

> *"We depend on technical devices; they even challenge us to ever greater advances. But suddenly and unaware we find ourselves so firmly shackled to these technical devices that we fall into bondage to them."*
>
> –Martin Heidegger

This new age of possibilities is distinctly different than the age preceding it in that human beings are no longer the subject in control of their destinies. Things are no longer regarded as objects but rather as "their ability to be used" (Heidegger, 1954/1977). Humans no longer stand apart as giving meaning as a subject in control of objects. Instead, humans become resource, and along with everything else, become "standing reserve" (Heidegger, 1954/1977). Human beings as standing reserve are neither subject nor object but rather a placeholder in an enframing scheme. Persons as placeholders are not only interchangeable but, in addition, the schematic itself becomes the ultimate affordance as offering an abstracted view of unlimited potential for flexibility or adaptability. For example, in the Westernized managed care medical model, the patient might be conceptualized as "the hip in room 209" or "one of the anticipated discharges for the day." In each example, goals—whether of profit or of care—can be lost within an unthinking and routinized yet efficient discharge of patients. The discharge routine becomes a thing unto itself, a structure without meaning other than a schematic of "available beds" on a supervisor's desk.

The technological style is about expediting, about furthering something else, about ensuring possibilities and unlocking the future. Everything that is summoned forth is put into a framework and is ordered, and can be reshuffled to extend possibilities (Heidegger, 1954/1977). Technology becomes organistic, a thing unto itself wherein meaning issues forth from the possibility of further reserves. The stem cell serves as the ultimate standing reserve. It represents total flexibility, standing by to become whatever we want it to be. We have resources that make possible "*endless* disaggregation, redistribution, and reaggregation *for its own sake*" (Dreyfus & Spinosa, 2004, p. 5). Thus, unwittingly, the reordering becomes the "for-the-sake-of."

According to Heidegger (1954/1977), the danger lies in the framework itself. In its organizing and reordering, the enframing becomes the style and thus is itself obscured from our view: There is no other meaning than future possibility. "We depend on technical devices; they even challenge us to ever greater advances. But suddenly and unaware we find ourselves so firmly shackled to these technical devices that we fall into bondage to them" (Heidegger, 1966, p. 54).

Ironically, as we depart from an age defined by human control over the world picture, we enter a world that threatens our control and, as Heidegger notes, "The will to mastery becomes all the more urgent the more technology threatens to slip from human control" (Heidegger, 1954/1977, p. 5). Yet Heidegger suggests that the answer to undoing the "grip of technology" is not in planning and calculation but rather in becoming receptive to what is going on: "The closer we come to the danger, the more brightly do the ways into the saving power begin to shine and the more questioning we become" (1954/1977, p. 35). The focus on technology in modern healthcare settings can cause students to forget the lifeworld of patients, yet patients and families engage caregivers through focal practices like birth that create a resistance to technology for its own sake.

CLEARINGS AND FOCAL PRACTICES

According to Heidegger (1927/1962), human beings are always in the world within situations. Understandings of being are opened in *clearings*, which Heidegger defined as disclosive spaces or situations of shared human practices, traditions, and language. Within a clearing, things show up in the light of our commonly held understanding of being so that individual interpretations have a "primordial familiarity" (Heidegger, 1927/1962). Clearings are situated so that they are always specific and therefore establish bounded possibilities. However, though "situated," individual clearings are not spatial, but rather "a moving center of pragmatic activity in the midst of a shared world" (Dreyfus, 1991, p. 164). Heidegger addressed local clearings as temporary worlds gathered around everyday things and activities concerning the thing (Dreyfus & Spinosa, 2004). These gatherings around typical things and events serve to focus and sustain us around what matters to us in our local world. Possibilities show up as appropriate and "what particular possibilities are relevant is determined by the situation itself" (Dreyfus & Spinosa, 2004, p. 11).

Borgmann (1984) extended Heidegger's notion of local clearings to the idea of focal practices, events gathered on a "thing" imbued with meanings from daily life events. A focal practice signifies an orienting place that discloses, clarifies, articulates, and sustains the things that matter to those who are participants. Focal things and practices create a center of socially embedded meanings that radiate from the practice.

In Borgmann's (1984) development of the notion of focal things and focal practices, the hearth is used as an exemplary focal thing. *Focus*, in Latin, means hearth. The hearth in Roman times was the gathering and centering place for family events. It was the site of daily practices as well as celebrations and religious rituals: in general, a focus of family activity. "The hearth sustained, ordered, and centered house and family" (Borgmann, p. 196).

Focal practices of family can be somber or celebratory. The following narrative, captured in the clinical journal of a nursing student, describes the particular focal practice of birth:

> *The first thing I noticed was that the patient was very calm, had an oxygen mask on, and seemed very concentrated on her task at hand. She didn't look up or even open her eyes at the sound of our voices, and appeared fairly relaxed and not in any outstanding pain at the moment. . . . We quickly found out that the patient was Spanish-speaking only, but her husband understood enough English to help us get by. They wholeheartedly agreed to us being in the room and reality struck me that I might actually witness a birth today. . . .*
>
> *After some time, the nurse performed a vaginal exam and decided to have her start pushing. . . . We instructed the patient on how to push and coached her through. . . . Her husband was very supportive and stayed at her head, offering a lot of encouragement and touch, while the nurse stayed at the foot of the bed. The patient continued to remain very calm and reserved throughout pushing, but it was evident that she was getting very tired. . . . She pushed through contractions for nearly two hours and started doubting herself and told her husband she couldn't do this anymore. . . . At this point, the baby's head was in view, but not crowning enough*

> to call the doctor in. It felt like we were stuck in the same spot for a long time. . . . I couldn't help but compare this birth to the birth of my daughter. I pushed for 20 minutes, and my daughter came into the world. I couldn't imagine pushing for two hours and still not being able to turn that last corner to the finish line. I could feel her pain, and I wanted so badly to push and breathe with her.
>
> It felt like an eternity, but the doctor eventually came in and asked the patient if she wanted assistance in getting the baby out. She agreed to vacuum extraction, and this decision really put things in motion! All of a sudden, the peaceful five of us turned into a buzzing 15+ people. . . . It took about three good pushes, and the baby's head came out, followed by the body. It almost felt like everything went into slow motion as the baby came out. . . . I could literally feel the relief from the mother as we heard some of her only words spoken the entire time . . . not just relief from the pushing and pain, but relief that she finally got to see her baby in person.
>
> They announced that it was a girl, and the new mom and dad were elated! Once the baby was stable, she was taken right to mom who immediately asked if she could put her on the breast. She held her and laughed, teared up, and looked at her husband. She was absolutely giddy with excitement, and couldn't get enough of her new baby. She passed her to dad, who beamed with absolute pride at the sight of his daughter.
>
> Later while the baby was receiving newborn care in the nursery . . . I noticed the father was trying to watch through the window, and I asked permission to tell him the weight and height and what would be happening next with his baby. . . . I asked if they had picked a name for her. He reached into his pocket and pulled out a piece of paper that his wife had written on: Bentazume. It was original to me, but special to them. I told him it was a beautiful name, congratulated him, and thanked him for the memorable experience.

One of the first things the student noticed was the patient's focused efforts on "her task at hand," evidenced by her lack of acknowledgement of the presence of others in the room, not responding to sounds. The patient's husband gave support by his nearness at the head of the bed, his touch, and his words of encouragement. Although the patient did not show signs of "outstanding" pain, after two hours of pushing, her doubts whether she would be able to birth the baby created more of a focus of concern. The student had been drawn into the focal practice and recalled an altered sense of the passage of time. Time felt like "an eternity." She drew a comparison between this birth and her own experience of birth—another focal clearing. She related to the physicality of pushing in labor, much like an athletic event in which one "turns the last corner to the finish line." She vicariously felt the patient's pain and seemed to want to merge in a bodily way with the patient to push and breathe together. Thus, rather than remain separated, the student maintained a position alongside. Similarly, she felt in an embodied way the physical relief of the patient following the birth.

The focal practice of birth seemed in jeopardy as "the peaceful five of us" turned into a "buzzing 15+ people" as additional medical personnel entered the room. However, the student's narrative remained focused on the birth, as the mother greeted her new baby. Here, one begins to experience the constituting of meaning of the new baby's "world" as an "elated" mother and father welcomed the announcement of a girl. The mother immediately sought to nourish the child; her emotions were heightened and abundant as she laughed, and then became tearful. We notice the sharing of the event as she turned to her husband, and then later physically passed the new family member to him as he smiled proudly.

The focal practices of birthing, recognition, and naming were continued in the nursery. The new family member was given a particular weight and height that would become part of the family's personal history of the birth event. Finally, the father produced a piece on paper on which had been inscribed the name of the child. The student acknowledged the name as unfamiliar to her, not a part of her world, yet she understood that the name had special meaning to the mother and father. The particular name, as well as the height, weight, gender, and time of birth will be part of the "always already" world of Bentazume.

The following narrative is an exemplar derived from another student's postconference account of a birth:

> *As Rebecca sat listening to report with the nurse she was to follow during her first day in labor and delivery, she realized that this was in fact a new world. Although she was in her sixth semester of a baccalaureate nursing program, what she heard in report might as well have been given in Russian. Words and phrases like "milliunits per minute," "shrom" [actually refers to the acronym for the spontaneous rupture of membranes, commonly known as the bag of waters breaking or leaking], and "montevideo" units were recalled as words in her theory book but had no meaning at this point in time. After report, the nurse explained to her that the patient, pregnant with her first baby, had been scheduled for an induction of labor since she was nearly two weeks past her due date. The nurse further explained that the patient had received serial ultrasounds during the pregnancy since the baby was "IUGR" [intrauterine growth restriction], and they were "starting the 'pit'" [pitocin administration to induce labor].*

> *As Rebecca and the nurse entered the room, the nurse suggested that Rebecca "ignore the machines since it's too much to explain" and "just focus on the family and support the patient in labor." Rebecca knew something about labor since she had coached her sister during the birth of her niece, and she had attended a childbirth class as part of her preparation for this semester's clinical focus. The patient was lying on her side with belts around her abdomen that seemed to tether her to the fetal heart monitor. Rebecca noticed two IVs infusing, but the patient seemed to not be in pain. The student noticed an older woman in the corner, eyes closed and lips moving as though muttering a prayer. The patient apologized, saying, "My mother is praying for the safe birth of my son." Rebecca remarked, "Oh, you know it's a boy?", and the patient proudly shared an ultrasound "photo" in a frame on the bedside table. "This is our first picture of Bharav," said the patient with a wide smile. It seemed as though the patient had attempted to bring "home" to the hospital. She was dressed in a floral chenille robe over her hospital gown, and there were matching furry slippers beside the bed. There were framed photos of family members, a floral arrangement, and wrapped presents on the bedside table; a bouquet of balloons tied to the bedrail; and a teddy bear on the rocking chair beside the bed. According to the patient, her husband was outside talking on the cell phone "since they don't allow cell phones in the room." He was talking to relatives in Sri Lanka that were also anxiously awaiting the newest family member.*

Whether by default or design, the nurse's instruction to focus on the family allowed the focal practice of birth within one family to emerge for the student. In part through the use of technologies such as cell phones, digital photos, and airplanes, the family is gathered and centered in the hospital room where the mother-to-be lies tethered to other technological devices. Technology has extended the range of this family's local world in both time and space. Even before birth, the yet-unborn child has been seen, gendered, and named; and the family is able to celebrate the birth with family in a distant country. The heightened sense of the importance of the event is represented in gifts and symbolically decorated balloons; ties to home are present in the warm and comforting slippers and robe; and the patient's mother summons God to bless the event.

Birth in the Age of Technology

Nursing students entering the clinical environment face the real possibility of confusion concerning the relative importance of technology and its devices in contrast to the local worlds and focal practices of patients. It is within the local world of a community of practice that the student takes up the practice of nursing. The community as well as the student dwells amidst a history and traditions that cannot be swept aside (Gadamer, 1975/2004). It is easy for the student to become confused in determining the "for the sake of" in a culture of medicine with one foot in Heidegger's modern age of technical rationalism, and the other in his postmodern age, threatened by enframement of possibility for its own sake. Still, the student cannot escape his or her own history and traditions that form the background of understanding in which the student's clearings are created.

What is important in nursing care that attends to the lifeworld is that the student seeks to understand the relevant meanings of birthing and birthing focal practices of the family. The student is apt to lean toward technological enframing as a result of the clinic and schooling. However, in addition to technology and post-modern self-understandings, birthing practices as biographical, relational practices also shape the possible clearings and often constitute the focal practices of birthing for the mother and family.

In the postmodern world of hospitals, technological devices (such as electronic fetal monitors and ultrasound machines) can lure and focus attention on performance and possibilities rather than the disclosive space of focal practices. The beguiling revealing of information can become activities that are self-defined and accounted for as mattering in a technical sense, rather than genuinely advancing the greater good of individuals and families. For example, surveillance devices such as ultrasound machines and fetal monitors have the potential to focus attention on information for its own sake and can distract the practitioner (doctor, nurse, or student nurse) from the patient as the focus of care. Within a technological understanding of medical care, there exists a danger of closing off the focal practices of the family around health, illness, and birth.

What is the self-understanding of the person who can have a focal practice of birth that incorporates technology? Rather than seeing the technological understanding of birth and the focal practices of birth as two worlds in collision, the two can be articulated as a fusion of horizons that provides a clearing. In the cited exemplars, one can interpret the background meanings of what matters to the people involved. For example, because these families have chosen to give birth in a hospital, they believe in the modern westernized medical model and the safety of hospitals. From the standpoint of the medical personnel, the use of technology within medical practice stems from the same assumptions of what it means to be a person that is thrown within a peopled world in which what matters is a safe, medically uncomplicated birth for mother and infant.

Instead of viewing technology and nursing as opposing forces, technology can be taken up in a different way. Technology can be viewed as aiding our practical engagement and taken up as part of our concern for the patient. It helps us understand differently: a qualitatively different view of technology as part of the focal practice of birth that creates a focal clearing for us. In this way, the technology "becomes embodied in practical activity" (Walters, 1995, p. 341). For example, as within the exemplar, the "baby photo" of the ultrasound (and thus the technology) was taken up as part of our concern for what matters to the patient while aiding the possibility of a safe birth.

The postmodern age affords nursing students access to devices (such as simulators) and the World Wide Web that can enhance their learning. As Borgmann (1984) observed, "Technology can fulfill the promise of a new kind of freedom and richness. If our lives are centered in a focal concern, technology uniquely opens up the depth and extent of the world and allows us to be genuine world citizens" (p. 248).

> *"If our lives are centered in a focal concern, technology uniquely opens up the depth and extent of the world and allows us to be genuine world citizens."*
> *–Albert Borgmann*

In the first exemplar, the student described how the patient's room was swiftly inhabited by more than 15 people after a medical device (the vacuum extractor) was applied to assist in the delivery of the baby. For many of the medical personnel in attendance, perhaps this had become merely a technological medical event with little regard for the particularly situated focal practices of the family. However, the student remained in a shared, disclosive space with the family, articulating and sustaining the local meanings and focal practices of birth.

In the second exemplar, the strange language and equipment of the labor and delivery environment had the potential to lure the student from her attentiveness to the focal practice and toward a commodified view of the patient as standing reserve. In this view, the patient would be nothing more than a notch on an experiential belt with perhaps some further information "gain" of the technical aspects of medicalized birth. However, the tradition of nursing practice strives to rescue, negotiate, and balance the focal practices and open the possibilities. Learning to strike the right balance is part of learning the practice. One does not discount technology, but rather takes up the technology in such a way that it doesn't edge out the focal practices.

The Possibility of Other Local Worlds

As clinical faculty and nurses, we need to reflect upon how we frame or open up clearings to students as they encounter the focal practices of patients and families from within today's culture of medicine. We need to keep open the possibility for other local worlds to show up alongside the dominant postmodern/technical paradigm. Gadamer (1975/2004) described our gaining understanding as the fusion of horizons:

> *Transposing ourselves consists neither in the empathy of one individual to another nor in subordinating another person to our standards; rather, it always involves rising to a higher universality that overcomes not only our own particularity but also that of the other. The concept of "horizon" suggests itself because it expresses the superior breadth of vision that the person who is trying to understand must have. To acquire a horizon means that one learns to look beyond what is close at hand—not in order to look away from it but to see it better, within a larger whole and in truer proportion. (p. 304)*

Gadamer's quote denies the personal subjectivity of empathy or the transposition of a mental representation, such as a standard. Instead, his statement suggests a breadth of vision informed by "that region of lived experience where the phenomenon dwells in recognizable form" (van Manen, 1997, p. 367).

A centering force can be retained in focal things and practices. Technology in its transparency can be extending and revealing of our world. Borgmann (1984) suggested that "We remember and realize more fully that the technological environment heightens rather than denies the radiance of genuine focal things and . . . we learn to understand that focal things require a practice to prosper within" (p. 196). A practice depends upon the practitioner's practical engagement within a situation of meanings and concerns of individuals.

Engagement means to participate in a dialog with a world. As such, "engagement means risking one's stance and acknowledging the ongoing liminal experience of living between the familiar and strangeness" (Schwandt, 2000, p. 207). Familiarity and strangeness speaks to the individual's particular thrownness within a tacit phenomenal field of shared meanings. New experiences expand our horizons of understanding. Experiential learning as a new experience of meaning involves the rupture of world toward the development of new understanding. Meaning is negotiated rather than constructed (Gadamer, 1975/2004) in a dialog between our prejudgments based upon the traditions into which we are thrown and the experiential "encounter with what is not understood" (Schwandt, 2000, p. 195).

The student exemplars presented here demonstrate the students' engagement or involvement with the Other within their focal practice of birth. In the first account, the student admits the strangeness of the newborn's name of Bentazume, yet growing up in a commonly experienced world of concerns allows her familiarity with the meaning of naming and particularizing a new being. The concrete experience of Being-With the patient and family allows the student to expand his or her horizon to include what at first seems strange. Although there may be different notions of care for different cultures, as human beings, we share the phenomenon of care (Heidegger, 1927/1962).

The potential exists to romanticize the language of focal practices and create a valorization or idealization in which one is a voyeur of someone else's experience. When reading the included exemplars, it is important to recall that focal practices are spontaneous and fleeting. They are gatherings focused in a particular event and things. These interpretive accounts are perspectival, always partial, and reflect particular situations in time and space. Heidegger used the term "temporal determinateness" (Heidegger, 1927/1962, p. 40) to describe how in a moment of time, a limited number of possible standpoints are disclosed.

Caring Practices in the Postmodern

Caring practices in our postmodern technocratic culture can be invisible and marginalized. Their nearness to our being can cause them to be taken for granted or ignored, especially in a world where ends often define means. Caring practices can be considered part of what Heidegger described as "the saving power" of the little or humble things. Benner (2000) considered this socially embedded practical knowledge as preserving human worlds:

> *All of the caring practices such as nursing, mothering, fathering, education, child care, care of the aged, social welfare, care of the earth may be potential saving practices even as they are threatened and marginalized by a society that creates myths about ever expanding possibilities to manage and control all aspects of life.* (p. 309)

Nursing education often includes formal classroom time spent on topics of cultural competencies, therapeutic communication, and formal ethical theory; however, "theory is necessarily a skeletal, simplified version of reality" (Benner & Wrubel, 1989, p. 20). The dynamism, uncertainty, complexity, and indeterminacy of the human world of practice cannot be captured in theory or isolable, context-free rules. Theory can provide an outline and a sense of "where to look," but details must be filled out by experiencing a range of particular cases

(Benner & Wrubel, 1989; Dreyfus, 1999). It is through the concrete experiences of Being-With patients and families that the student can rise to Gadamer's (1975/2004) higher universality and reach a superior breadth of vision.

Learning everyday ethical comportment occurs through Being-With the Other and staying open to an understanding of their focal practices as a centering force of what matters in their particular world. In the clinical environment, the nursing student should be encouraged to remain open to the things that matter, the possibilities that people project onto their futures, and the ways in which they interpret the past. One of the challenges of nursing as a caring practice is to attend to the human experience of being ill or injured, giving birth, growing old, or facing death while skillfully using technology to create human possibilities and relationship. Artful use of technology will open up worlds or at least hold them open, rather than close them down and usurp the human significance of vulnerability, birth, growth, and death.

References

Benner, P. (1997). A dialog between virtue ethics and care ethics. *Theoretical Medicine, 18*, 47-61.

Benner, P. (2000). The quest for control and the possibilities of care. In *Heidegger, coping, and cognitive science: Essays in honor of Hubert Dreyfus* (Vol. 2, pp. 293-309). Cambridge, MA: The MIT Press.

Benner, P., Tanner, C., & Chesla, C. (1996). *Expertise in nursing practice: Caring, clinical judgment, and ethics*. New York: Springer.

Benner, P., & Wrubel, J. (1989). *The primacy of caring: Stress and coping in health and illness*. Menlo Park, CA: Addison-Wesley.

Borgmann, A. (1984). *Technology and the character of contemporary life: A philosophical inquiry*. Chicago: University of Chicago Press.

Dreyfus, H. L. (1991). *Being-in-the-world: A commentary on Heidegger's being and time, Division 1*. Cambridge, MA: The MIT Press.

Dreyfus, H. L. (1994). Preface. In P. Benner (Ed.), *Interpretive phenomenology: Embodiment, caring, and ethics in health and illness* (pp. vii-xi). Thousand Oaks, CA: Sage.

Dreyfus, H. L. (1999). *What computers still can't do: A critique of artificial reason*. Cambridge, MA: The MIT Press.

Dreyfus, H. L., & Spinosa, C. (2004). *Highway bridges and feasts: Heidegger and Borgmann on how to confirm technology*. Berkeley, CA: Regents of the University of California.

Dunne, J. (1997). *Back to the rough ground*. Notre Dame, IN: University of Notre Dame Press.

Gadamer, H. G. (2004). *Truth and method*. London: Continuum. (Original work published 1975).

Heidegger, M. (1962). *Being and time*. (J. Macquarrie & E. Robinson, Trans.). New York: Harper & Row. (Original work published 1927).

Heidegger, M. (1966). Memorial address. (J. Anderson & E. Freund, Trans.). In *Discourse on thinking* (pp. 43-57). New York: Harper & Row.

Heidegger, M. (1977). The age of the world picture. In *The question concerning technology and other essays* (pp. 115-154). New York: Harper & Row. (Original work published 1952).

Heidegger, M. (1977). The question concerning technology. (W. Lovitt, Trans.). In *The question concerning technology and other essays* (pp. 3-35). New York: Harper & Row. (Original work published 1954).

Lave, J., & Wenger, E. (2006). *Situated learning: Legitimate peripheral participation*. New York: Cambridge University Press.

MacIntyre, A. (1984). *After virtue* (2nd ed.). Notre Dame, IN: University of Notre Dame Press.

Merleau-Ponty, M. (2006). *Phenomenology of perception*. (C. Smith, Trans.). New York: Routledge. (Original work published 1945).

Nagel, T. (1986). *A view from nowhere*. NY: Oxford University Press.

Schon, D. (1983). *The reflective practitioner: How professionals think in action*. New York: Basic Books.

Schwandt, T. A. (2000). Three epistemological strategies for qualitative inquiry: Interpretivism, hermeneutics, and social constructionism. In N. K. Denzin & Y. S. Lincoln (Eds.), *Handbook of qualitative research* (2nd ed., pp. 189-214). Thousand Oaks, CA: Sage.

van Manen, M. (1997). From meaning to method. *Qualitative Health Research*, 7(3), 345-369.

Walters, A. J. (1995). Technology and the lifeworld of the critical care nurse. *Journal of Advanced Nursing, 22*, 338-346.

CHAPTER 3
Distal Nursing
RUTH E. MALONE

> The only space where the moral act can be performed is the social space of 'being with,' continually buffeted by the criss-crossing pressures of cognitive, aesthetic, and moral spacings. In this space, the possibility to act on the promptings of moral responsibility must be salvaged, or recovered, or made anew; against odds—sometimes overwhelming odds—the responsibility must exchange its now invalidated or forgotten priority for the superiority over technical-instrumental calculations. . . . If it happens, it will happen only as an accomplishment. There is not and there will never be any guarantee that it will indeed happen. But it does happen, daily and repeatedly—each time that people care, love, and bring succour to those who need it. (Bauman, 1993, p. 185)

> No practices can survive for any length of time unsustained by institutions. (MacIntyre, 1984, p. 194)

INTRODUCTION

Interpretive phenomenology as method points to consideration of embodied experience and human practices. But such practices cannot be understood except within a context of place and space. Philosophers of phenomenology have suggested that *place* has an ontological primacy and may be grasped through narrative, while *space* is a more abstract conceptualization. This paper presents an example of a secondary theoretical analysis of spatial dynamics in nursing practice, drawing on primary interpretive phenomenological studies to illustrate how power relationships embedded in hospital-based spatial-structural practices disrupt nursing's proximities to patients.

Reprinted from *Social Science and Medicine*, 56, 2317-2326 Author Ruth E. Malone, Distal Nursing, Copyright 2003, with permission from Elsevier.

All human relationships have spatial aspects. This is true not only because we are material beings with bodies that move and have volume, but because our proximity to or distance from others and from places have meaning for us. When we are sick, these often-taken-for-granted proximities and distances become revealed to us in our experience of displacement—from familiar routines and places, but also often from our own bodies, which we may experience as having betrayed or even abandoned us (van Manen, 1998). Leaving behind the place of *home* and entering into the unfamiliar institutional spaces of the hospital, our understandings of intimacy and distance are challenged by intrusive examinations, loss of private space, the threatened foreshortening of our life horizons, and the need to depend upon the kindness of strangers as we seek not only wellness, but re-emplacement in our bodies and our lives. In hospitals, nurses are among the strangers to whom we turn.

Nursing as a human practice also has spatial aspects. Because relationship with the patient is considered central to nursing practice, nursing depends at least in part upon sustaining some meaningful *proximity* to patients. This paper considers the spatial-structural dynamics of nurse-patient relationships within hospitals under conditions of organizational restructuring. Hospital nursing, I argue in this paper, is increasingly constrained by spatial-structural practices that disrupt nursing's relations with patients by reducing or eliminating heretofore taken-for-granted proximity.[1] Three "nested" kinds of proximity are threatened: physical, narrative, and moral. Examining these proximities through a place-space lens suggests that structurally, nursing is becoming increasingly "distal" to patient care.

The plan of the paper is as follows: First, I situate the paper within several perspectives on space and place; next, I discuss three types of "nested" proximity that characterize nurse-patient relationships; third, I describe spatial-structural changes under conditions of hospital restructuring within the United States and show how these reduce proximity and constrain nurse-patient (as well as nurse-nurse) relationships. I conclude with a discussion of the potential implications of this loss of proximity for nursing and, drawing on social theories of spatial production, the power relations "distal nursing" conceals and reinforces.

THEORETICAL PERSPECTIVES: SPACE AND PLACE

At least two broad strands of discourse are relevant to this discussion: Phenomenological perspectives on space and place in philosophy, which suggest that place grounds our subjective, embodied experience and can only be understood through experience (Casey, 1993; Malpas, 1999), and critical geographical and historical perspectives which draw attention to the power relationships instantiated in places and spaces (Foucault, 1963/1975; Foucault, 1979; Lefebvre, 1992/1974; Massey, 1994, 1995).

Very roughly, the former focuses more closely on the "micro" level of experience and subjectivity as shaped by place and space and the latter on "macro" structures that shape the possibilities for spatial relationships between groups. Each of these perspectives can be useful in considering the spatial dynamics of hospital nursing.

For some phenomenologists, place has a special ontological primacy. Malpas (1999) argues that understanding of place is grasped through narrative, while Casey suggests it is grasped more directly through bodily experience as "persons-in-places" (Casey, 1993, p. 30). For both, *place* is experience-near, characterized by a sense of unity and coherence, while *space* is more abstract, a conceptualization we are even able to develop only because we first understand ourselves *as* emplaced. In this perspective, it is because we are *not* disembodied subjects set over against a separate background or environment, but persons-in-place, that proximity and distance have relevance in our relations with others.

Another strand of space/place theory concerns itself with power relationships and how they shape and are shaped by spatial relationships. This perspective emphasizes that space is neither neutral nor passive (Lefebvre, 1992). Rather, it is shaped by human social activities. The social construction of 'space' and 'place' is characterized by tension and conflicts between the 'global' and the 'local,' the material and the metaphorical; the boundaries between these are fluid, and the very identity of places as such is constantly at issue (Massey, 1994, 1995). Material changes shaped by power inequities may reconfigure places and spaces and with them, the power relations they instantiate. Foucauldian perspectives on power are also relevant to this discussion. Power, as Foucault shows us, not only conceals itself, but conceals through spatial forms that reinforce power relations (Foucault, 1963/1975; Foucault, 1979; Rabinow, 1984).

NESTED PROXIMITIES IN NURSING

Within nursing, Liaschenko (1994; 1997) was perhaps the first to suggest that geographical concepts are relevant to understanding the nurse-patient relationship at all levels. Liaschenko argued that although ethical concerns are commonly considered to arise out of the local, intimate aspect of nurse-patient relationship, they often originate at a larger structural scale. Liaschenko suggested that patients, by virtue of their social positions, have different spatial vulnerabilities, and that this was at least partially due to nursing's "gendered" spatiality. In this paper, I seek to extend this work by proposing that hospital nursing is itself spatially vulnerable insofar as it depends upon a taken-for-granted proximity to patients that is acutely threatened by the localized spatial and power dynamics of macro-originated economic and ideological pressures.

At least three types of proximity are at issue: *physical proximity*, which I define as a nearness within which nurses physically touch and care for patients' bodies; *narrative proximity*, in which nurses come to "know the patient" (Tanner, Benner, Chesla, & Gordon, 1993) by hearing and trying to understand (and, in turn, transmit to one another) the patient's "story" (of the illness for him/her, of his/her particular life); and *moral proximity*, in which nurses encounter the patient as Other, recognize that a moral concern to "be for" exists, and are solicited to act on a patient's behalf. These proximities are nested: physical proximity sets up the possibility for dialogue with the patient and family through which aspects of the patient's narrative may be grasped, and it is through understanding the patient as a person with a life (Liaschenko, 1995) that nurses are able to begin to appreciate the moral significance of issues for him/her and to act accordingly on his behalf when he/she is unable to do so.

Physical proximity between nurses and patients is so taken-for-granted that nurses' subordinate social status has been attributed to the physical nature of nurses' contact with the diseased body and its effluvia. Learning how to wash the body, how to assist with toileting, and how to prevent skin breakdown during long illnesses are part of every nurse's basic educational preparation, and clinical knowledge includes learning how to provide physical comfort through positioning the body. In addition, assessment of patient condition through direct physical contact, such as touching the patient to assess the warmth, moisture, and texture of the skin, is basic to hospital nursing. However, the relationship of physical proximity is not merely one of application of technique, as van Manen has pointed out. Physical contact, such as washing, may also be part of inviting a "reuniting" or "re-emplacing" of the patient in a "livable relation with his or her body" (van Manen, 1998, p. 9).

Narrative proximity in nursing has two aspects: coming to "know the patient" (Tanner et al., 1993) through hearing directly or piecing together from family and other sources a story of what the illness means in his or her life, and respectfully transmitting this knowledge in narrative form to others who care for the patient. The latter aspect has implications for both the care of this particular patient and for the transmission within nursing of socially embedded knowledge, as Benner's work on nursing practice has shown (Benner, Hooper-Kyriakidis, & Stannard, 1999; Benner, Tanner, & Chesla, 1992; Benner, Tanner, & Chesla, 1996; Benner & Wrubel, 1989).[2] In using the word narrative, I mean "a more or less coherent written, spoken, or (by extension) enacted account of occurrences" (Hunter, 1996, p. 306) rather than narrative in any formal linguistic or literary sense. Through listening to patients and telling each other stories about *particular*[3] patients within the context of the local situation, nurses impart informal but important knowledge of how to make qualitative distinctions between particular patients and their experiences (Rubin, 1996), a point to which I will return.[4]

Nursing, as the profession most charged with bearing witness to the patient's distress or healing on a day to day, hour by hour basis, also involves a kind of moral proximity. It is in our direct, face to face encounter with the Other, as Levinas has noted (Levinas, 1981), that we are solicited to act, that recognition arises that there are both mutual vulnerabilities (Malone, 2000) and power inequities in the caregiving relationship. Gadow (1980) has asserted that nursing's heart is "existential advocacy," a being-for patients. One cannot "be for" an abstract class of patients in this way; one is called upon to be for *this* patient, at this moment, in all his or her complexity.

That moral proximity is nested within physical and narrative proximity is illustrated through drawing on an example from Benner's work. Benner cites the narrative of a nurse who cared for a 60-year-old African American man who was quadriplegic from a previous accident, disfigured by radical neck surgery for cancer, admitted to the hospital from a long term care facility with severe respiratory problems and put on ventilator support. The physicians' rather bleak assessment of the patient's quality of life, based on their more experience-distant perceptions of the clinical features of the patient's condition, led them to discuss withdrawing ventilator support and letting the patient die. The nurse, however, argued strenuously against this:

> I think we could have made a decision on not treating [George] fully, based upon what he looked like and what we thought he was. And I really stood up for him. I don't think some people ever got beyond just looking at him and saying, "This man is disfigured and not able to take care of himself. . . ."He was an incredible fighter . . . even withdrawn, he was actively withdrawn. . . . I don't think they [the physicians who wanted to withdraw ventilator support] stood with him and looked at him or gave him a Pepsi, or saw him watch the ball game [on television]. He really derived a lot of pleasure from living. . . . I think it was more a case of their perception of quality of life versus our perceptions of George's quality of life as we got to know him more, and what he was like at the skilled nursing facility. . . .He was a spokesperson for the patients, he helped people who had alcohol and drug problems. He had a girlfriend there who was also wheelchair-bound, and they used public transportation together. They were the Valentine King and Queen. I think

the doctors just looked at him and saw, "This is as good as it gets, and this is really depressing, and he is really depressed, so why continue?" (Benner Tanner, & Chesla, 1996, p. 21)

What is important to notice in this narrative is its focus on situating the patient in his particularity and how this is accomplished by means of proximity. The nurse contrasts the doctors' "just looking at him" (in an objectifying, biomedically focused way) with "standing with him" or "seeing him watch the ball game" in day by day interactions. Learning more about the patient's situatedness in his everyday life—establishing a narrative proximity that was possible only due to their ongoing physical proximity—the nurses were able to see past his dismaying functional impairment to his personhood, his emplacement in a life. Through narrative proximity, nurses gain moral proximity, as they stake out the particular and the local as essential to decision making and transmit the message that it is insufficient to consider only general clinical features in an abstract sense; in a sense, the patient must be *emplaced* (as a person-in-place) in a life context in order to interpret what is a moral course of action.[5]

Another important element to notice in this narrative relates to the interrelationship between proximity and *time*. This nurse was able to make her case not merely because she had been physically near to the patient—which, of course, the physicians also had been—but because she had been near long enough to "get to know him." Proximity is thus not merely spatial, but temporal as well.

Certainly, nurses do not sustain all three types of proximity in their relationships with every patient. When circumstances are unambiguous and routine, or hospitalizations are brief and uncomplicated, the nurse-patient relationship may likewise appropriately be brief and routine, requiring minimal proximity. But, increasingly, as will be discussed below, only patients with the most complex and potentially complicated conditions qualify for admission to hospitals, suggesting a need for more nurse-patient proximity rather than less. I shift now to considering some of the recent macro-level changes that have altered nurse-patient proximities.

Structural Spatial Changes Affecting Proximities

During the past decade, an unprecedented cluster of structural changes has occurred within the health care sector in general; the effects of these changes have been especially pronounced within United States hospitals (although similar scenarios are unfolding across Canada and Western Europe as cost-cutting pressures increase) and upon nurses specifically (Norrish & Rundall, 2001; Sochalski, Aiken, & Fagin, 1997). Discussion of the larger, interrelated economic and social factors that have shaped these extensive changes is beyond the scope of this paper; the aim here is to call attention to their local spatial-structural effects on nurse-patient relationships within hospitals, which are considerable. The changes to which I refer include but are not limited to: shifts toward treatment of patients in outpatient and home settings, reduced length of stay for hospitalized patients; work redesign strategies aimed at reducing costs; use of so-called "flexible" staffing, which involves using more part-time and temporary staff; certain efficiency measures, including changes in charting and reporting practices; and an emphasis on abstract classification systems and "standardization" of care.

Collectively, these changes reduce nurse-patient proximity in several ways. First, and most obviously, they reduce time available for direct physical contact between nurses and patients. As noted above, proximity involves not only spatial but temporal nearness. As patients leave hospitals more quickly and work redesign strategies redistribute nurses' work to lower-paid, lower-skilled workers, nurses become "care managers," positioned distally as overseers rather than proximally as direct care providers. Nurses thus have less time to spend with any particular patient as they spend more time on administrative and general clinical oversight and/or are replaced by non-nurse administrative staff (Aiken & Fagin, 1997; Wiener, 2000).[6] Instead of nurses, patients may have "care partners" or "service partners," who may have as little as two weeks of orientation for their new roles (Wiener, 2000).[7] The increased reliance on "flexible" staffing likewise means that a patient may have a different nurse each day as hospitals turn to registries for temporary staff. This minimizes possibilities for the sustained engagement with patients that is required to develop narrative proximity, or knowledge of the patient's story. The changes also reduce proximity among nurses themselves, as fewer nurses are spread more thinly as supervisors of lower-cost workers.

Certain traditional practices requiring physical proximity and long regarded as basic to good nursing care have also been jettisoned in "redesigning" nursing work. For example, the back rub, a way to assess patients' hydration, nutritional and circulatory status as well as a comforting tactile practice that allowed patients access to a nurse's uninterrupted attention, is no longer a part of routine nursing care in most institutions (Connelly, 1999; Meintz, 1995). The back rub, usually provided as part of evening or bedtime routine, was a few moments of comforting physical contact between nurse and patient that was often accompanied by dialogue between nurse and patient. As with the bed bath (van Manen, 1998), the backrub opens a space within which a healing relationship may take form. Backrub conversation thus often consisted of more than mere small talk: it provided an opportunity for coaching, non-threatening teaching, and development of a more fine-grained, situated understanding of this particular patient—an important part of understanding the patient in the "place" of his life outside. As nurse staffing decreased, such practices were identified as nonessential functions and eliminated in many facilities (Meintz, 1995).

Because, as discussed above, physical proximity is necessary for development of narrative proximity in the nurse-patient relationship, these changes also have implications for nurses' role as hearers and bearers of the patient's story. However, it is not only the loss of physical proximity that is involved (and with it the opportunities for hearing the patient's story), but also the loss of organizationally supported modes of communication through which such stories might be transmitted among nurses.

For example, 25 years ago, nursing notes in patient charts actually took the form of short narratives, written by the nurse caring for the patient on each shift. While some institutions structured these according to various parameters, such as using different colored inks to denote the different shifts of work, they were, for the most part, relatively free-form written accounts of the patient's day that included whatever the nurse felt might be relevant to those who would be caring for the patient in the following hours or days. These notes might, for example, include notations about who visited the patient, situating the patient in a context of relationships; about how the patient was coping with the demands of treatment; about complaints of and treatment for pain; or about specific questions or fears voiced by the patient. Sometimes the notes offered synopses of discussions or direct quotations from patients or family members.[8]

During the late 1970s and 1980s, many institutions began requiring more highly structured forms of nurses' notes, such as SOAP (subjective, objective, assessment, plan) charting. Though their purpose was to provide an organizing framework, minimize redundancy and make the notes more efficiently usable, such schemes also had the consequence of restricting individual nurses' prerogative to choose the way in which the patient/nurse relational narrative would be conveyed. Today, in order to minimize the time the preparation of nursing notes requires, many institutions structure nurses' notes in the form of care plan check-off boxes or computer-assisted algorhythms, which use a standardized format.

While such "charting by exception" (that is, only noting that which does not appear to follow a standard expected course) can be helpful in some respects, it also systematically truncates and structures the communication about patients that is shared in written form between nurses. Check-off boxes simply cannot accommodate narrative forms of communication. The selection of what it is important to note and how to note it are no longer the purview of the individual nurses caring for the patient, but are now prescribed in advance as a standard classification scheme in which individual nurses' interpretations may be viewed as usually unwelcome or technically aberrant deviations. The structuring of nurses' written communications into such distally determined forms reinforces the perception that nursing itself is an activity that can be reduced to a series of discrete tasks or points on such a prespecified "clinical pathway" (which is in turn, congruent with the spatially redesigned role of nurse as distally located "manager" of others who carry out such tasks).

Finally, the abovementioned cluster of interrelated changes in hospital settings disrupt moral proximity in nurse-patient relationships, by constituting patients in terms of their classification within abstract systems and constituting care as consisting of the abovementioned distally directed, standardized tasks rather than direct human engagement. Here I include the well-intentioned movements within nursing management toward defining and implementing abstract classification systems that could be used for "outcomes research," as well as the interconnected emphasis on standardized care plans or standardized "pathways" for biomedically defined conditions. Bowker and Star (1999) make the point that such abstract systems can never entirely capture what is important to know and do in a particular patient's case. Some specifications remain irretrievably implicit, and, as they observe, "what is left implicit becomes doubly invisible: it is the residue left over when other sorts of invisible work have been made visible" (p. 247).

Benner, who has perhaps developed the strongest critique of such abstracting strategies to describe nursing practice, cautions that "once nursing practice [is] defined as isolated units of behavior, diagnoses, and interventions without the significance of those actions (the in-order-to's, and for-the-sake-of's, for-that-purpose, to-that-end), there is no way to get back to everyday integrative clinical knowledge that always entails engaged reasoning in particular clinical situations. Thus, articulating nursing knowledge into the available economic and scientific language creates conflict and incongruities with the knowledge and ethos embedded in the actual caring practices of nurses." (Benner, 2000, p. 296). The effort to become increasingly explicit in defining discrete interventions based on abstractions from aggregated data paradoxically fuels a flight from the particularity and complexity of actual patient situations.[9]

The problem for nurse-patient moral proximity is that such distally directed, abstracting approaches either trivialize or ignore the profound contingency within any human interaction, contingency that permits the Other to emerge in all his or her particularity, soliciting our moral responsibility.[10]

Distal Nursing: Dangers

There are potential dangers in making nursing distal, not the least of which is that as nurses lose their proximities with patients and with one another, and see their work in terms of fulfilling extralocal demands for categorical and procedural efficiency and uniformity, they will likewise lose their sustaining narrative and moral traditions and will take up their work as mere technicians. This may reshape nursing as a "we're just running the trains" occupation (Lifton, 1986, p. 400). Under such circumstances, caring begins to stand out as something unusual and ultimately deviant.

In a study of emergency room nurses and patients (Malone, 1995, 1998, 2000), I talked with an emergency nurse who had counseled a sobbing, drug addicted woman about a treatment program. "I took about 15, 20 minutes *out*—and I really talked with her," she said. It is significant (and not, in my experience, atypical in contemporary hospitals) that the nurse understood herself to be taking time "out" to provide this kind of support for a patient, even though it was an entirely appropriate and needed intervention. Such humane support is implicitly seen as *external* to the "real" nursing work of managing the technical tasks necessary for discharge production.[11] Caring practices may be reduced to such snatched moments of near-covert connection, morally satisfying but risking possible sanction and carried out in the absence of institutional recognition and support.

Frank argues, drawing on the work of Dorothy Smith, that the move to the generalizing extralocal perspective means that patients are regarded as instances of a category and that, in the process, there is an "erasure" of suffering from the illness experience that can increase suffering (Frank, 2001). Earlier research on nursing practice seems to bear out this idea. Rubin (1996) studied nurses who appeared clinically "disengaged," identified by their head nurses as experienced but not expert, and found that a striking feature of these nurses' practice was their inability to remember particular details about their patients. That is, these nurses did not have at their disposal the narratives about patients that other nurses did.

"Not only could they not describe a critical incident that had made a difference in their practice; most could not even remember the specifics of a particular case, even the most recent," observed Rubin (Rubin, 1996, p. 172). For example, Rubin discusses a nurse who told a story about ending a patient's life through her own administration of an injection that slowed and eventually stopped the patient's breathing.

Nurse: I'll tell you one that I'm sure you've heard before about someone who . . . was admitted on a Saturday and had a chronic illness and was elderly and had lost her home and was being asked to move into a nursing home and she had to give up her pets and so on. And by Sunday, she . . . had changed her mind, was ready to die and was dying and there wasn't a lot that could be done to prevent it anyway unless she wanted to be intubated and have a long course and probably die anyway, and opted not to be intubated and to take—what did she take?—some minor Valium or something. I've forgotten what, and stopped breathing, basically (Rubin, 1996, p. 172).

The nurse, Rubin notes, seemed not to recognize the enormity of the life changes thrust upon this woman except in terms of an abbreviated list of nonspecific, categorical conditions: "elderly," "chronic illness," "give up pets," "and so on." The rapidity with which the decision to die was made is not questioned, and, as Rubin discusses, the nurse does not describe engaging in any serious discussion or deliberation about other measures or alternative scenarios—in fact, these are quickly dismissed ("probably die anyway"). The nurse's description (which Rubin describes more fully and contrasts with the highly detailed, situated narratives of nurses in the same study who were identified as clinical experts), does not include acknowledgment of the patient's suffering; it characterizes the situation in terms of a choice made independently and autonomously by the patient, wherein the nurse's role is merely one of instrumentality, of providing the technical means.

These nurses, Rubin argues, "assume that the objective features of the situation . . . have only one meaning and that that meaning is the same for everyone" (p. 176). They are unable to make the kinds of qualitative distinctions among patients that narrative and moral proximities encourage. They are, it could be argued, perfect "distal nurses"—disengaged from patients as persons, regarding the work of patient care as technical management and efficient production, unlikely to perceive or raise difficult issues based on the particularity of any individual patient. Table 3-1 contrasts this "distal" view of nursing with the "proximal" perspective that is associated with nursing's particularistic narrative traditions. Distal nursing is a highly rationalized, abstract representation of what nurses do that makes perfect sense within a perspective distant from actual care situations.

Table 3-1   Distal and Proximal Perspectives on Nursing

Distal	Proximal
Hospital as institutional space	Hospital as healing place
Hospital as place of business	Hospital as place of care
Concern with abstract and general	Concern with particular
Illnesses as diagnoses	Illnesses as narratively understood
Practice as technical management	Practice as human engagement
Diagnoses as objective	Diagnoses as socially negotiated
Subjectivity as interior, suspect	Subjectivity tied to particular places

continues

Table 3-1 Distal and Proximal Perspectives on Nursing *(continued)*

Distal	Proximal
Knowledge as objective	Knowledge as situated
Meaning as irrelevant and personal	Meaning as shared and essential to healing
Values as outside scope	Values as reflected in practices
Nurses as managers	Nurses as healers

From this even-more-distal perspective, patients are meaningful only in the aggregate, the hospital is itself understood only as institutional space, and the knowledge that counts is generated based on abstractions from the aggregate. In contrast, proximal nursing understands patients as particular persons situated within social worlds, works to shape the hospital as a place of healing, and privileges knowledge derived from the patient's life and the experience of providing care.

Spatial-Structural Power Dynamics

Distal nurses fit perfectly within a spatial-structural ordering for health care that preserves and reinforces existing economic and power relations. Scholars from Heidegger (Heidegger, 1977) to Foucault (Foucault, 1963/1975; Foucault, 1979; Rabinow, 1984) and others have called attention to the technologically totalizing and rationalizing character of modernity, which emphasizes an instrumental "ordering for ordering's sake." Malpas (2000) describes how this technological understanding tends toward revealing or presenting to us things and relations in terms of objectified commodities or available resources. The spatial-structural power dynamics at work in U.S. healthcare increasingly favor construction of all aspects of healthcare in terms of commodity exchange (Malone, 1999). Nursing becomes a technical means for transforming illness and injury into consumption of services. Switching bedside nurses to distal managers serves the commodification process by constituting nursing care as a cheaper product that, in turn, frees up funds for consumptive acquisition of technological equipment and administrative and information systems, both of which reinforce commodification—the equipment as commodity and the systems as ways to efficiently manage commodity acquisition and distribution.

Human practices such as proximal nursing that undermine classification and commodification (through insistence on narrative, particularity and subjective experience, for example) constitute sources of resistance and thus must be tightly controlled.[12]

Foucault's notion of "dividing practices" comes to mind. These are "modes of manipulation that combine the mediation of a science (or pseudo-science) and the practice of exclusion" (Rabinow, 1984, p. 8). The spatial-structural separation of nurses from patients, the truncation of nurses' traditional narrative modes of communication in favor of institutionally sanctioned fragments, and the bureaucratic emphasis on classification and standardization may be considered dividing practices, the aim of which is to order, objectify, and control.

It is also useful to consider Lefebvre's (Lefebvre, 1992/1974) distinction between *representational spaces*, or space as directly *lived* by its inhabitants, which I equate with nurses' proximal, narratively structured "re-emplacing" relations with patients; and *representations of space*, or abstract *space* as conceived by healthcare managers, policymakers, and planners, which I equate with the rationalizing character of modernity. "In spatial practice," argues Lefebvre, ". . . the reproduction of social relations is predominant. The representation of space, in thrall to both knowledge and power, leaves only the narrowest leeway to representational spaces, which are limited to works, images, and memories whose content . . . is so far displaced that it barely achieves symbolic force. . . . Within this space . . . lived experience is crushed, vanquished by what is 'conceived of'" (Lefebvre, 1992/1974, pp. 50-51).

However, Lefebvre argues that there are inherent contradictions in such abstracting spatial-structural power relations. Because one of the characteristics of this rationalizing power is the elimination of differences, practices that demand consideration of particularity set up a tension that highlights the failure of abstract spatial structures to honor human experience. This creates the possibility for more holistic spatial relations. Such a new or reformed space, according to Lefebvre, "will put an end to those localizations which shatter the integrity of the individual body, the social body, the corpus of human needs, and the corpus of knowledge" (Lefebvre, 1992/1974, p. 52).

Proximal nursing thus emerges as a powerful form of spatial resistance that reveals, sustains, and creates alternative ways of constructing illness, care, and relationship. Proximal nursing is a practice of resistance precisely because it resists abstraction and commodification and because its commitment to the face to face care of persons re-emphasizes particularities that create contradictions and difficulties within dominant representations of space. It is, therefore, no surprise that the discourses of embodiment, narrative, and situational ethics have recently become so urgent within nursing and other healthcare disciplines. These are discursive efforts to sustain corresponding dimensions of physical, narrative, and moral proximity in relations between patients and healers.

CONCLUSION

This paper has argued that spatial-structural ordering procedures at work in U.S. hospitals increasingly reshape nursing as a "distal" practice, disrupting nurses' physical, narrative, and moral proximity to patients. Loss of proximity threatens loss of nursing's traditional appreciation for the particular in clinical and moral decisionmaking and may create a distanced, "we're just running the trains" mentality. Nursing's power lies in its honoring of the particular and relational; it is thus important to understand that "proximal" nursing is a source of human resistance to modernity's tendency toward abstract, commodified ordering and a challenge to existing power relations.

A major shortage of hospital nurses now exists, most acutely in states such as California where these changes in healthcare were first widely adopted.[13] While the demographics of an aging nursing workforce, wider career opportunities for the young women who still make up the majority of nurses, and other factors play a role, I would argue that the departure of experienced nurses from hospitals may also have to do with their discomfort in the role of "distal nurse" and the tensions involved in resisting it or reconciling it with their narratively developed understandings of practice. If we want educated practitioners who engage with us on a human level, as opposed to merely processing our bodies, we must consider how spatial-structural power relations further or obstruct relationships between patients and healers.

ACKNOWLEDGMENTS

Work on this paper was supported by a residential research fellowship at Irvine, California funded by the University of California Humanities Research Institute (HRI). I would like to express my appreciation to HRI director David Goldberg; assistant director Debra Massey Sanchez; and the HRI staff who helped make our visit such an intellectually renewing and productive experience. My gratitude also to the members of the HRI group: Carolyn Cartier, Edward Casey, Sharon Kaufman, Jeff Malpas, Sara Shostak, Nancy Stoller, and to Terry Sayre, whose support made the HRI experience possible.

FINAL COMMENT

"Seeing" the taken-for-granted spatial aspects that constrain possibilities in nursing practice, as interpretive phenomenology encourages, is critical for understanding nursing as a practice of resistance to modernity's tendency toward an abstract, commodified ordering for ordering's sake. Nursing's power lies in its honoring of the particular and relational. This analysis shows how primary interpretive phenomenological work can be used to inform theorizing about the broader positioning of nursing within dominant representations of space.

References

Aiken, L. H., & Fagin, C. M. (1997). Evaluating the consequences of hospital restructuring. *Medical Care* (35), 10.

Aiken, L. H., Sochalski, J., & Anderson, G. F. (1996). Downsizing the hospital nursing workforce. *Health Affairs, 15*(4), 88-92.

Bauman, Z. (1993). Social spaces: Cognitive, aesthetic, moral. In Z. Baumann (Ed.), *Postmodern ethics* (pp. 145-185). Oxford, UK: Blackwell.

Benner, P. (2000). The quest for control and the possibilities of care. In M. A. Wrathall & J. Malpas (Eds.), *Heidegger, coping, and cognitive science* (Vol. 2, pp. 293-309). Cambridge, MA: The MIT Press.

Benner, P., Hooper-Kyriakidis, P., & Stannard, D. (1999). *Clinical wisdom and interventions in critical care: A thinking-in-action approach*. Philadelphia: Saunders.

Benner, P., Tanner, C., & Chesla, C. (1992). From beginner to expert: Gaining a differentiated clinical world in critical care nursing practice. *Advances in Nursing Science, 14*(3), 13-28.

Benner, P., Tanner, C., & Chesla, C. (1996). *Expertise in nursing practice: Caring, clinical judgment, and ethics.* New York: Springer.

Benner, P., & Wrubel, J. (1989). *The primacy of caring: Stress and coping in health and illness.* Menlo Park, CA: Addison-Wesley.

Blum, L. (1991). Moral perception and particularity. *Ethics, 101,* 701-725.

Bowker, G. C., & Star, S. L. (1999). *Sorting things out: Classification and its consequences.* Cambridge, MA: The MIT Press.

Burns, J. P. (1998). Performance improvement with patient service partners. *Journal of Nursing Administration, 28*(1), 31-37.

Casey, E. S. (1993). *Getting back into place: Toward a renewed understanding of the place-world.* Bloomington, IN: Indiana University Press.

Connelly, J. (1999). 'Back rub!': Reflections on touch. *Lancet, 354*(Suppl 3), SIII2-4.

Foucault, M. (1975). *The birth of the clinic.* New York: Random House. (Original work published 1963).

Foucault, M. (1979). *Discipline and punish.* (A. Sheridan, Trans.). New York: Vintage Books.

Frank, A. W. (2001). Can we research suffering? *Qualitative Health Research, 11*(3), 353-362.

Frankford, D. M. (1994). Scientism and economism in the regulation of health care. *Journal of Health Politics, Policy and Law, 19*(4), 773-799.

Gadow, S. (1980). Existential advocacy: Philosophical foundation of nursing. In S. F. Spicker & S. Gadow (Eds.), *Nursing: Images and ideals/Opening dialogue with the humanities.* New York: Springer.

Gadow, S. (1995). Narrative and exploration. *Nursing Inquiry, 4*(Dec 2), 211-214.

Gadow, S. (1999). Relational narrative: The postmodern turn in nursing ethics. *Scholarly Inquiry for Nursing Practice, 13*(1), 57-70.

Gilligan, C. (1982). *In a different voice.* Cambridge, MA: Cambridge University Press.

Heidegger, M. (1977). *The question concerning technology*. (W. Lovitt, Trans.). New York: Harper and Row.Hunter, K. M. (1996). Narrative, literature, and the clinical exercise of practical reason. *Journal of Medicine and Philosophy, 21*, 303-320.

Lefebvre, H. (1992/1974). *The production of space*. Oxford, UK: Blackwell.Levinas, E. (1981). *Otherwise than being or beyond essence*. The Hague, Netherlands: Martinus Nijhoff.

Liaschenko, J. (1994). The moral geography of home care. *Advances in Nursing Science, 17*(2), 16-26.

Liaschenko, J. (1995). Ethics in the work of acting for patients. *Advances in Nursing Science, 18*(2), 1-12.

Liaschenko, J. (1997). Ethics and the geography of the nurse-patient relationship: Spatial vulnerabilities and gendered space. *Scholarly Inquiry for Nursing Practice: An International Journal, 11*(1), 45-59.

Lifton, R. (1986). *The Nazi doctors: Medical killing and the politics of genocide*. New York: Basic Books.

MacIntyre, A. (1984). *After virtue* (2nd ed.). Notre Dame: University of Notre Dame Press.

Malone, R. E. (1995). Heavy users of emergency services: Social construction of a policy problem. *Social Science and Medicine, 40*(4), 469-477.

Malone, R. E. (1998). Whither the almshouse? Overutilization and the role of the emergency department. *Journal of Health Politics, Policy and Law, 23*(5), 795-832.

Malone, R. E. (1999). Policy as product: Morality and metaphor in health policy discourse. *Hastings Center Report, 29*(3), 16-22.

Malone, R. E. (2000). Dimensions of vulnerability in emergency nurses' narratives. *Advances in Nursing Science, 23*(1), 1-11.

Malpas, J. E. (2000). Urbanity, modernity and the technological. In H. Bott, C. Hubig, F. Pesch, & G. Schroeder (Eds.), *Stadt and kommunikation im digitalen zeitalter* (pp. 211-226). Frankfurt: Campus Verlag.

Malpas, J. E. (1999). *Place and experience: A philosophical topography*. Cambridge, UK: Cambridge University Press.

Massey, D. (1994). A global sense of place, *Space, place, and gender* (pp. 146-156). Oxford, UK: Polity Press.

Massey, D. (1995). The conceptualization of place. In D. Massey & P. Jess (Eds.), *A place in the world? Places, cultures, and globalization* (pp. 46-85). Oxford, UK: Oxford University Press/The Open University.

Meintz, S. (1995). Whatever became of the back rub? *RN, 58*(4), 49-50, 53, 56.

Nightingale, F. (1969). *Notes on nursing: What it is and what it is not*. New York: Dover Publications.

Norrish, B. R. & Rundall, T. G. (2001). Hospital restructuring and the work of registered nurses. *Milbank Quarterly, 79*(1), 55-79.

Rabinow, P. (Ed.). (1984). *The Foucault Reader*. New York: Pantheon Books.

Rubin, J. (1996). Impediments to the development of clinical knowledge and ethical judgment in critical care nursing. In P. Benner, C. A. Tanner, & C. A. Chesla (Eds.), *Expertise in nursing practice: Caring, clinical judgment, and ethics*. New York: Springer.

Sochalski, J., Aiken, L. H., & Fagin, C. M. (1997). Hospital restructuring in the United States, Canada, and Western Europe: An outcomes research agenda. *Medical Care, 35*(10), OS13-OS25, *Supplement*.

Stone, D. (1999). Care and trembling. *American Prospect, 0*(43), 61.

Tanner, C. A., Benner, P., Chesla, C., & Gordon, D. R. (1993). The phenomenology of knowing the patient. *Image: Journal of Nursing Scholarship, 25*(4), 273-280.

van Manen, M. (1998). Modalities of body experience in illness and health. *Qualitative Health Research, 8*(1), 7-24.

Wiener, C. L. (2000). *The elusive quest: Accountability in hospitals*. New York: Aldine de Gruyter.

Footnotes

[1] It is important to note that "nursing" can encompass a wide variety of activities performed by a wide variety of persons, from unlicensed caregivers to nursing assistants to licensed vocational/practical nurses and registered nurses with varying levels of educational preparation. In this paper, I will be primarily concerned with registered nurses practicing in United States hospitals, specifically with those nurses who are or have been engaged in direct bodily care of patients (as opposed to those in various educational, research, administrative or supervisorial roles). Interrelated spatial dynamics and narrative forms may be very different in other settings where nursing is practiced.

[2] Benner is not alone in calling attention to narrative as important to ethical nursing practice. See also the work of Sally Gadow (Gadow, 1995, 1999).

[3] By *particularity*, I mean this individual patient's unique, irreducible, and irreplaceable life, as contrasted with viewing the patient as a category of something—a type, a diagnosis, or a cluster of symptoms or characteristics. When people speak of wanting to be "treated like a human being," they seem to be making this distinction even though they must rely on some shared understanding of humanity to do so. My use of *particularity* should not be confused with Cartesian notions of radically free, autonomous subjects. Even such a pioneer of systematic observations and statistics as Florence Nightingale emphasized appreciating particularity as essential to nursing: "One likes to suffer out all his suffering alone, to be looked after as little as possible. Another likes to be perpetually made much of and pitied, and to have someone always by him" (Nightingale, 1969, p. 117). Nightingale also argued that nursing concerned not "nursing sickness" but "nursing the sick," drawing attention to a focus on the situated person rather than the patient's medical diagnosis or set of symptoms (Nightingale, 1969).

[4] In emphasizing narrative proximity, I am not suggesting a sentimentalized vision of nursing that ignores the social complexity of the role. Nursing requires practitioners to draw on a wide range of knowledge and skills, and this discussion should not be misinterpreted as dismissing nursing's technical and scientific knowledge base as unimportant. However, nursing since Nightingale has emphasized a holistic conception of care and healing that extends beyond the biomedical to encompass the patient as a person within a life context.

[5] This understanding is reminiscent of Gilligan's (1982) descriptions of moral reasoning from particulars rather than from abstract principles. Gadow (1995) suggested that the difference between this kind of knowledge about patients in their particularity and the abstract, "objective" knowledge also used in hospital work is like the difference between "colonial and local knowledge about what it is like to live here. 'Here' is the place where a particular patient and nurse find themselves together, a place that is fully concrete, a lived situation" (p. 8, author-supplied hard copy). Gadow described nursing practice in terms of an explorer's journey to a strange country. Although a map may be helpful, it cannot help one understand what it is like actually to live there. Being "here" with patients, then, requires the willingness and ability to sustain proximity.

[6] Nursing personnel employed in U.S. hospitals declined by 7.3% nationally between 1981-1993 (after adjusting for case mix); there was a 46% increase in non-nurse administrative staff (Aiken, Sochalski, & Anderson, 1996).

[7] During these two weeks, "service partners" presumably master "guest relations, food handling, food and nutrition services skills, unit orientation, housekeeping skills, cardiopulmonary resuscitation, infection control, admitting/discharge procedures, activities of daily living, and safety/body mechanics" (Burns, 1998, p. 35).

[8] Interestingly, even then, nursing's narrative contributions to the written representation of the patient's hospitalization experience were apparently regarded as having no lasting value; these nurses' notes were commonly discarded after the patient left the hospital (and the physician's notes remained the primary if not only recorded representation of what took place). Nursing's written narratives within hospitals have in many respects always been at the margins, dominated by the discourse of medicine, giving rise to nursing's strong oral tradition of sharing stories.

[9] Benner's work has also explicated the value of narrative in communicating nursing knowledge between clinicians at different levels of expertise. See, for example, (Benner, 2000; Benner et al., 1999; Benner et al., 1992; Benner et al., 1996; Benner & Wrubel, 1989).

[10] Lawrence Blum (Blum, 1991) has argued that an appreciation of particularity is the essential prerequisite to acting morally in a situation. A "particularistic attitude" means "being alive to the ways that a given situation might differ from others (to which it might be superficially similar), not being quick to assume that a noted feature of a situation correlates with others with which it has been correlated (within one's experience) in the past, not being quick to assume that a principle which has been conclusive in similar situations will be conclusive in the current one, and the like" (p. 720). Knowing moral principles is not sufficient, as Blum and others have argued, because one must first recognize or be solicited by a situation in moral terms.

[11] Deborah Stone (Stone, 1999), describing home care workers she studied, found similar patterns in which nurses and other care workers reported that they were required by their employers to focus their care more and more narrowly on specific medical problems and provided "social care" on their own time because relationship-sustaining activities were not regarded as part of the business of care. Stone also argues that policymakers ought to worry about the "displacement" of such relationships.

[12] Also see Frankford (Frankford, 1994) for an excellent discussion of the ordering character of scientism and economism in health policy discourse.

[13] As this paper went to press, California had just passed AB 394, which requires that hospitals meet minimum nurse-patient ratios. The California Nurses' Association, which sponsored the bill, argues that improved staffing ratios may bring more nurses back into hospital practice. Whether they will be "proximal" or "distal" nurses remains to be seen.

CHAPTER 4

Research and Ontology: Neurology and Parkinson's Disease Sufferers' Lived Experiences of Embodiment and Dwelling in Lifeworlds

HELENA SUNVISSON

BACKGROUND

Phenomenological research studies contribute to the body of knowledge by articulating the complexity of being human, of experiencing embodiment, and of dwelling in a world organized by interests and concerns for persons with illnesses such as Parkinson's disease (PD). Caregiving and coping with PD requires knowledge of the lived experience regarding ways in which PD pathophysiology affects the lived body and is embodied and managed by persons with varying lifeworld interests and concerns that are related to the illness experience. In disciplines that deal with caring about human beings, knowledge gained from various theories and research studies must be used in the best interest of a particular person even though the knowledge is grounded in various general ontological understandings of human beings.

According to Merleau-Ponty (1945/1962), the visible and movable body is captured in a net that holds together self, others, things, and the world. The meeting between body and the world gives birth to meaning to possible world variants of this world. This means that lifeworld is both sensuous and situated and the lived body is a situated *intertwining* of intentionality and materiality. As our bodies are our access to the world, most bodily changes render into a changed access to and experience of that world. According to Leder (1998), notions of disease should thus involve existential *and* biological terms that are concerned with care and treatment. And scholars such as Benner (2000) and Meleis (1997) claimed that care is inappropriate without this intertwining.

> *"If nurses do not have a good grasp of the science of pathophysiology and medical and nursing interventions, then they can make neither good ethical or good clinical decisions, because they cannot know what it is good to do in the particular situation."* (Benner, 2000, p. 16)

Consequently, this chapter will situate PD experiences into a phenomenological framework and will discuss ways in which these experiences might be understood from a neurological perspective. The intention is to then compare research within neuroscience with lifeworld research on a PD-afflicted person's lived experience of embodiment and environmental influences and explore ways to use research outcomes that are grounded in various ontologies to best serve persons afflicted with PD.

For a deeper understanding of environment, Casey (2001) investigated the ontological meaning of *place* and how it relates to human being's lived experience; he then took a stand on human as *habitus*. In his interpretation, habitus becomes habitude and open for innovation. Casey references this statement to Bourdieu (1972/1977). Understood in this way, habitus becomes the mediating link between, for example, consciousness and body, nature and culture, self and others—elements that continuously becomes entwined, uniting us with the world in which we live.

Performance mirrors social and cultural patterns, and it is as *habitus* that humans exist and act in relation to the place they inhabit. A core of habits that embodies and constitutes what is experienced thus constitutes *self*. World as place is then sensed and perceived and experienced and actively lived (ibid.). The body reaches out for the world as place and stores impressions and experiences from other familiar places. Impressions from a place may remain a long time after a place is left. Stored impressions come alive when they are aligned with certain present experiences. As a *thirdspace*, place is simultaneously social, historical, and spatial (ibid.; Soja, 1996): It links human beings, place, and time into an experience that rises from attention being paid to a situation in which a human being is involved. "The world is not what I think, but what I live through. I am open to the world, I have no doubt that I am in communication with it, but I do not possess it; it is inexhaustible" (Merleau-Ponty, 1945/1962, p. xvii).

PERSPECTIVES ON CHANGED LIFEWORLD CAPABILITIES

The following studies focused on people living with PD and on environmental factors that they experienced because of changing capabilities for performing daily habits (Habermann, 1996, 1999; Sunvisson 2006; Sunvisson & Ekman, 2001; and Van Der Bruggen & Widdershoven, 2004). Here are some exemplars:

> *I would put my hand up to wave good-bye and I'd put it up and it wouldn't wave. And that was a peculiar feeling. I could lift it, and it wouldn't be automatic—and I'd think wave. Oh, yeah, I had to consciously do it. Scrambling eggs for reason: "How do you do this?" And then I could think it through and do it. (Habermann, 1996, p. 403)*

> *But it's like I must be much more systematic nowadays for instance, when I'm cooking or something. It's really hard work to prepare a meal because I have to make so many small, odd decisions. Nothing goes by itself. Every single decision must be preceded by a discussion in my mind. (Sunvisson & Ekman, 2001, p. 45)*

> *I fumble when distance is short. If I see a glass there, and I intend to grab it, I sometimes have problems with estimating distance. (Sunvisson, 2006, unpublished quotation)*

These people with PD consciously guide movements into single sequences, and this deliberate, focused movement slows their actions. By concentrating, they move their bodies toward an object of intent and force their hand to grasp it. With this introverted concentration, feeling for the room and relationships to things in the room become vague. And inborn, smoothly flowing body rhythm—in its motor intention—is weakened.

This focus on the body (e.g., guiding the hand to grab a glass and not having the glass in focus) makes distance hard to distinguish. Things are no longer ready-at-hand. Tempo turns static, and adjusting to unexpected demands becomes increasingly difficult. Consequently, altered physical capability results in changed body rhythms.

> *Professionally, I'm worth nothing now. I can't follow the evolution at the office any more. I've become rigid in body and mind. I'm afraid of everything new. I can't cope with the time pressure any more—the high speed at which all work must be done.... (Van Der Bruggen & Widdershoven, 2004, p. 298)*

In addition, the people with PD find it increasingly difficult to rapidly change focus while doing activities or making decisions. The need to compensate for a no-longer fluidly moving body creates a need to structure activities within a slow rigid rhythm, and this makes it difficult and usually impossible to adapt to another person's rhythm and timing (Sunvisson, 2006, Sunvisson et al., 2009). When with others, who act in a faster rhythm, the rhythmical being and attunement for the person with PD become disrupted—sometimes so disrupted that it isn't possible to act at all. All stakeholders also need to know about individual PD sufferers' abilities to sometimes get around or break immobility episodes, as illustrated here:

> *For example, if I'm in the post office and have to sign something. I cannot write. I just can't. There is no point in trying, I start with big letters and then they become so small and the whole paper becomes entangled. But if I really concentrate on what I'm doing and let my leg go instead of my hand, then I can write. (Sunvisson, Habermann, Weiss and Benner 2009, p. 10)*

> *When I get an art brush in my hand and it's like this [showing how she trembles], I can calm down a little bit and then start painting. And it doesn't become smeared. I think that I manage to get my feelings and my thoughts to go out through my arm. I think that is the way that it works. (Sunvisson, 2006, p. 95)*

Experiences of environment, situations, and meetings with other persons can significantly influence PD afflicted persons' abilities to act in a situation. Feeling stress, feeling questioned, and being uncertain could render into a reaction with tremor and sudden immobility.

> *For example, the other day, when I met that lady coming from my hairdresser. I felt so lively and healthy as I walked along the street. I thought I walked so well and quite straight. And then I met an elegant lady who said, 'Oh dear, oh dear, how will this work? Do you think you will find your way home, poor little thing?' Obviously, she felt sorry for me staggering along; then it really became visible that I had problems with walking straight, but I hadn't noticed it before she came. And then I couldn't finish the errands that I had planned. She broke me down. There was no need for more. (Sunvisson, 2006, p.95)*

In contrast, being full of expectation; feeling happy, optimistic, or amused; or being involved in an engaging way could enable an expansion of own abilities in unexpected ways.

> *Good Lord, how strong that feeling and that experience [the compliant attitude of leaders and participants] must have been. I've been into churches many times you see, but never anything like this … And I didn't know about it, you see, until I came home. Then I understood, because I felt OK the whole week. (Sunvisson and Ekman, 2001, p. 46)*

A dialectical interplay between the experience of involvement in the situation *and* the ability to intentionality experience oneself embodied, demonstrates the embodied, sentient capacities of acting by being directed toward the world. Conversely, *not* experiencing involvement caused problems for these people with PD in their intentional, habitual being. Physical surroundings are also important for mobility:

> *It's fantastic when I walk in the forest. My posture really changes; I'm totally relaxed. You should see me when I'm out shopping. People probably think that I'm really drunk. My gait is so unsteady. (Sunvisson, 2006, p. 95)*

These people with PD experienced an alteration between an intentional being toward the world—when the body is the vehicle for intentions—and a direction toward the world *through* the body, with use of concentration on constructing their movements, which was not always a successful strategy (cf. Merleau-Ponty 1945/1962, pp. 129-185).

Within the phenomenology framework, this can be discussed as a reasonable condition for an altered way of performance and living place. As per Merleau-Ponty's philosophy—as Gallagher (1986) noted—several body schemata operate in a tacitly lived space on a preconscious level. According to Gallagher (2001), Merleau-Ponty suggested that these body schemata work best when perceptually transcending one's own body. As a system of motor programs, body schemas "operate *below* the level of self-referential intentionality" (Gallagher, 2001, p. 150), which makes posture and motility attunement to the environment possible without need for constant body attention or even excessive focus on a familiar environment.

> "The possession of the body implies the ability to change levels and to understand space"
>
> **Merleau-Ponty**

With this suggestion, body schema isn't a pure cortical representation but reflects oriented attunement of the body to its environment. Casey (2001) argued that spatial and temporal living bodies don't work in place but rather inhabit place in an oriented way. This supports Merleau-Ponty's contention that "the possession of the body implies the ability to change levels and to *understand* space" (1945/1962, p. 251). The phenomenal body moves within this prereflective *understood* space. When reaching out a hand to catch something, the hand is moved, and posture is attuned to gearing the body in an intentional way toward the object (cf. Burleigh-Jacobs, Horak, Nutt, & Obeso, 1997; Merleau-Ponty, 1945/1962; Sudenow, 1993). Further, in reaching out as an intention, *the thing reached for shapes the intention*. Things and the world catch up with the phenomenal body.

Thus, people with PD can experience themselves intentionally moving toward the world when experiencing the surroundings *calling* for them. For example, walking in the forest or climbing up stairs is much easier than walking along a plain corridor that might feel like walking in deep water. A command, a rhythmic beat, or something thrown in front of their feet can interrupt an immobility episode (see examples from the neurological part of this chapter).

According to Merleau-Ponty

> The object which presents itself to the gaze or the touch arouses a certain motor intention which aims not at the movements of one's own body, but at the thing itself from which we are, as it were, suspended. (1945/1962, p. 317)

The lived body acts within a spatiality of *situation* as an orientation in space is to act within a projection of a prereflective horizon of meaning. (Merleau-Ponty, 1945/1962, p. 100) Accordingly, it seems as though people with PD experience a break in this oriented space—a disturbance in the projection of the body—as if the virtual habitual body and the actual body don't mesh. When not experiencing this orientation in space, movements must be consciously guided in such a way that they lose their rhythm and precision. Or put another way: When not being able to move within oriented space, no prereflective horizon is spread out, and no access to build habitual movements is present for actively meeting challenges in situations or events. When people with PD move smoothly and skillfully, these experiences are actively attuned to the moods, tones, emotions, and special condition of events and place. When no such special conditions are experienced for bringing about new motor intentions, motor actions must be self-consciously constructed—and these are slow and fumbling actions.

Habermann (1996, 1999), Andersson and Sidenvall (2001), Sunvisson & Ekman (2001), Sunvisson (2006) and show that people with PD experience themselves as living with unpredictable motility, which according to the previous discussion, is to live with ongoing, change-oriented attunement of the body to its environment. According to Sunvisson and colleagues (2009) this means that PD sufferers' capacity to respond with fluid movements in certain situations fails when their motility gets locked up. In these moments, their awareness of the present movement (because of readjustment of the previous level of awareness) fails because adjusting capabilities for attuning to the present field are impossible to achieve in an embodied, spatially oriented way (cf. Merleau-Ponty, 1945/1962, pp. 248-290). The ways they are *in* the situation have importance for involvement experiences and for their ability to carry things out.

Neurological perspectives on the interconnection of environment and embodied movement

As shown by Sunvisson and colleagues (2009) neurological research offers a limited number of studies that specifically focus on how the environment affects persons with PD, excluding studies concerning risk factors, exposures, and toxins (Strickland, 2005). Neurological research on PD is extensive, and this presentation is rough and very limited. The clinical picture of PD is usually described with these main physical symptoms (Gelb, Oliver, & Gilman, 1999):

- *Bradykinesia* (movement poverty with delayed and slow execution and decreased capacity for simultaneous movements)

- *Rigidity* (muscular stiffness)

- *Rest tremor* (trembles in arms and legs—sometimes also in chin—when in rest)

Short, shuffling steps and decreased or absent arm swings characterize a PD sufferer's gait. Problems with starting, moving, and sudden unforeseen stops become obvious with time (Jancovic, 1987).

Cognitive decline also occurs (e.g., visuospatial deficit) and is described as indistinctness for distance in the narrow space with influences on cognition and locomotion (Parnetti & Calabresi, 2006). *Bradyphrenia* (slowed thought processes—another cognitive symptom) affects quick decision-making, and cognitive signs as attention and apathy relates indirectly to immobility phases during the day when medical treatments are not optimal. (Zgaljardic, Borad, Foldi, & Mattis, 2003). Also seen is an increased sensitivity to stress (Ellgring et al., 1993). Although no cure exists, symptomatic therapy mainly relieves symptoms, at least in the early years (Miyasaki et al., 2002).

In neurological research, PD is related to rapid cell degeneration in the *substantia nigra pars compacta*, a core in the basal ganglia area in the brain where the main part of the dopamine producing neurons are located (Jellinger, 1998). Delayed initiation of voluntary movements, decreased execution of automatic and repetitive movements, absence of movement execution, and problems with maintenance of internal gait rhythm are all causally connected to the progressive degeneration of the basal ganglia area (Morris, Iansek, Matyas, & Summers, 1996).

With time, people with PD show an increasing reliance on external sensory information to initiate and execute movements (such as being able to walk when the floor is line-patterned). Abbruzzese and Berardelli (2003) suggested that this guidance of movement is attributable to a deficit in proprioceptive regulation.

It has also been found that cues of various kinds can improve PD sufferers' mobility. Use of cognitive cues that sometimes can eradicate immobility is a known phenomenon that relates to internal prompting through self-instruction (Nieuwboer, Feys, de Weerdt, & Dom, 1997). Use of visual or auditory cues (Jiang, 2006) or listening to rhythms can also improve mobility (Holten, 2005). When people with PD are concentrating on cues, walking is no longer an automatic task that must be processed through the defective basal ganglia (Morris et al., 1996). Praamstra, Stegeman, Cools, & Horstink (1998) suggested that use of visual cues improves mobility in activation of the cerebellar visual-motor pathway. Reasons why gait improves with rhythmic auditory stimulation are still unclear, however (Rubinstein, Giladi, & Hausdorff, 2002). Interesting—but poorly understood—is the relationship between PD sufferers' expectation that a new drug will improve motor performance and actual physical function improvement after placebo administration (Lidstone, de la Fuente-Fernandez, & Stoessi, 2005).

These results are within the framework of the neurological understanding of mobility, which means that movement production depends upon a complex motor circuit that starts with a cognitive decision to move, or is a reflexive reaction on stimuli that starts the organizing of motor schemata in various levels, which involve the *substantia nigra*, basal ganglia, subthalamic nucleus, thalamus, and the cerebral cortex (Ghez & Krakauer, 2000). Information from the highest level is transported via self-organizing systems of neural networks to lower levels in the motor-control hierarchy (Kohonen, 2001). On lower levels, the specific body position needed for the movements gets structured; and those movements needed for the intention—for example, reaching out for a glass—become organized for use. The body starts to gear itself for moving forward; the arm stretches; and simultaneously, the fingers begin to stretch out and form a useful grip shape before the hand closes around the glass. The movements become purposeful and specific as interpretation of incoming information (provided by receptors in muscles, tendons, joints, skin, hearing systems, and eyes) corrects and reorganizes the commanding of the movements (Shumway-Cook & Woollacott, 2001).

Research as Conditional Truth

In the medical paradigm, humans are understood as having a body that orients itself in an objective space. This understanding of motility is grounded in the Cartesian division of consciousness from the external world (the abstract self and the body's belonging to the object world), which emphasizes environmental sensitivity as an extra-personal space orientation (Merleau-Ponty, 1964/1968; Parr & Butler, 1999). Table 4.1 displays a comparison of ontological concepts within phenomenology and neuroscience with focus on motility and environmental influences.

Table 4.1 Ontological Concepts within Phenomenology and Neuroscience, Attributable to Motility and Environmental Influences

Phenomenology	Neuroscience
A human being is a body subject	A human being has a body
Experienced situations shape action	Action starts from position
Movement is intentional (*for itself*)	Cognitive decision or reflection executes movement (*in itself*)
Body schemata	Motoric schemata

The objective of neuroscience research is to develop theories of the brain and nervous systems and, optimally, to discover cures for certain diseases: for example, using surgery techniques, medical treatment (drug or gene therapy), or vaccination. Limitations are its reduction of people to parts and subsequent dehumanization (Gordon, 1988; Parr & Butler, 1999).

The objective of lifeworld research is to illuminate the world as it is lived and experienced with certain phenomenon in focus: for example, the meaning of health and illness that is shaped by individual concerns and demands. Limitations include, for instance, inability to make prognoses; its usefulness is limited by the relatively small body of life-world research studies about certain phenomena, such as PD.

Table 4.2 illustrates outcomes from both types of research discussed to this point.

Table 4.2 Outcomes from Neuroscience and Lifeworld Research on PD (Sunvisson, Habermann, Weiss & Benner, 2009)

Living and experiencing PD	Objective signs of PD
Conscious guiding of movement sequences. Forced to be focused and concentrated when doing things. Rigid physical ability; forced to structure and live in a slow, rigid rhythm of time. Ongoing changing abilities between being toward the world and being toward the world through the body. Living in imbalance; feeling uncertain about abilities. Changed experience of time and place.	Bradykinesia: movement poverty, delayed and slow execution, decreased capacity for simultaneous movements. Muscular rigidity. Resting tremor. Bradyphrenia: slowness in thinking. Increased stress sensitivity. Visuospatial deficit: distance indistinctness during orientation in the narrow space

Although these results come from various ontological concepts, there are many broad connecting points. Here are some suggestions:

- Bradykinesia *might be experienced* as decreased physical capabilities—with a need to be focused and concentrated when doing things.

- Muscular rigidity and decreased capacity for simultaneous movements *might be experienced* as a changed way of living and of experiencing time and place.

- Increased sensitivity to stress and bradyphrenia *might be experienced* as living in imbalance and being uncertain about one's abilities.

- Visuospatial deficit *might be experienced* as increased need for conscious guidance of movement sequences when performing certain actions and such.

Consider results from lifeworld research as a contribution to increased understanding of the complexity of being human and of the experienced *self* in the world. Consider results from neuroscience research as a contribution to increased understanding of the biophysical body of living creatures. Keeping in mind the sensed, experienced ways that we live, medical understanding must be further developed to *also* involve lifeworld dimensions and reflection upon its meaning for a particular person in front of us—to use this knowledge in the best interest of this person.

> "Medical understanding must be further developed to *also* involve lifeworld dimensions and reflection upon its meaning for a particular person in front of us—to use this knowledge in the best interest of this person."

The Challenge to Intertwine the Chiasm

Through a living relationship with oneself, others, and the world, human beings assign meaning to experiences. In this living relationship, things (including self and others) matter. Letting things matter is part of being human and one of life's challenges (Benner, 2001). When experiencing illness, the habitual living in a homelike world is disrupted. During the illness experience, the *I* becomes forced to confront the fact that this *I* is a body and that this *I* is in the world as a lived body. So if *my* way of understanding life, meaning, and concerns fails, this renders into experiences of being *de-situated* (Benner & Wrubel, 1989). Illness experiences challenge the embodied way of understanding life and the lived body's access to the world. The desire to find this access to the world (when incapable of finding it on own terms) drives the search for care and treatment (Sveen, 1997). Because the lived body bestows meaning, experiencing new sensations may open or close possibilities and therefore transform the person—and as such, become a part of oneself in the realm of the lived world.

> [C]onsciousness projects itself into a physical world and has a body, as it projects itself into a cultural world and has its habits: because it cannot be consciousness without playing upon significances given either in the absolute past of nature or in its own personal past, and because any form of lived experience tends towards a certain generality whether that of our habits or that of our 'bodily functions.'
>
> These elucidations enable us clearly to understand motility as basic internationality. Consciousness is in the first place not a matter of "I think that" but of "I can." (Merleau-Ponty, 1945/1962, p. 137)

This means that habitual structures are not to be thought of as causal, but rather as motivational. Because the lived body is meshed with the world, places also become lived in an altered way, for example, because of illness or disability (cf. Sacks, 1991, pp. 343-44; Toombs, 2001). Some specific condition or experience might also harbor new meaning regarding experience of time—altering the way time is lived (Benner & Wrubel, 1989, p. 217). Understanding the lived body as a way in which the world comes to be (Leder, 1998) means that we must ask individuals how they live in a situation, experience body rhythm, live within an immobility episode, and experience uncertainty when they doubt their abilities.

Understanding the lived body is, then, crucial when attempting to meet patients' needs because it

- Sets the stage for what to perceive

- Cultivates openness and attentiveness in a certain direction

- Governs methods of interpretation and understanding

- Enables sensitivity to patients' ways of living their illnesses and to emotions and concerns in the situation (Benner, 2000)

One example might shed light on this. Many of us who have met people with PD might find it hard to understand when a patient reacts to a suggestion with a rigid, rejecting body. Maybe we find this person obstinate; or maybe we just let the incident pass, waiting for another time that might better suit the patient. If we can understand this person's way of living place and time—and that a sudden interruption might mean a disruption of this person's rhythmical being (resulting in diminished drive)—then we can use more sensitivity when making suggestions. If the lived rhythm of time becomes slow and an opportunity to hurry things along isn't there, then we, as professionals, must adjust to the patient's rhythm. Then, it might be possible for them to open up (or keep open) capabilities for involvement and activity. If not, the resulting effect might be that these people lose their orientation in space and time, and we see these locked-in persons as *unwilling* to cooperate (cf. Sacks, 1991).

> "If the lived rhythm of time becomes slow and an opportunity to hurry things along isn't there, then we, as professionals, must adjust to the patient's rhythm."

CONCLUSION

Having PD is to live with a neurological disorder for which medications are available. Medical treatment is incredibly important. Without it, health, well-being, and survival after disease onset are extremely threatened. However, the lived body is an *intertwining* of intentionality and materiality (Merleau-Ponty, 1945/1962, pp. 130-155), and notions of disease should involve existential and biological concepts related to care and treatment (Leder, 1998). When caring for people with PD, neurological knowledge about PD must be used in a way that becomes comprehensive and meaningful for *each* PD sufferer, which is why caregivers must ask people with PD about their lived experiences and self-understanding. This interaction must occur, regardless of the purpose of the meeting between a health care professional and the person with PD.

Referring to this discussion, I want to state even more emphatically than Merleau-Ponty that "(o)ur concern in this preliminary outline was only to catch sight of this strange domain to which interrogation, properly co-called, gives access. . . . " (1964/1968, p. 140).

Much research remains to be done to broaden and deepen understanding of living with a progressive illness such as PD as well as of intertwining the chiasm of the biological body and the person's lived body in the world and the bodying forth of the self in the world.

ACKNOWLEDGMENTS

Gratitude is expressed to Jan-Edvin Olsson, professor in Neurology, for fruitful discussions about the neurological part of this chapter. Gratitude is also expressed to Dr. Judy Petersen for her linguistic revision and copyediting of this chapter.

References

Abbruzzese, G., & Berardelli, A. (2003). Sensorimotor integration in movement disorders. *Movement Disorders*, *18*(3), 231-240.

Andersson, I. & Sidenvall, B. (2001) Case studies of food shopping, cooking and eating habits in older women with Parkinson's disease. *Journal of Advanced Nursing*, *35* (1), 69-78.

Benner, P. (2000). The roles of embodiment, emotion and lifeworld for rationality and agency in nursing practice. *Nursing Philosophy*, *1*, 5-19.

Benner, P. (2001). The phenomenon of care. In K. Toombs (Ed.), *Handbook of phenomenology and medicine* (pp. 351-369). Dordrecht, Netherlands: Kluwer Academic Publishers.

Benner, P., & Wrubel, J. (1989). *The primacy of caring, stress, and coping in health and illness*. Menlo Park, CA: Addison-Wesley.

Bourdieu, P. (1977). *Outline of a theory of practice*. (R. Nice, Trans.). Cambridge, UK: Cambridge University Press. (Original work published 1972).

Burleigh-Jacobs, A., Horak, F., Nutt, J., & Obeso, J. (1997). Step initiation in Parkinson's disease: Influence of levodopa and external sensory triggers. *Movement Disorders*, *12*(2), 206-215.

Casey, E. (2001). Between geography and philosophy: What does it mean to be in the place-world? *Annals of the Association of American Geographers*, *91*(4), 683-693.

Ellgring, H., Seiler, S., Perleth, B., Frings, W., Gasser, T., & Oertel, W. (1993). Psychosocial aspects of Parkinson's disease. *Neurology*, *43*(Suppl. 6), 41-44.

Gallagher, S. (1986). Body image and body schema: A conceptual clarification. *The Journal of Mind and Behavior*, *7*(4), 541-554.

Gallagher, S. (2001). Dimensions of embodiment: Body image and body schema in medical contexts. In K. Toombs (Ed.), *Handbook of phenomenology and medicine* (pp. 147-175). Dordrecht, Netherlands: Kluwer Academic Publishers.

Gelb, D., Oliver, E., & Gilman, S. (1999). Diagnostic criteria for Parkinson disease. *Archives of Neurology*, *56*, 33-39.

Ghez, C., & Krakauer, J. (2000). The organization of movement. In E. Kandel, J. Schwartz, & T. Jessell (Eds.), *Principles of neural science* (4th ed., pp. 653-673). New York: McGraw-Hill Education.

Gordon, D. (1988). Tenacious assumptions in Western medicine. In M. Lock & D. Gordon (Eds.), *Biomedicine examined* (pp. 19-55). Dordrecht, Netherlands: Kluwer Academic Publishers.

Habermann, B. (1996). Day-to-day demands of Parkinson's disease. *Western Journal of Nursing Research, 18*, 397-413.

Habermann, B. (1999). Continuity challenges of Parkinson's disease in middle life. *Journal of Neuroscience Nursing, 31*(4), 200-207.

Holten, S. (2005). Music therapy for people with Parkinson's. In M. Ebadi & R. F. Pfeiffer (Eds.), *Parkinson's disease* (pp. 809-818). Washington, DC: CRC Press.

Jancovic, J. (1987). Pathophysiology and clinical assessment of motor symptoms in Parkinson's disease. In W. Koller (Ed.), *Handbook of Parkinson's disease* (pp. 99-126). New York: Marcel Dekker.

Jellinger, K. A. (1998). Neuropathology of movement disorders. *Neurosurgery Clinics of North America, 9*(2), 237-262.

Jiang, Y. (2006). Effects of visual and auditory cues on gait initiation in people with Parkinson's disease. *Clinical Rehabilitation, 20*, 36-45.

Kohonen, T. (2001). *Self-organizing maps* (3rd ed.). Berlin: Springer.

Leder, D. (1998). A tale of two bodies: The Cartesian corpse and the lived body. In D. Welton (Ed.), *Body and flesh. A philosophical reader* (pp. 117-129). Oxford, UK: Blackwell.

Lidstone, S., de la Fuente-Fernandez, R., & Stoessi, J. (2005). The placebo effect in Parkinson's disease In M. Ebadi & R. F. Pfeiffer (Eds.), *Parkinson's disease* (pp. 623-640). Washington, DC: CRC Press.

Meleis, A. (1997). *Theoretical nursing: Development and progress* (3rd ed.). Philadelphia: Lippincott.

Merleau-Ponty, M. (1962). *Phenomenon of perception*. (C. Smith, Trans.). London: Routledge & Kegan Paul. (Original work published 1945).

Merleau-Ponty, M. (1968). *The intertwining—the chiasm*. In C. Lefort (Ed.), *The visible and the invisible* (pp. 130-155). (A. Lingis, Trans.). Evanston, IL: Northwestern University Press. (Original work published 1964).

Miyasaki, J. M, Martin, W., Suchowersky, O., Weiner, W. J., & Lang, A. E. (2002). Practical parameter: Initiation of treatment for Parkinson's disease: An evidence-based review. *American Academy of Neurology, 58*, 11-17.

Morris, M. E., Iansek, R., Matyas, T. A., & Summers, J. J. (1996) Stride length regulation in Parkinson's disease. Normalization strategies and underlying mechanisms. *Brain, 119*, 551-568.

Nieuwboer, A., Feys, P., de Weerdt, W., & Dom, R. (1997). Is using a cue the clue to the treatment of freezing in Parkinson's disease? *Physiotherapy Research International, 2*(3), 125-132.

Parnetti, L., & Calabresi, P. (2006). Spatial cognition in Parkinson's disease and neurogenerative dementias. *Cognitive Processing, 7*(Suppl. 5), 77-78.

Parr, H., & Butler, R. (1999). New geographies of illness, impairment and disability. In R. Butler & H. Parr (Eds.), *Mind and body spaces* (pp. 1-24). London: Routledge.

Praamstra, P., Stegeman, D. F., Cools, A. R., & Horstink, M.W. (1998). Reliance on external cues for movement initiation in Parkinson's disease. Evidence from movement-related potentials. *Brain, 121*, 167-171.

Rubinstein, T., Giladi, N., & Hausdorff, M. (2002). The power of cueing to circumvent dopamine deficits: A review of physical therapy treatment of gait disturbances in Parkinson's disease. *Movement Disorders, 17*(6), 1148-1160.

Sacks, O. (1991). *Awakenings*. London: Pan Books Ltd.

Shumway-Cook, A., & Woollacott, M. (2001). *Motor control*. Philadephia: Lippincott Williams & Wilkins.

Soja, E. (1996). *Thirdspace. Journeys to Los Angeles and other real-and-imagined places* (pp. 310-320). Oxford: Blackwell.

Strickland, D. (2005). Rural environment and Parkinson's disease In M. Ebadi & R. F. Pfeiffer (Eds.), *Parkinson's disease* (pp. 63-71). Washington, DC: CRC Press.

Sudenow, D. (1993). *Ways of the hand*. Cambridge, MA: The MIT University Press.

Sunvisson, H., Habermann, B., Weiss, S. & Benner, P. (2009). Augmenting the Cartesian medical discourse with an understanding of the person's lifeworld, lived body, life story and social identity *Nursing Philosophy, 10*, 241–252.

Sunvisson, H. (2006). Stopped within a track: Embodied experiences of late-stage Parkinson's disease. *International Journal of Qualitative Studies on Health and Well-being, 1*, 91-99.

Sunvisson H., & Ekman S.-L. (2001). Parkinson's disease and environment: Patient experiences from environmental influences. *Nursing Inquiry, 8*(1), 41-50.

Sveen, K. (2000). *Det kultiverade lidandet* . (The cultivated suffering). (O. Hellström, Trans.) Göteborg, Sweden: Daidalos.(Original work published 1997).

Toombs, K. (2001). Reflections on bodily change: the lived experience of disability. In TK. Koombs (Ed.), *Handbook of phenomenology and medicine* (pp. 247-261). Dordrecht, Netherlands: Kluwer Academic Publishers.

Van Der Bruggen, H., & Widdershoven, G. (2004). Being a Parkinson's patient: Immobile and unpredictably whimsical. Literature and existential analysis. *Medicine, Health Care and Philosophy, 7*, 289-301.

Zgaljardic, D. J., Borad, J. C., Foldi, N. S., & Mattis, P. (2003). A review of the cognitive and behavioral sequelae of Parkinson's disease: Relationship to frontostriatal circuitry. *Cognitive and Behavioral Neurology, 16*(4), 193-210.

CHAPTER 5

Health, Disorder, and the Psychiatric Enterprise: Reclaiming Lost Connections

CYNTHIA STUHLMILLER

In this chapter, I describe why Benner's insights on human experience are important for understanding psychiatric phenomena. Her stance critiques narrow decontextualized views of what constitutes illness and honors the experiences of individuals and communities who confront and live through challenges. In psychiatry such experiences that become problematic are most often reduced to a list of symptoms, disorders, and technical terms and can obscure personal and collective coping possibilities.

In this chapter, diagnoses of Post-Traumatic Stress Disorder (PTSD), Seasonal Affective Disorder (SAD), and schizophrenia are used to illustrate the dangers of classification systems generally—and why the interpretive approach developed by Benner and colleagues paves the way to restoring human connections that can preserve dignity and worth that is necessary for health and healing.

The research excerpts spotlighted in this chapter point to the iatrogenic nature and trend of the diagnostic culture of psychiatry. Undoubtedly, diagnoses can bring meaning to experiences and join individuals in suffering. However, they can also serve to disconnect individuals and communities when the meanings are based on the deficit view of the person or persons. This view undermines personal and collective strength and cultural resilience and coping practices.

Ian, a disaster rescuer in the United States, stated in an interview:

> I felt good about what I did because I performed a service to many of the people's families. My job is to save lives..... . I felt high in helping somebody, and when there is no hope of helping that person, the only thing I can do is get the bodies out. I take a lot of pride in my job. I thought I did a good job. (Stuhlmiller, 1992; 1996a, p.120)

As the interview continues, tears well up in Ian's eyes, and he begins to tremble as he takes out of his wallet a tattered checklist for symptoms of stress that he received at the disaster site. He blurts out

> But I feel horrible for not having had a normal reaction to an abnormal situation. [As the checklist reads,] You have just been exposed to a life threatening event and it is normal and likely that you will experience one or more of the following [negative] psychological symptoms. (ibid.)

Ingrid, a research participant in Tromsø, Norway described living in long periods of light and dark. When asked about emotional changes during darktime that denote depression, a marker of seasonal affective disorder, she replied

> Oh yes, we experience those thoughts during winter months but we do not call it depression, we call it blue thoughts and consider them to be a source of life's richness. They are important to understanding the dark reflective side of self and the fullness of our lives. . . . But it is a problem if ordinary life is going to become a diagnosis. (Stuhlmiller, 1995, p. 22)

Simon, a consumer activist and man living in Australia with schizophrenia for over 30 years describes the injustice, stigma, and neglect of people who experience a mental illness. He challenges what he refers to as the dominant psychiatric paradigm—the medical model.

> Traditionally mental health consumers have been talked about, our realities and lives described for us, out voices suppressed, turned into case studies or ignored in the interest of the dominant paradigm. (Champ, 2000, p. 17-18)

As an artist and writer Simon says:

> In sharing my writing and art I politicize the personal in representing my reality as a person with a psychiatric disability. I try to give voice to personal realities that are often misrepresented or stereotyped. (ibid.)

He explains further

> Often professional and consumers view situations and needs differently. A good example is how, when professionals describe what are the most distressing aspects of living with schizophrenia, they suggest that these are hallucinations or delusions. However, a consumer experiencing the illness may actually prioritize loneliness, stigma or feeling of hopelessness as the most

disabling aspect of living with the condition. Listening to either view perhaps suggests different responses to and treatment of the condition. (ibid. p.167.)

The voices in this chapter describe profound existential feelings of uniqueness and isolation that develop in response to altered functioning and are deepened through self- or social alienation and medical trivialization. We are reminded that restoring health involves finding meaning in experience and reclaiming connections that have become disrupted or lost.

The intent of this chapter is to contribute to the dialogue about the foundation of and intentions of mental health nursing. And while mainstream psychiatric nursing scientists and practitioners focus on the exciting developments in neurobiology, the human genome project, and newer and more effective psychotropic medications—all important endeavors—it is encouraged here that mental health nursing reclaim its place within nursing philosophy (patient-centered caring and respect), nursing theory (interpersonal nursing and a health orientation), and nursing practice (working with client strengths, enhancing activities of daily living) (Horsfall & Stuhlmiller, 2000, p. 5). The paradigms that underpin these divergent philosophies—pathogenesis and salutogenesis—are explored as they affect mental illness and health.

CONNECTING THE OBJECTIVE/SUBJECTIVE DIVIDE

The study and practice of nursing have traditionally straddled two paradigms. One paradigm focuses on the causes and effects of disease or breakdown—*pathogenesis*. The other paradigm—*salutogenesis*—focuses on that which contributes to health and wellness.

The pathogenic paradigm supports the notion that objective data is contained in the body that provides confirming evidence for a particular alteration or disease. When the identified problem is treated or removed, the disease is expected to diminish. This model, based upon reductionistic science, has long been the central focus of Western medicine. From this premise, when a person is exposed to a pathogen or negative event, he is at risk to develop disease or breakdown with symptoms that can further impair the person. The terminology derived from pathogenic paradigm uses a language of inability, vulnerability, risk, disorder, deviation, and disability. The person is thereby rendered somewhat helpless in the face of the pathogen.

Based on the definition of Antonovsky (1979), the salutogenic paradigm focuses on discovering and promoting the healthy aspects of persons—their coping abilities, strengths, and resiliencies even in the midst of disease and suffering. Knowledge from this paradigm is derived from understanding the world of the person. The language of salutogenesis is one of positive possibilities and acknowledges that people have achievements, capacity, and constructive potential. Deficits are viewed as challenges and opportunities that can lead to growth and learning.

For example, disaster survivors and rescuers, while exposed gruesome and horrific life-threatening situations, may develop distressing reactions such as nightmares and flashbacks and experience anxiety for a long time. However, they also describe positive changes and discoveries such as a reaffirmation of things they like about themselves, the importance of relationships, a renewed or re-evaluated sense of purpose and goals in life, strengthened values, and newfound skills and confidence. New lessons are learned and old ones are rediscovered (Stuhlmiller, 1996).

The following statements from a variety of disaster survivors and rescuers illustrate a range of possible positive outcomes.

> The event gave me a chance to really take an inventory of things.
>
> I discovered I am getting older and it is probably time to think of doing something else that is more rewarding.
>
> You should enjoy yourself in life because you don't know what is going to happen.
>
> I realize I should slow down a little bit and not worry about little things so much.
>
> It taught me to believe in God more, I mean it made me stronger.
>
> I learned a lot about people, the way I look at people, the way I look at myself.
>
> It made me more confident in my abilities.
>
> For myself, I sure do enjoy my life a lot more.
>
> It was by far and away, in that short period of time, the most enlightening and exhilarating experience in my life.
>
> (Stuhlmiller, 1996).

Nurses typically learn about disorders and psychological and emotional changes that occur during life transitions and health alterations. This information provides the necessary background for understanding disease trajectories and general responses. Nurses use this knowledge to investigate the person's experience of illness to help discover what is possible for that person in terms of coping. This requires the nurse to learn about the person's interpretation of the situation and his specific sources of concern, discomfort, distress, suffering, and well-being.

Although the distinction between pathogenic and salutogenic paradigms helps locate the focus of medicine and nursing, the story from the ground up is far more complicated. Benner and colleagues (Benner, 1984; Benner, Tanner, & Chesla, 1996; Benner & Wrubel, 1989) have long recognized that the pathogenic paradigm fails to capture the fullness of human experience. Theoretical learning from formal lists of standardized symptoms, techniques, and interventions is a useful starting point. However, care guided by this paradigm overlooks and diminishes the critical personal, situational, and relational aspects that constitute illness and make health and recovery possible. At the same time, suggesting that experiences that cannot be directly observed or measured are subjective, idiosyncratic, and personalized (and therefore cannot be made explicit) is to ignore that humans inhabit a common world and, therefore, share in accessible meanings. Care informed from this paradigm also falls short when the common connections between the care giver and the care recipient remain unacknowledged.

Drawing upon the work of Heidegger, Kierkegaard, Dreyfus, and others, Benner opened up understanding of the lived experience through phenomenological inquiry. From this perspective, Cartesian dualism is challenged because it cannot account for the whole experience of the person. The reason that disease or health can be understood and grasped is because we are commonly linked as humans and connected to each other more or less with practical know-how gained from being in the world and growing up in a specific culture and tradition.

An examination of the psychiatric enterprise illustrates how individuals who experience social and psychological disconnection can be afforded relief and even connection through a diagnosis. However, social and psychological disconnection will deepen if attention to preserving and rebuilding strength, capacity, and understanding through meaningful personal, occupational, cultural, and societal connections is not the focus of health restoration. As will be pointed out, psychiatric disorders are conceptualized and based upon historical, political, cultural, social, economic, professional, and contextual issues—and must therefore be dealt with in those terms.

> *"Effective caregiving requires more than intent or sentiment. It requires skill and knowledge and being in relation with others in ways that foster mutuality, empowerment, and growth"* (Benner, 1994, p. 45).

POST-TRAUMATIC STRESS DISORDER: CHALLENGING PERSONAL AND OCCUPATIONAL MEANINGS

As a psychiatric diagnosis, PTSD made its debut in the *Diagnostic and Statistical Manual of Mental Disorders*, 3rd edition (American Psychiatric Association, 1980). Motivated by a political agenda to acknowledge the long-endured suffering of Vietnam War veterans (Stuhlmiller, 2003), this nosology created meaning and legitimization for the psychological wounds experienced by not only survivors of war but others exposed to life-threatening events, such as disaster, violence, and the Holocaust. Although this long-awaited classification was welcomed as a source for understanding the aspects of extreme experiences shared by soldiers and others, its placement in a manual of mental disorders ushered in the acknowledgment of a new disability with an accompanying set of expectations. Additionally, because of the underlying belief that the effects of trauma such as created by war are universal, the recognition of the actual dynamics that lead to its development—the social, cultural, historical, financial, and political climate of the time—were left unexplored.

This nosology also generated assumptions pertaining to future events. For example, the ubiquitous nature of all extreme threats could now be considered traumatic, and soon the need for a cadre of professionals to mitigate the inherent risk from expected psychological fallout was needed. The steamroller of the trauma industry was born. Whereas taking care to not minimize suffering resultant from tragic events, the leveling of experiences and application of a one-size-fits-all intervention known as the "psychological debrief" failed to make room for alternate experiences and consequences for victims, such as newfound skills, confidence, or values (Stuhlmiller & Dunning, 2000b).

As illustrated in the introduction of this chapter, Ian did not fit an expected pattern of response and therefore felt alienated from others. He did not share the "requisite" guilt or remorse expected. Rather, he interpreted the absence of symptoms to mean, "I am not normal." Interestingly in this case, to be normal is to be "disordered" and included in a book of pathology. As was found in this study, extreme events do shatter assumptions about personal and collective safety, control, and invincibility; however, how they are experienced is based upon both common meanings of an occupation and culture as well as the unique aspects of the person in the specific disaster situation.

Benner's (1984) early work demonstrated that applying interventions based upon narrow definitions of stress and the application of predictive models can induce further stress to individuals. She found that in a study of mid-career men, work stress and satisfaction was based upon a web of person-in-situation context that involved personal concerns, commitments, and involvement. Some individuals found work to be a source of stress, but others sought comfort and meaning in work as a positive coping resource. Thus, removing a person from work because work has become stressful could lead to more stress for the individual who derived value and worth from the work itself. Similarly, for a person who finds work meaningless, his removal from work will do little to restore meaning. This discovery called into question the popular stress-distancing techniques. Instead, Benner rightly claimed, the expected cause of the stress—that is, work, disease, loss—was not itself the issue but, rather, the meaning that it held for the person. From this premise, she defined stress as "the disruption of meanings, understanding and smooth functioning so that harm, loss and challenge are experienced" (p. 412). Flowing from this definition, "coping is the restoration of meaning" (Benner & Wrubel, 1989, p. 408).

Ian, who felt that he did a good job, took pride in his work. He had trained extensively for rescue work, and this was his call to duty. His occupational socialization and experience provided pre-understanding of the value of saving lives. When allowed to conduct his practice, stress was not felt. However the post-event intervention of comparing himself against a symptom checklist, which was aimed to normalize acute symptoms of stress, diminished his experience of success. Stress became that which challenged his sense of accomplishment and defined him as different from others. When professionals miscalculate and/or assign meanings that do not ring true for the person(s), stress is generated, and well-being compromised. Coping for Ian was to realign his own understanding with that which he experienced.

Similarly, in investigations of emergency workers of earthquakes, floods, fires, riots, mudslides, murders, and rail disasters (Stuhlmiller, 1996b; 1997), stress was found to have little to do with theoretically defined threats to safety, gruesomeness, death, and destruction. Experienced rescuers have well-developed skills to deal with these routine aspects of their work. Rather, stress resulted from interferences in getting the job done: namely, equipment failure, poor interagency communication, and bureaucratic delays.

The essential problem with PTSD, as well as other diagnoses of the reductionistic model, is that the offending pathogen—trauma—is considered to be an outside objective agent. The trauma assaults, violates, and disconnects the person from his usual world of understanding. Because trauma is considered an attack from the outside, responsibility for healing is also therefore considered to be needed from an outside and professional intervention (Stuhlmiller & Dunning, 2000a). This conceptualization is faulty and may be why no evidence supports that psychological debriefing has any effectiveness and can even be iatrogenic. The Bennerian perspective provides counterbalance to this view, suggesting that trauma can be defined only in terms of personal, situational, and cultural contexts—and, therefore, healing can be derived only from honoring those sources.

SEASONAL AFFECTIVE DISORDER: CHALLENGING PERSONAL AND CULTURAL MEANINGS

In the mid-1980s, Rosenthal defined SAD as a form of depression that varies with seasons and also involves recurring episodes of fall/winter depression that alternates with hypomania in spring/summer. Other depressive symptoms include excessive sleep, appetite increase, carbohydrate craving, weight gain, dysphoria, anxiety, irritability, social withdrawal, decreased libido, difficulty concentrating, and problems with interpersonal relations (American Psychiatric Association, 1987; 1994). The physiological explanation involves suppression of melatonin and disruptions to circadian rhythms and neurohormones attributable to the absence of sunlight. The treatment for SAD is sitting in front of a light box and antidepressant drug therapy. Light box therapy involves sitting in front of a box that gives off bright light that mimics the natural outdoor light. This exposure is thought to alter circadian rhythms and the body's natural release of melatonin.

In 1993, I commenced a study of SAD in Tromsø, Norway, located 400 miles north of the Arctic Circle. As a researcher living in a culture different from my own, many of my taken-for-granted ways of life were challenged. For example, the Northern Norwegian society—rich in tradition—exposes its people to philosophy in primary education: They are taught *how* to think in addition to *what* to think. This stands in contrast to the U.S. system, which tends to focus on teaching facts and figures or received knowledge (Stuhlmiller, 1992).

Northern Norwegians also possess a deep sense of and respect for nature: Nature and culture are closely connected concepts. In fact, nature—considered a national icon—is central to discussions of "Norwegianess" as expressed in the notion "When nature is more important than culture" (Gullestad, 1992). Norwegian people dwelling in this rugged and dramatic environment live in harmony with nature without attempting to control it or conquer it—as some might in the United States. As one informant said, "We belong to nature and don't try to stand outside of nature as all-powerful engineers" (Stuhlmiller, 1992).

Activities of work and social life are thus lived in concert with nature, seasons, and seasonal change. Celebrations and rituals such as the month-long event of Julebord (Christmas feasts and gatherings), when the sun leaves, political rallies, and frequent parades were found to mitigate the experience of darktime as problematic. Although people described a life that corresponded to seasonal change and features of SAD, research participants asserted that it is considered part of life and not to be medicalized. "It is a problem if ordinary life is going to become a diagnosis" (Stuhlmiller, 1995, p. 22). To be out of sync with nature is to lose your connection to your cultural identity.

During the course of the study, a newspaper headline read "Darktime is Dangerous" (Holte, 1993). The accompanying article suggested that because winter darkness disrupts sleep patterns, not only would social relations be impaired from fatigue, but that people were at additional risk of job accidents. Upon investigation, I discovered that the effort to problematize responses to seasonal change was driven by the local university psychology department in an effort to fulfill an agenda. The psychology department advertised help in the form of antidepressants and light therapy, and the department chair held a franchise to sell light box equipment. While the campaign to generate clients continued, the counterargument of cultural mitigating practices generated from my study opened up lively community debate.

Although research findings, conducted by the same psychology department, did not support the theory of widespread prevalence of SAD in Tromsø, within a year of my departure from Norway, a major conference about SAD was held at the university. The conference was sponsored by a pharmaceutical company that makes antidepressant medications. Although it is difficult to estimate the impact of introducing the notion of SAD to a community, treatment for SAD has increased in Tromsø since that time as reported by my research informants (personal communications, 1995, 1996, 1997). Problems once attributed to everyday living are now considered to be a result of SAD. Instead of joining at a local gathering spot for a traditional meal, appointments are kept for light therapy. In effect, cultural understandings of seasonal change have shifted from individuals to experts who diagnose and treat. Time-tested rituals and connecting practices are being replaced with technological fixes that disconnect people from each other and their culture (Stuhlmiller, 1998).

Ingrid (introduced earlier in the chapter) suggested the importance of darktime in allowing for reflections that do not occur at other times of the year. This does not mean that symptoms of SAD do not exist. However, disrupted sleep brings time for reflection on the dark side of self, which ultimately brings richness and fuller understanding to life. Summer time is full light: action time, with little time for reflection. As Ingrid comments

> *Social life is best in winter. We must be in our homes and we make some good things. We have celebrations and so on. There is very much of that in the dark period but in the light period we can use the nature so, we are not so social then.* (Stuhlmiller, 1998, p.154)

Another research participant, Ellen, cogently explains the dangers of diagnosis:

> *The first time I heard of this [SAD] was the research at the psychiatric hospital and it said what you should do to avoid darktime problems. . . . We get the advice*

> *as children but it was part of the ordinary life and it was another thing when a doctor says do this and that. If you are getting a diagnosis you don't think you can do anything for yourself. It does not mean we are sick but it does mean something to us (Stuhlmiller, 1998, p.155).*

Not only does this study point out the undermining of a cultural understanding that can result from medicalizing everyday life situations but also the challenge to self-efficacy. Reconnecting individuals to themselves and each other is an age-old practice that cannot be supplanted by technological means.

SCHIZOPHRENIA: CHALLENGING PERSONAL AND SOCIETAL MEANING

People with schizophrenia experience problems related to perceptions, thoughts, feelings, and behaviors. These people often have perceptions that do not correspond with consensus views of reality; communication does not make sense; emotions are extreme and debilitating or behaviors that are harmful or troublesome. It is as if the self disconnects from the self, others, and society. Almost worse is the stigma attached to the diagnosis, which raises questions about personal adequacy and autonomy.

Like PTSD and SAD, the diagnosis of schizophrenia provides a means of understanding aspects of experiences that are shared by others and serve as shortcuts for knowing the person. Diagnoses also impact on how others respond to the diagnosed person and ultimately influence their self-concept. As pointed out by Hall (1996), psychiatric labels have life-eroding effects that do not consider societal and self-defined goals or meanings; ingrained patterns of oppression and discrimination; and positive aspects and strengths of the person. She claims that the assumption of diagnostic certainty and cure is misleading and that the narrow view of the person leads to stereotyping and humiliation.

Champ (2000) provides insight into how psychotic illnesses alter perceptions which beg for increased patience, understanding, and reconnection of and with others:

> *During my first admission to the psychiatric ward, the nurse who was taking me to be showered became a guard leading me to the gas chambers in a concentration camp of my delusions own making. I was not being showered but lead to my death. . . .it was not a fantasy but my reality. . . . .Beyond the more radical changes in perception of nurses that I have experienced because of psychotic symptoms nurses*

have not always been seen by me as they intended because of my interpretation of their role. In the early years of my recovery, sometimes in the journals I kept nurses were referred to as the 'soul fuckers' who dispensed what I would call 'mind death'. Nurses did indeed seem to me to be interfering with my very soul with medications that significantly changed my emotions and sense of being in the world. I thought of my illness as a special sensitivity and often saw society as for more out of touch with reality than I was. At such times the healing role of the nurses seemed secondary to a perceived role that they were indeed agents of social control, repressing original thought and enforcing a narrow conception of reality supported by the status quo . . . that made me believe a powerful system was intent on repressing me. . . . For me a good nurse can recognize when a consumer has developed a strange belief about them and restore the consumers perceptions of themselves as they truly are. (p. 331)

It is no doubt that the diagnosis of schizophrenia fits Simon. However, it is also easy to see from his description why in his state of altered perceptions, the meaning of everyday practices of nurses (showering, and dispensing medication) take on additional meaning during his illness, which in fact may not be too far from the intentions of the nurse to control behavior, repress emotion and thought, and support the treatment plan or status quo. As Simon pointed out, nurses who fail to acknowledge the concerns of clients or explore how their help is being perceived are likely to be misunderstood and thus create more anxiety. As a diagnosis, schizophrenia removes Simon from 99% of the population who, according to statistics, do not experience schizophrenia (APA, 1994, p. 886). The illness separates him further from himself and his world. In the struggle to find a place to stand in the midst of uncertainty and rejection, Simon eloquently explains the importance of reconnection which captures the focus of this chapter.

For me schizophrenia severely ruptured the relationship that I had enjoyed with myself prior to the illness. My sense of being in the world, my thought processes, and indeed the very way senses perceived the world would go through involuntary changes. I was plunged at times into a confusing and frightening world ruled by my own paranoia and delusions. Living with the ever changing experience of schizophrenia over 23 years has changed my relationship with myself many times and in many ways . . . the nurses I valued most at the time were those who rather than imposing their reality on me, helped me to explore where reality and wellbeing might exist for me. . . I have come to see that one does not simply patch up the self one was before developing schizophrenia, but one has to recreate a concept of who one is that integrates the experience of schizophrenia . . . the best professionals involved

> *in my care, like me, have opened themselves to the mystery that is schizophrenia. They have gained trust, sharing, and support my inner search for meaning and for an understanding of the relationship between myself and the illness. (Champ, 1998, p.57-58)*

Simon described a shattered sense of coherence and the out-of-control feelings of confusion, fear, and ruptured sense of self. Recovery for him is in searching, questioning, re-creating, reconciling, and integrating the changes that he has experienced into a coherent sense of self. He locates the importance of the nurse in dwelling with the frightened and confused person, working toward a discovery of meaning to make sense of the disconnection of self with the world. To explore with Simon "where reality and wellbeing might exist" for him, the nurse joins in searching for clues to help him make sense of, manage, and find meaning in his experience. The nurse also helps Simon connect his private illness experience with the wider range of available meanings that include the continuum of pathological and nonpathological understandings.

While scientists continue to further isolate causes and effects of diagnoses such as PTSD, SAD, and schizophrenia, disorder prevention and recovery as so vividly pointed out by Ian, Ingrid, and Simon does not come in the form of technological interventions such as pills or talk therapy. Rather, it is based on honoring the experience of the person and helping them find their particular sources of meaning—not undermining or prescribing meanings.

ETHICS AND RESPONSIBILITY

From time immemorial, humankind have survived traumatic events, thrived in environments of extended light and dark, and dwelled in worlds of frightening altered perceptions. How then have these facts of life come to be considered pathologized states demanding medical and psychiatric intervention? From the mid-nineteenth century, deviant behavior became the purview of "mad" doctors. Because of the value placed upon scientific understanding and academic training, doctors became the knowers of what constitutes sickness, what can be done about it, and who is at risk (Stuhlmiller & Dunning, 2000a & 2000b). Over time, with the quest for social order, prediction, and control, sources for understanding life shifted from traditional and spiritual authority to technological, political, scientific, and professional authority (Stuhlmiller, 2003).

In the 1990s, the touted "decade of the brain," (Bush, 1990) new frontiers in psychiatry were forged through identification of specific brain chemicals and genomes linked to mental illness. This neurological determinism has provided increasing explanation of diseases and ailments of contemporary living, including social phobia, attention deficit/hyperactivity disorder, chronic fatigue, compassion fatigue, anorexia, alcoholism, and so on. Neurological determinism, however, minimizes social, psychological, and situational explanations, which also change biochemistry. The depersonalized, desituated person is merely a mass of stimulus and response—or as Shorter (1997) has suggested, a symptom pool through which distress is experienced and expressed.

Unfortunately, the diagnostic culture of symptom-categorizing dominates health care in the United States today. Exploration of personal and collective coping abilities, strengths, and resilience takes a back seat to the more expedient medical, surgical, and pharmaceutical interventions. Symptoms are not embraced as meaningful signals to be understood, nor are they acknowledged as powerfully shaped by cultural and particularly medical expectations. Instead, symptoms and emotions are to be reduced or eliminated. The quick-fix of a pill is the fast-food alternative to a thoughtfully prepared ritual of a shared, sit-down meal. Psychiatry has become little more than a drive-through, "dope 'em up and ship 'em out" practice that is endorsed and furthered by the capitalistic excess need to reward pharmaceutical and insurance companies. Lost from this approach is understanding, learning from struggles—and, ultimately, personhood (Stuhlmiller, 2000).

As pointed out by Ian and Ingrid, in the diagnostic culture, life experiences are reshaped and redefined to meet the genetically and neurologically determined expectation of professional authority. In effect, the experiencing person is no longer the author or authority of his own life. Simon, on the other hand, illuminated the significance of client-focused care that respects and honors the experience of the person regardless of his illness trajectory. Benner and Wrubel (1989) referred to this as "presencing" or "engaged care." Recovery for Simon was assisted by the persons who stood alongside and did not impose their reality upon him but, rather, joined him in his search for his meaning. Joining and connecting practices, based upon a foundation of mutual trust and respect, pave the path for recovery.

Nurses have long drawn upon the healing power of human connections that transcend all other scientific explanations, expectations, and interventions. The placebo effect provides convincing evidence. Even Nightingale (1859/1946, p. 111) claimed that only through engagement can ways to maintain or bring back health be discovered. She stated, "Pathology teaches the harm that disease has done. But it teaches nothing more. We know nothing of the principle of health . . . except from observation and experience [of the person]." Nightingale instructs to nurses to "find out the fancies of the patients." They are the most valuable indication of what is necessary for their recovery.

Nurses have also long been involved in helping people regain a sense of coherence (manageability, meaningfulness, and comprehensibility) over what is occurring to them—be it a result of trauma or some other form of physical or mental distress. With events such as 9/11, the ongoing death and destruction in the Middle East, and large-scale national and international disasters and massacres, the line in the sand becomes deeper between good and evil, sane and insane, and right and wrong. If culture provides a meaningful source of connection, it can become a double-edged sword, as to be part of society is to participate in the shortcut of labels, stereotypes, and politics of difference that involves discounting and alienating others. These labels neatly package and cover over personal collective human potentials, goals, and aspirations of those identified as other. As I see it, the growing dilemma for nurses will be in our own ability to help others find meaning as threats, dangers, insecurities and self-questioning become a growing reality for us too. Even when meaning is not readily apparent, finding meaning in meaninglessness becomes an important charge.

Nurses dwell with and among persons in the margins of life. As firmly stated in our code of ethics, we deliver services with respect to human needs and values without prejudice while acknowledging the basic right to self-determination (American Nurses Association, 2001). Nurses do not withhold care from perpetrators or those considered by others as less worthy. Rather, nurses seek to connect and understand so that we can help those alienated to reconnect and join with.

Connectedness is about shared humanity. Although we may all be different, we are more alike than unlike. And because we are not made from the same cookie cutter, diagnostic labeling and standardized approaches can never capture the lived experience or determine care that is best. The pathogenic paradigm provides essential background knowledge for understanding basic commonalties, but the practice and ethical demand of nursing is to deliver oneself into the hands of others and take care of the lives of those who are placed in one's hands (Logstrup, 1997). This requires interpersonal skill learned from practical experience and is driven by a genuine concern for the other. It entails a responsibility to do right by the other (Weiss, Malone, Merighi, & Benner, 2002).

From this stance, there are no certitudes or absolutes (Benner, Hooper-Kyriakidis, & Stannard, 1999). As argued, "Snap judgments, tunnel vision, overgeneralization, and fixation on certain problems to the exclusion of others are all possible sources of poor judgment" (ibid. p. 5). Disease trajectory and clinical pathways are only useful guides to inform skilled ethical comportment. The art and craft of the nurse is derived from unearthing the wisdom and expertise of the person being nursed. As Simon cogently expressed, it involves the search for meaning and understanding of the relationship between the person and their illness.

Expert nurses do not rush in to define situations with a predetermined set of protocols. Rather, they stand with, observe, and respectfully engage by attending to the cues and lead of the person (Stuhlmiller, 1996). This approach guards against iatrogenic outcomes that can be witnessed from a psychiatric enterprise that ignores personal, occupational, cultural, and societal meanings. The widespread assumption that trauma can lead to long-term, persistent negative psychological consequences can create a self-fulfilling prophesy. To suggest that people will be worse off as a result of trauma is to shortchange them from the possible strengths, capacities, and growth that can emerge (Stuhlmiller & Dunning, 2000a). To medicalize a deeply embedded understanding of seasonal change without consideration of sociocultural consequences is irresponsible. To discredit and undermine cultural values and rich traditions that promote cultural resilience is unethical (Stuhlmiller, 1998). To close off to, ignore, and silence the interpretations and expressions of a person with a psychosis is to demean the authenticity of that person's experience (Champ, 2000).

Nursing is at its finest when the nurse as a person and the person nursed come to know, explore, and respond as collaborators in discovering possibilities of health, illness, and healing. Benner, like Nightingale, has provided countless nurses of our generation with the language, tools, and bright light to illuminate the irreplaceable importance of the human endeavor known as nursing.

References

American Nurses Association. (2001). *Code of ethics for nurses with interpretive statements.* Retrieved November 11, 2009, from: www.nursingworld.org/MainMenuCategories/ThePracticeofProfessionalNursing/EthicsStandards/CodeofEthics/CodeofEthics.aspx

American Psychological Association. (1980). *Diagnostic and statistical manual of mental disorders* (3rd ed.). Washington, DC: American Psychological Association.

American Psychological Association. (1987). *Diagnostic and statistical manual of mental disorders* (revised 3rd ed.). Washington, DC: American Psychological Association.

American Psychological Association. (1994). *Diagnostic and statistical manual of mental disorders* (4th ed.). Washington, DC: American Psychological Association.

Antonovsky, A. (1979). *Health, stress and coping.* San Francisco: Jossey-Bass.

Benner, P. (1984). *Stress and satisfaction on the job: Work meanings and coping of mid-career men.* New York: Praeger.

Benner, P. (1994). Caring as a way of knowing and not knowing. In S. Phillips & P. Benner (Eds.), *The crisis of care: Affirming and restoring caring practices in the helping professions* (pp. 42-63). Washington, DC: Georgetown University Press.

Benner, P., Hooper-Kyriakidid, P., & Stannard, D. (1999). *Clinical wisdom and interventions in critical care: A thinking-in-action approach.* Philadelphia: Saunders.

Benner, P., Tanner, C., & Chesla, C. (1996). *Expertise in nursing practice: Caring, clinical judgment, and ethics.* New York: Springer.

Benner, P., & Wrubel, J. (1989). *The primacy of caring: Stress and coping in health and illness.* Menlo Park, CA: Addison-Wesley.

Bush, G. (1990). Project on the Decade of the Brain: Presidential Proclamation 6154. Retrieved November 11, 2009, from http://www.loc.gov/loc/brain/proclaim.html [Filed with the Office of the Federal Register, 12:11 p.m., July 18, 1990]

Champ, S. (1998). A most precious thread. *The Australian and New Zealand College of Mental Health Nursing, 7,* 54-59.

Champ, S. (consumer contributor) (2000). In J. Horsfall, & C. Stuhlmiller, *Interpersonal nursing for mental health* (pp. 17-18, p. 167, p. 331). Sydney, Australia: MacLennen & Petty.

Gullestad, M. (1992). The art of social relations: Essays on culture, social action, and everyday life in modern Norway. Oslo, Norway: Scandinavian University Press.

Hall, B. (1996). The psychiatric model. A critical analysis of its undermining effects on nursing in chronic mental illness. *Advances in Nursing Science, 18*(3), 16-26.

Holte, A. (1993, nd.). Morketid er farlig [Darktime is dangerous]. *Nordly's,* p.1. Horsfall, J., & Stuhlmiller, C.M. (2000). *Interpersonal nursing for mental health.* Sydney, Australia: MacLennan & Petty.

Logstrup, K. (1997). *The ethical demand.* Notre Dame, IN: University of Notre Dame Press.

Nightingale, F. (1859). *Notes on nursing: What it is and what it is not.* London: Harrison and Sons. (Facsimile edition, J. B. Lippincott Company, 1946).

Shorter, E. 1997. *A short history of psychiatry: From the era of the asylum to the age of Prozac.* New York: Wiley.

Stuhlmiller, C. M. (1992). *An interpretive study of appraisal and coping of rescue workers in an earthquake disaster: The Cypress collapse.* Dissertation abstracts international, 52, 09B p. 4671. (University Microfilms No. 9205240).

Stuhlmiller, C. M. (1995). The construction of disorders: Exploring the growth of PTSD and SAD. *Journal of Psychosocial Nursing and Mental Health Service, 33*(1), 20-23.

Stuhlmiller, C. M. (1996a). *Rescuers of Cypress: Learning from disaster.* (Book #2 of the International Healthcare Ethics Series). New York: Peter Lang Publishing.

Stuhlmiller, C. M. (1996b). Studying the rescuers. *Sigma Theta Tau International Reflections, 22*(6), 18-19.

Stuhlmiller, C. M. (1997). A nursing perspective on Thredbo and other disasters. *Nursing Matters,* 14, 5-6.

Stuhlmiller, C. M. (1998). Understanding seasonal affective disorder and experiences in Northern Norway. *Image: Journal of Nursing* Scholarship, *30*(2), 151-156.

Stuhlmiller, C. M. (2000). *Mental as anything: Dope 'em up & ship 'em out.* Keynote address to Emergency Nurses & Mental Illness Conference Ausmed Publications, Sydney, NSW.

Stuhlmiller, C. M. (2003). Trauma, culture and meaning: Central concerns for mental health nurses. *International Journal of Mental Health Nursing, 12,* 1-2.

Stuhlmiller, C. M., & Dunning, C. (2000a). Challenging the mainstream: From pathogenic to salutogenic models of posttrauma intervention. In J. Violanti, D. Paton, & C. Dunning (Eds.), *Posttraumatic stress intervention: Challenges, issues, and interventions* (pp. 10-42). Springfield, IL: Charles Thomas Publishers.

Stuhlmiller, C. M., & Dunning, C. (2000b). Concerns about debriefing: Challenging the mainstream. In B. Raphael & J. Wilson (Eds.), *Stress debriefing: Theory, practice and evidence* (pp. 305-320). Cambridge, UK: Cambridge University Press.

Weiss, S. Malone, R., Merighi, J., & Benner, P. (2002). Economism, efficiency, and the moral ecology of good nursing practice. *The Canadian Journal of Nursing Research, 34*(2), 95-119.

CHAPTER 6

Understanding End-of-Life Caring Practices in the Emergency Department

DEVELOPING MERLEAU-PONTY'S NOTIONS OF INTENTIONAL ARC AND MAXIMUM GRIP THROUGH PRAXIS AND PHRONESIS[1]

GARRETT K. CHAN

INTRODUCTION

Phenomenology as a methodology to understand how emergency department (ED) clnicians' caring practices for dying patients can help overcome the sense of loss of self-understanding, sense of alienation, moral dilemmas, and loss of social integration for clinicians, patients, and families (*see* Benner & Wrubel, 1989). This reclaiming of understanding allows us to see and understand more fully the caring and even potentially healing practices of clinicians for patients and families in crisis that constitute the foundation of nursing and medical practices. Interpretive projects can illustrate notions of good practice and the knowledge embedded in advanced levels of practice. By articulating these practices, we can confirm good practices, explore additional possibilities, and use them as a basis for new visions of practice (Benner & Wrubel, 1989). This chapter is a philosophical examination of end-of-life care in the ED in an effort to help us understand how core medical and nursing values are embodied as care practices and ethical comportment. This chapter integrates Aristotle and other philosophers' notions of *phronesis* and *praxis* with Merleau-Ponty's ontological notions of *intentional arc* and *maximum grip* in the context of the culture and practices at the end-of-life in emergency care.

Reprinted from *Nursing Philosophy* (2005), with kind permission from Wiley-Blackwell. Minor edits were made for this book.

The emergency department (ED) is a fast-paced environment where patients present suddenly and unpredictably with life-threatening illnesses or injuries, and clinicians function with sub-optimal levels of information (Chan, 2004; Iserson, 1996). Despite heroic efforts, many people die in the ED (McCaig & Ly, 2002). Current end-of-life care models proposed by national educational initiatives (Emanuel, von Gunten, & Ferris, 1999; Ferrell and Grant, 2001) and the Institute of Medicine (IOM) (Field & Cassel, 1997) are based upon chronic illness trajectories of dying that may be difficult to apply to ED end-of-life caring practices (Chan, 2004).

Care of the patient and family at the end-of-life has been identified by both the American Nurses Association (ANA) and the American Medical Association (AMA) as an important core value in their respective professions (American Nurses Association, 2001; American Medical Association's Council on Scientific Affairs, 1996; American Medical Association, 2002). In addition, attention to end-of-life issues continues to be a national priority for research and funding according to the IOM and the National Institutes of Health (NIH) (Adams & Corrigan, 2003; National Institute of Nursing Research, 2004). Poor end-of-life care is an issue for American society that must be improved (Lunney et al., 2003a). Previous studies have focused on the epidemiology of death, provision of or lack of end-of-life care in the intensive care unit, descriptions of palliative care (e.g., symptom management, advance care planning, spiritual care), and the experience of clinicians' moral distress when caring for patients who are dying (Corley, 1995; Lunney et al., 2003b; SUPPORT Investigators, 1995; Timmermans, 1999). In critical care, national research priorities are focused on identifying and measuring processes, quality, and outcomes of end-of-life care (Clarke et al., 2003; Rubenfeld & Randall, 2001). However, reducing and testing these empirical indicators of the construct of "good end-of-life care" requires that scientists continue down an epistemological path that ignores the ontological and complex life worlds of human actions, caring, and concerns.

End-of-life scholars have spent less time talking about how philosophy could help interpret care at the end-of-life. A philosophical approach may help us understand how core medical and nursing values are embodied as care practices and as ethical comportment. The goal of this paper is to explore Merleau-Ponty's notions of the *intentional arc* and *maximum grip* as a source of influence on praxis and phronesis in embodied ED end-of-life care practices. First, however, an orientation to the ontological notions of what it is to be a clinician will be presented, followed by a description of Merleau-Ponty's two concepts. A case exemplar will be used to illustrate different aspects and perceptions of the same phenomenon.

PHILOSOPHICAL NOTIONS ON WHAT IT IS TO BE A CLINICIAN

There are many philosophical notions that underlie one's understanding of what it is to be a person and a clinician that have been described by philosophers such as Martin Heidegger, Hubert Dreyfus, Charles Taylor, Patricia Benner, and Judith Wrubel. In examining these phenomenological philosophical notions, one can understand how they intertwine and support one's assumptions about being, knowing, knowledge and practice.

Praxis, Phronesis, and Embodiment

The notions of *praxis* and *phronesis* were first described by Aristotle. The Aristotelian scholar, Joseph Dunne, elucidates praxis as the

> conduct in a public space with others, in which a person, without ulterior purpose and with a view to no object detachable from himself, acts in such a way as to realize excellences that he has come to appreciate in his community as constitutive of a worthwhile way of life.... [Praxis is] an activity that both involved one with other people and at the same time was a realization of one's self, praxis engaged one more intimately, or afforded one less detachment (Dunne, 1997, p. 10).

Praxis is the activity that is publicly intelligible and is held in common with other practitioners. There are singular universals and commonalities that are understood by other practitioners, such as, "assess and treat Airway, Breathing, and Circulation first," and "Give the patient as much autonomous choice as possible based on one's cultural beliefs." The practitioner is engaged in the activity, is *unreflective* about the praxis (i.e., it is without rational calculation), and actualizes notions of good practice that are held by local and larger groups of professional practitioners (Benner, 2000). Praxis is not a private, an idiosyncratic, nor a subjective habit where the only person to comprehend the practice is the practitioner him or herself.

While praxis or a practice is the public conduct, the person embodies a knowledge that is socially embedded in a practice that is gained through experience. Aristotle called this type of knowledge phronesis (Dunne, 1997). The clinician caring for a patient is involved in a practice. This practice is influenced by his or her moral agency, experiential or practical knowledge, perceptiveness to the particulars of a situation, and skillful comportment. Understanding the end-of-life experiences in the ED requires an appreciation for clinicians' actions or practices (*praxis*), and their embodied knowledge (*phronesis*).

The notion of embodiment, based on the works of philosophers such as Heidegger (1927/1962), Merleau-Ponty (1945/2001), Dreyfus (1991), Benner &Wrubel (1989), and Benner (2000) is central to a phenomenological view of what it is to be a person. These philosophers counter the Cartesian and Kantian representations of a mind-body dualism, that include mental representations and the notion that a person sits over and against a world of which he or she is not a part. In contrast, the notion of embodiment is a "social, sentient sensori-motor embodied person [who] dwells in a human world of relationships, concerns, and [common] meanings" (Benner, 2000, p. 6).

Contrary to the Cartesian notion of indubitable knowledge generated from rational calculations, Benner (2000) has described a type of certainty that clinicians develop from experiential knowledge. Development of qualitative distinctions in particular cases and the development of perceptual acuity through contrasting whole cases from past experience open possibilities and understandings of the patient for the clinician. Skillful clinicians who have experienced caring for dying patients use their senses to perceive and understand the real lifeworld of the person for whom they are caring. This understanding of the patient's real lifeworld with all of the events, consequences, and relationships by a phronetic clinician is a form of embodied realism. In other words, a sensing, embodied knower can apprehend and know the world of the patient (Benner, 2000). However, Benner also notes that phronetic knowledge is dialogical with experience and is always open to correction and improvement.

Experience, Virtue, and Ethical Comportment

Gadamer (1960/1989) has described experience as perceptions of a person that are open and dialectical with new experiences that may negate previous experiences. These experiences are not an end, or *telos*, but rather a process that is grounded in the history of the person. Experiences, or perceptions, constitute phronesis that are neither fully transparent nor fully available to the person (Dunne, 1997).

The relationship between experience and phronesis is dynamic. It is a continual refining process that shapes and influences one's lifeworld and experiences from which we draw or evolve one's knowledge and skill. Insights are gleaned from past experiences that enrich one's skilled know-how and theoretical knowledge (Dreyfus, Dreyfus, & Benner, 1996). Over time, this continual dialogue between experience and knowledge develops expertise in the practice. This is illustrated by Dunne:

> Now when a person is experienced we might say that the virtue through which he or she exploits that experience or puts what has been learned from it

to work—and in the process learns more and so further develops and refines his or her experience—is phronesis. Phronesis is what enables experience to be self-correcting and to avoid settling into mere routine or universalizing. . . .. Phronesis does not ascend to a level of abstraction or generality that leaves experience behind. It arises from experience and returns into experience. It is, we might say, the insightfulness—or using Aristotle's own metaphor, "the eye"—of a particular type of experience, and the insights it achieves are turned back into experience, which is in this way constantly reconstructed or enriched. And the more experience is reconstructed in this way, the more sensitive and insightful phronesis becomes—or, rather, the more the experiencer becomes a phronimos. (Dunne, 1997, p. 292-293)

Virtue is central to phronesis. According to Dunne (1997), the virtue of a person is developed, often painstakingly, by experiential knowledge. Virtue is understood to be an embodied comportment that is unreflective and egoless (i.e., free of mental content) rather than as a possession (Dreyfus et al., 1996). In other words, the world and situation that is socially and experientially constituted solicits or calls to the person to act in a way that is meaningful and good rather than virtues being possessed by a person who will apply these good virtues to a situation—and, therefore, the outcome is good.

The virtuous character and lifeworld are inextricably linked and reciprocal. Being a part of one's lifeworld affords us experiences that belong to one's lifeworld. Through experiencing different situations in one's lifeworld, we acquire and enrich phronesis. This knowledge-skill acquisition is an important part of phronesis. "[Phronesis] is natural . . . not innate but rather what is acquired by experience. . . ." (Dunne, 1997, p. 279).

However, knowledge, virtue, and skill are iterative or circular. Background meanings, practices, skills, and habits are learned by living in and moving around in a world with shared traditions and knowledge. While some skills and practices are taught through theoretical or predictive models, clinicians encounter situations that do not fit these context-free theories. A clinician who is connected and involved responds to each unique situation with experience-based intuition as a guide for ethical comportment (Dreyfus et al., 1996). As the clinician acts in the situation, the experiential knowledge informs current and future action yet avoids routinization and universalization. Experiential knowledge changes one's interpretation and proto-interpretation of the world (Taylor, 1985). Dreyfus et al. (1996) summarize this concept in the following quote:

> When an individual becomes a master of his culture's practices or a professional practice within it, he or she no longer tries to do what one normally does, but rather responds out of a fund of experience in the culture and in the specialized practice. This requires having enough experience to give up following the rules and maxims dictating what anyone should do, and instead, acting upon the intuition that results from a life in which talent and sensibility have allowed learning from the experience of satisfaction and regret in similar situations. Authentic caring in this sense is common to . . . Aristotelian phronesis. (p. 274)

Aristotle advocates that "we ought to attend to the undemonstrated sayings and opinions of experienced and wise older people or of *phronimoi* not less than to demonstrations; because experience has given them an eye they see aright" (Aristotle, as cited by Dunne, 1997, p. 280). The *phronimoi* have encountered a multitude of experiences that allows them to develop virtues and phronesis associated with practice.

Perception and "Ultimate Particulars"

While experience and phronesis are so closely intertwined, it is important to discuss the influence that intuition or perceptiveness (*nous*) and the "ultimate particulars" (*eschaton*) have on phronesis (Dunne, 1997). It is these ultimate particulars of similar yet distinct experiences that round out the knowledge in different ways, leading to a more robust understanding of the world. As mentioned above, the relationship between experience and knowledge is dynamic. Repeated exposures to similar experiences allow for the recognition of resemblances, similarities but also the qualitative distinctions, nuanced differences, particularities, and patterns to show up for the practitioner (Benner, Hooper-Kyriakidis, & Stannard, 1999; Benner, Tanner, & Chesla, 1996). Expertise is cultivated. In order for phronesis to develop, one needs to be open to these insights in the particulars of the experiences and intuit (or be attentive to) the differences before they become incorporated into a habitus or sedimented pattern of experience (Dunne, 1997; Merleau-Ponty, 1945/2001).

Skillful Comportment, Style, and Situated Freedom

In practice, action is pervasive. Phronesis is constituted by experiential knowledge that influences one's embodied comportment and is precognitive and nonrational. Benner et al. (1999) describe this embodied way of knowing as "thinking-in-action" and "skilled know-how" (p. 12-13). Skilled know-how is the skillful performance of expert, embodied clinicians in clinical situations. Thinking-in-action is the practical reasoning that moves the skilled, embodied clinician to a "clearer understanding and resolves contradiction or confusion" (Benner et al., 1999, p. 10). Skilled clinical know-how combined with clinical wisdom and good judgment is more apparent in expert clinicians in crisis situations when there are life-threatening events (Benner et al., 1999).

In skill acquisition, Benner and colleagues (1999) described two skillful comportments that are central to clinical wisdom: clinical forethought and clinical grasp. However, before one can understand clinical grasp and clinical forethought, one must examine the notion of wisdom.

According to Meacham (1990) and Weick (2001), wisdom is a delicate balance of what is known, what is not known, the realization that the knowledge is fallible, and doubt. As Meacham so eloquently wrote

> [T]he essence of wisdom . . . lies not in what is known but rather in the manner in which that knowledge is held and in how that knowledge is put to use. To be wise is not to know particular facts but to know without excessive confidence or excessive cautiousness. . . . [T]o both accumulate knowledge while remaining suspicious of it, and recognizing that much remains unknown is to be wise. . . . The essence of wisdom is in knowing that one does not know, in the appreciation that knowledge is fallible, [and] in the balance between knowing and doubting. (1990, pp. 185, 184, 210)

Meacham's definition of wisdom acknowledges that a wise person has knowledge and continually critiques and refines the knowledge, all the while recognizing that the knowledge could be wrong. This understanding of wisdom allows for the practitioner to anticipate that the knowledge is a blend of what has been known, presumed, and coherent in the past with the possibility that in the present, sudden discoveries of difference, uncertainty, or the unexpected might challenge the assumptive set (i.e., preconceptions) (Benner et al., 1999; Merleau-Ponty, 1945/2001).

Another aspect in understanding wisdom that is important to note is that one understands events and actions retrospectively while one lives life and acts in the present and moves forward (Weick, 1999). The philosopher Kierkegaard commented, "It is perfectly true, as philosophers say, that life must be understood backwards" (Kierkegaard, 1843/1967). However, Gardiner offered an insightful addition, ". . . but they [philosophers] forget the other proposition, that it [life] must be lived forwards" (as cited by Weick, 1999, p. 134). Interpretation, justification, and meaning are attached after the action has been completed.

A skillful, embodied practitioner draws upon past experiential knowledge and the requisite theoretical knowledge and uses his or her perceptual skill to get a good grasp of the clinical situation (Benner et al., 1999). A wise, expert clinician is attuned to the clinical situation and uses perceptual skill to detect when the patient's condition is changing or not responding as expected. This expert, reflective clinician is capable of improvising and adapting interventions in the present situation based upon the experiential and theoretical knowledge of the past.

Expert clinicians are also able to anticipate likely clinical events based upon previous experiential and theoretical knowledge. Benner and colleagues (1999) describe the combination of thinking-in-action with anticipation as clinical forethought. Clinical forethought is shaped by the clinical grasp of the phronetic practitioner and is derived from the nuanced particulars of the situation. In expert practice

> [C]linical forethought is crucial to recognition of early changes in the patient, because it prepares the nurse to 'see' or recognize what is likely to transpire, and to act based on these early changes. The most effective clinical forethought is based on both scientific understanding and experiential learning of clinical trajectories (Benner et al., 1999, p. 65).

In addition, clinical forethought allows for the possibility that expectations can be confirmed or disconfirmed based on the perception of the skilled clinician.

Merleau-Ponty (1945/2001) has described the relationship between an individual's history and psychological structure having an influence on a person's "style." This style allows people to open up possibilities, but it also limits the individual from seeing things in other ways that do not fit into the style or routine:

> All explanations of my conduct in terms of my past, my temperament and my environment are therefore true, provided that they be regarded not as separable contributions, but as moments of my total being, the significance of which I am entitled to make explicit in various ways, without its ever being possible to say whether I confer their meaning upon them or receive it from them. I am a psychological and historical structure, and have received, with existence, a manner of existing, a style. All my actions and thoughts stand in a relationship to this structure. . . . The fact remains that I am free, not in spite of, or on the hither side of, these motivations, but by means of them (Merleau-Ponty, 1945/2001, p. 455).

In the preceding quotation, Merleau-Ponty also describes the notion of *situated freedom*, or the freedom to act based on one's shared and mutually accessible perceptions of the world and based on one's own culture, background, language, meanings, perspectives and sets of habits (Benner & Wrubel, 1989; Taylor, 1979). Benner & Wrubel (1989) contrast situated freedom from the notion of *radical freedom*, whereby people can "choose all their meanings all the time" (p. 54). From within situated freedom, situated possibilities open up for people; and these situated possibilities are shaped by those meanings, perspectives, personal concerns, and local practices of the profession.

MERLEAU-PONTY'S INTENTIONAL ARC AND MAXIMUM GRIP

According to Dreyfus and Dreyfus (1999), there are two concepts that are rarely discussed in Merleau-Ponty's *Phenomenology of Perception* (1945/2001): the *intentional arc* and the notion of *maximum grip*. These two concepts are central to perception, skill acquisition, and comportment.

Intentional Arc

Merleau-Ponty describes how the relationship between an involved, embodied being perceives and copes with objects and situations in the world as an *intentional arc* (1945/2001, p. 136). Dreyfus and Dreyfus (1999) describe the intentional arc as

> . . . the tight connection between the agent and the world, viz. that, as the agent acquires skills, these skills are "stored," not as representations in the mind, but as more and more refined dispositions to respond to the solicitations of more and more refined perceptions of the current situation.

The intentional arc is the embodiment of the interconnection of skillful action and perception, and there are three ways one's embodied skills determine the way things show up for us and therefore call us to act in certain ways: innate structures, general acquired skills for coping, and specific cultural skills (Dreyfus & Dreyfus, 1999).

The innate structures of one's body and one's own abilities help shape the possibilities for action. For example, *where* the mountains are passable or not passable is a function of one's climbing ability and not based on one's intention to pass through the mountains. One's embodied skills of going through a mountain pass are possible by the innate structures and capacities of the human body of whether one can ambulate or must use a wheelchair.

General acquired skills for coping are refined by the situations and things to which one is exposed. Situations and things show up as soliciting skillful responses as one encounters them more and more. However, situations and things cannot solicit these general acquired skills without being grounded in a cultural world that affords a context. For example, a family member who has never had an experience seeing or working with a cardiac monitor will not know what action needs to be taken if the alarms start ringing, other than calling for the nurse.

The involved, embodied agent immediately sees a situation or an object from a perspective, and those situations or objects afford some action. One's skills are refined through experiential learning that can include trial and error attempts, by imitation, or through application of theoretical knowledge. The intentional arc feedback loop of the embodied agent and the perceptual world calls for responding and refining perceptions of the current situation.

Maximum Grip

The concept of maximum grip is not explicitly described by Merleau-Ponty in *Phenomenology of Perception* but rather is an interwoven concept with distinct allusions to the notion of attaining an optimal gestalt in situations and with objects. Dreyfus and Dreyfus (1999) organized and explicated this Merleau-Pontian notion and called the concept *maximum grip*. Maximum grip is "the body's tendency to respond to these solicitations in such a way as to bring the current situation closer to the agent's sense of an optimal gestalt" (Dreyfus & Dreyfus, 1999). The following three passages from *Phenomenology of Perception* illustrate the concept of maximum grip.

Human beings are always tending towards getting a maximum grip on their situation or perceiving an object. Merleau-Ponty described this ability to experience the detail of an object in the following quotation, where he describes how the tensions around the object fluctuate and when the tensions are minimized or solved, the details of the object come into focus.

He offers the following example:

> For each object, as for each picture in an art gallery, there is an optimum distance from which it requires to be seen, a direction viewed from which it vouchsafes most of itself: at a shorter or greater distance we have merely a perception blurred through excess or deficiency. We therefore tend towards the maximum of visibility, and seek a better focus as with a microscope. . . .

> The living body itself appears when its microstructure is neither excessively nor insufficiently visible, and this moment equally determines its real size and shape. The distance from me to the object is not a size with increases or decreases, but a tension which fluctuates around a norm. . . . There is one culminating point of my perception which simultaneously satisfies these . . . norms, and towards which the whole perceptual process tends. (pp. 302-303)

From this fluctuation around a norm, the embodied agent seeks to reduce the "tension" of the deviation from the norm and move towards equilibrium. This new equilibrium potentially opens up new possibilities or ways of perceiving the situation or object:

> Whether a system of motor or perceptual powers, our body is not an object for an 'I think,' it is a grouping of lived-through meanings which moves towards its equilibrium. Sometimes a new cluster of meanings is formed; our former movements are integrated into a fresh motor entity, the first visual data into a fresh sensory entity, our natural powers suddenly come together in a richer meaning, which hitherto has been merely foreshadowed in our perceptual or practical field, and which has made itself felt in our experience by no more than a certain lack, and which by its coming suddenly reshuffles the elements of our equilibrium and fulfils our blind expectation. (Merleau-Ponty (1945/2001), p. 153)

Maximum grip, however, is not attained through some cognitive process but rather is an embodied perception of a given object or situation at any given moment:

> The constitution of a spatial level is simply one means of constituting an integrated world: my body is geared onto the world when my perception presents me with a spectacle as varied and as clearly articulated as possible, and when my motor intentions, as they unfold, receive the responses they expect from the world. This maximum sharpness of perception and action points clearly to a perceptual ground, a basis of my life, a general setting in which my body can co-exist with the world (Merleau-Ponty, 1945/2001, p. 250).

In the preceding quotation, Merleau-Ponty suggests that maximum grip is dependent upon one's perceptual ground, which forms the background of one's world. He writes that one organizes the field through one's maximum grip and it seems to be a reciprocal or co-produced process. This field is one's background from which one notices or overlook things or events, and therefore can make choices, navigate, and understand the world.

Maximum grip is fluid and is always being refined and influenced by new perceptions, understandings, and experiences. It is not an ultimate, static endpoint. One can sense if one is getting closer or further away from the optimum (Dreyfus and Dreyfus, 1999). Involved, skillful coping is a steady flow of skillful activity in response to one's sense of equilibrium or disequilibrium of the situation and is dependent on what skills have already been acquired through previous experiences (Dreyfus & Dreyfus, 1999).

Merleau-Ponty (1945/2001) describes several levels of one's background: A general background, cultural background, and an individual background. According to him, everything happens on a background, such as making choices and co-producing one's world from the natural world. One's world both constitutes us and is constituted by the person. One is thrown into a particular lifeworld complete with background meanings and practices that are shaped by one's concerns, relationships, culture, language, and practices. Through one's lived experiences and the history developed around the experiences in one's world, one's background, one's access and grip of situations within one's world are continually shaped and changed. One's world creates and limits horizons for the person. With maximum grip, there is intentionality without a mental representation of an ultimate goal or intention. In other words, absorbed and skillful coping is a response to one's sense of the situation as opposed to always requiring a purpose. Dreyfus and Dreyfus (1999) have described this skillful coping as being *purposive* without the agent requiring a *purpose*.

According to Dreyfus and Dreyfus (1999), the intentional arc is enriched and refined through the body's tendency toward maximum grip. To improve one's skills, one must be involved with situations and get a lot of practice.

Case Exemplar

Mrs. Gonzales (all names are pseudonyms) is a 68 year-old Hispanic, Spanish-speaking woman who came into our ED with severe shortness of breath secondary to widespread metastatic cancer. Fortunately, the physician, a respiratory therapist, and I spoke Spanish almost fluently. Mrs. Gonzales had very little hair, and the hair that she had was very brittle and sparse. She had a drawn, tight look about her face and body, and her color was ashen. Her skin was paper-thin and hung loosely on her body. She had a smell of old urine and an unwashed body. Her oxygen saturation ranged from 82 to 90% on 15 liters per minute oxygen via non-rebreather mask. She told us that she had cancer of the ovaries, uterus, and breast for about 10 years and had undergone multiple cycles of radiation and chemotherapy. She stated that she finished her last round of chemotherapy about four months previously. Mrs. Gonzales decided that she did not want any more chemotherapy, nor did she want to continue to live. Her wishes were to die at home, and she stated that her family activated the Emergency Medical Service against her wishes. We concluded based on the answers she provided to our questions and her following commands appropriately; she appeared to understand what was happening to her. We explained some of the options such as pain management and anxiolytics that would be available to her in terms that she would be able to understand. She repeated that she did not want to live and she was ready to die.

Then Mrs. Gonzales' family arrived. The large extended family consisted of her husband, eight children, and six grandchildren as well as friends who arrived to our ED in small groups. Her husband and four of her children met with our physician and told us to do everything that we could to save their loved one. The family members said that the oncologist told them that everything would be fine, and that the oncologist never led them to believe that she was not doing well.

While the physician was meeting with the family outside of the room, Mrs. Gonzales became asystolic. Two other nurses, two respiratory therapists, and I just stood there, wondering what we should do. Could we trust her judgment when she was so hypoxic? We decided to intubate and start cardiopulmonary resuscitation (CPR) while the physician came back in the room; however, everyone was moving at a slow pace. We gave her the minimal amount of epinephrine by Advanced Cardiac Life Support standards, and it had no effect. I slowly gave her another round of epinephrine, and her heart started beating again with a pulse. I felt terrible because I felt we were going against her wishes. The physician went out to speak with the family to explain that her heart stopped beating and what the family wanted to do if that happened again. They continued to say that they wanted "everything" done for her. She arrested again, and we started chest compressions at a slow rate but gave no medications. I decided to have the family come in the room to show them what "everything" meant. Once they saw the ventilator and the ED staff perform chest compressions, what CPR really entailed, they told us to stop the code.

Once the physician announced the time of death, I asked the family if they wanted to sit and be with her. As I lowered the gurney side rails down, I encouraged those family members who wanted to touch or hold Mrs. Gonzales to do so. I brought the family members coffee, water, and facial tissue. I turned down the lights to the room and brought chairs in for the family members to sit. Fortunately, there were few other patients in the ED, so there was time and room to allow the family to stay as long as they wished. The family members stayed with Mrs. Gonzales for about 3 hours, and then they left the ED. The husband and one of the daughters of Mrs. Gonzales thanked me for letting them have that time with their wife/mother. As they left, I told them how sorry I was for their loss. They thanked me for trying to help their wife/mother. I never saw them again.

INTENTIONAL ARC, MAXIMUM GRIP, AND PRAXIS/PHRONESIS IN THE ED

In everyday practice, ED clinicians encounter dying people and death. The skills and habits of caring for people near the end-of-life become incorporated into the clinician's body through lived-through experiences. When a dying person, or a person who is dead but receiving resuscitative efforts, comes to the hospital, ED clinicians perceive that the person is dying. Through multiple encounters with people dying in the ED, the ED clinicians develop an anticipation or are set to cope with the person at the end of their life often sooner than the person or person's family. According to the Centers for Disease Control (CDC), approximately 374,000 people died in EDs throughout the United States in the year 2000 (McCaig & Ly, 2002). Through this repeated exposure to a background in which death occurs, little by little, ED clinicians incorporate death and caring for dying people as being part of their background.

The ED is one world that clinicians join and share with each other. On a cultural level, ED clinicians share experiences and therefore develop local background meanings, practices, and expectations. The ED is a microculture that exists within clinicians' other worlds with both loose and demarcated boundaries between those worlds. ED clinicians have a sense of time, perceptions of illness and dying, and promises of technology shaped by their background experiences, habits, and practices. Merleau-Ponty (1945/2001) elucidated this "link" between one's perception and the incorporation of one's skillful, sentient bodies into one's "perceptual field" or background.

While there is technical knowledge of resuscitation (e.g., chest compressions, intubation and ventilation, vasopressor administration), the skillful comportment and character of the clinicians is to apply the knowledge while being attentive to the particulars of the situation (e.g., success rates of CPR in terminally ill cancer patients, wishes of the patient, family wishes and desires) that allows a situation to "unconceal its own particular significance" (Dunne, 1997, p. 306).

Patients and families who come to the ED also come with their backgrounds that are shaped by their own lifeworlds and lived experiences. The patients and families may or may not be familiar with the ED microculture; or, if they are familiar with the ED culture, they have different perceptions of illness, death and dying, and promises of biomedicine. This can also happen when patients or family members are healthcare professionals. There are local practices and knowledge that are specific to the ED culture that are not shared by other specialties in medicine and nursing. These lived experiences influence the intentional arc of the patient and family.

Chan (2004) describes the ED as a place of transition. It is a fast-paced, highly stressful environment where patients stay for a short period of time and are either discharged home or transferred to an impatient unit. ED clinicians may function with suboptimal levels of information. These ED cultural characteristics open certain possibilities and close down others (Benner et al., 1999). For example, technological care and attempts at reviving and stabilizing patients for transfer to an inpatient unit takes priority over caring and healing practices that bear witness to death and dying as the closing of a human life (Chan, 2004).

Kaufman (2002) notes that health providers' and even the healthcare institution's perspectives on the care of a dying patient can come into conflict with a family's perspective on what is possible, or even what is hoped for a particular patient. She gives an example of a healthcare team taking care of a patient whom they understand is dying, yet the family is convinced that the patient will be sustained by medical technologies. The family hopes that the organ-system failure will be reversed by these technologies. Therefore, the family refuses to withdraw any treatments. In her research, Kaufman (2002) discovered that while healthcare professionals have their own understandings about good dying practices in the hospital setting, families are "preoccupied not with good dying, but with other concerns, especially their hopes for the patient's recovery, their long-standing relationship with the patient, and their sense of overwhelming responsibility for critical decision making" (p. 36). However, in another scenario, Kaufman (1998) describes examples in the intensive care unit (ICU) where healthcare professionals employ aggressive treatment techniques and focus on biological indicators of life in an attempt to stave off the inevitable death. In these cases, the human being lying in the bed is ignored, and there is no attempt to attend to the closing of a person's life.

Shared practices and meanings of the biomedical culture may be taken up differently when the dying experience is actually lived (as in the case of the patient or family with a dying member) or is imagined (as in the case of healthcare professionals). Halpern (2001) describes clinical empathy as the ability of a clinician to resonate emotionally with patients and for the clinician to be able to imagine how it feels to experience something in order to "unify the details and nuances of the patient's life into an integrated affective experience" (Halpern, 2001, p. 88). Clinical empathy allows clinicians to access the lived experience of others. An important distinction, however, is that the clinician imagines the experience in a genuine way yet does not live through the actual experience. Benner and Wrubel (1989) describe notions of expert nursing practice as a negotiation between being neither intrusively or oppressively close or involved, nor being too detached and distant.

In the case exemplar, before Mrs. Gonzales' family came to the ED, there was tension around Mrs. Gonzales' condition. Mrs. Gonzales was *in extremis* (or in extreme distress) because she was very short of breath. In these times of extreme distress, as a clinician, my perception fluctuates around what is possible for this patient. Mrs. Gonzales could get better through different treatments I could provide (e.g., intubation with mechanical ventilation on a ventilator, medications to attempt to reverse the pathophysiology present), or she could die from the advanced stage of the natural disease process. I perceived that Mrs. Gonzales was dying, based on assessing her clinical condition using my senses of sight, touch, and listening to the things she said to me. From past experience, I have seen some people face their imminent death and say, "I am going to die," and they do die. So in the beginning of the case exemplar, I perceived that Mrs. Gonzales was going to die, yet the tension of whether she was going to die or live fluctuated until I could get a maximum grip on her condition and situation. Mrs. Gonzales did not want further intrusive therapies and expressed this to me.

I believe that I was able to see the detail of Mrs. Gonzales' condition because the fluctuations around the norm were minimized quickly due to my previous experience with other dying patients and my background. In a time of high stress and in a fast-paced environment, my body is transparent to me. That is, body is inextricably intertwined with my individuality, background, perceptions, experience, and world. I do not have a mental representation or make a conscious decision about each individual action. My body is set to act from phronetic knowledge. Merleau-Ponty describes this embodiment an "inextricable tangle" (1945/2001, p. 454).

Refinement of phronetic knowledge can come from being perceptive in situations and of people, reflective and checking out assumptions and interpretations in order to learn directly from patients and families (Benner, 2000). By being present with a person and perceiving them through one's own senses (e.g., touch, smell, sight, and hearing) and having the experiential knowledge, we are called to act in a moral way by being attuned to the situation. The embodied realism of touching a body of a person who has paper-thin skin and smells of stale urine and an unwashed body; and seeing a look of distress, discomfort, and terminal disease; combined with hearing the sounds of ragged respirations revealed to those clinicians involved that death was imminent for Mrs. Gonzales. The situation called to the ED clinicians to act in a meaningful and good way. In the perception that death was imminent, the ED clinicians' care priorities and ethical comportment were on pain and symptom management and bearing witness to the human passage of a life.

The perception that death is a part of life influences the possibilities ED clinicians perceive for a person. Many people come to the ED and are unknown to the ED clinicians. This lack of relationship shapes the background from which possibilities can be for the person. Malone (2003) described three kinds of proximity that are central to relationships between nurses and patients: physical, narrative, and moral. Physical proximity aids nurses in providing direct clinical care, nurses understand the patient as a person through narrative proximity, and moral proximity assists in ethical comportment and decision-making on behalf of patients who cannot speak for themselves. These proximities are threatened or not attained in a fast-paced ED with limited relationships with patients and families. In the exemplar, I sought to understand the moral particulars through a hurried narrative proximity (e.g., the patient wanting to die and the family wanting to save her). Despite this truncated narrative proximity, I still held on to the narrative proximity as a way to achieve moral proximity.

Importantly, this example should not suggest that ED clinicians allow every person to die in the ED. Heroic efforts are frequently performed to attempt to stave off death. These heroic efforts are ethically and clinically defensible when the patient actually has a chance for survival at an acceptable quality of life and gives consent to the therapies. The mandate of the profession of nursing is to engage in caring practices; nurses are concerned with the human experiences and responses to birth, health, illness, and death (American Nurses Association (ANA), 1995). However, ED clinicians need to carefully balance the heroic, resuscitative care of the dying patient that includes painful and undignified procedures with the bereavement care of the family who might cling to the comforting thought that the person died despite the healthcare team's heroic efforts. These comforting thoughts may help survivors in their bereavement.

According to Jameton (1984) and Rushton (1992), moral distress occurs when clinicians are unable to turn their moral choices into moral action. In the case exemplar, I felt moral distress because I perceived that the patient was dying despite any resuscitative interventions that I or anyone could have done. My background as a nurse and the patient's imploring requests to allow her to die motivated me to care for the patient in a certain way: to help her and her family pass through this stage of life in the most comfortable and peaceful way possible. Because I perceived that the only outcome for the patient was death, I could not support performing aggressive and assaulting interventions (e.g., chest compressions and defibrillation [electricity to the body]) as these would not help and would go against her wishes. I felt horrible perhaps because my maximum grip on the situation was being distorted through the wishes of the family. As the family wanted to try and "fix" the problems of death, I felt that the personhood of Mrs. Gonzales recessed into the background and the process of "fixing" the illness came to the foreground and objectified Mrs. Gonzales. My habitus, or the background that is built and incorporated in one's body (Bourdieu, 1980/1992), was being thwarted making me *feel* terrible.

I was also conflicted about the patient's own clarity and capacity for autonomy. I believed her when she said that she wished to die. However, I was not clear regarding her having decision-making capacity when she said this. However, her perception that she was dying matched my own perception that she was indeed dying. Benner, Hooper-Kyriakidis and Stannard (1999) note that "forcing activity against [the patient's] will is an ethical violation of [the patient's] rights and safety" (p. 27). To resolve the conflict, I had the family come into the room and witness how their abstract ideas of "everything" compared with the violent futile medical particulars of "doing everything."

In contrast to ED clinicians, patients and families often have very limited experience with dying. The family may have perceived the patient's condition differently (i.e., been given information contradictory to the clinical picture). Because the family was Hispanic, the cultural background shared not only with each other as a family, but also part of the larger Hispanic culture, opens certain possibilities to the family while closing down others. Families may see the person and grieve over their loss and be thrown into a crisis that shapes their perceptual field and the possibilities available to them. Therefore, intentional arc is partially shaped by these interpersonal perceptions within the situation that are a part of individual and cultural backgrounds. These influencing backgrounds allow possibilities from which people cope with the situation.

The continual refinement of one's perceptions (i.e., maximum grip) combined with one's experiential knowledge and a moral agent who advocates for good are ED clinicians who strive to practice in an ethical manner. There is a risk, however, that ED clinicians are set to an optimism that allows for the clinicians to perceive themselves as always having the maximum grip; yet with incomplete or perhaps misinformation, they may not have the maximum grip. Additionally, maximum grip is threatened in situations that are infrequent or have never before been encountered; therefore, experiential knowledge is missing. There is no infallible knowledge about when one has the absolute maximum grip. This grip is perceptual, experientially gained in the situation, and is continually refined, corrected, and improved through one's senses and through real events as they unfold.

In this case, the family is prevented from having a maximum grip of the patient's clinical condition by their lack of medical understanding; their desire for the patient to live; possibly religious or cultural values; and the lack of knowledge or experience to see that a person who has those signs and symptoms of a failing body (i.e., an ashen color; difficulty breathing; a drawn, tight look to her body; advanced illness) is near death.

Perhaps during a crisis situation, the family may retreat into a more familiar ground. The expectation of continued survival and that familiarity and wish/dream may become so powerful that the family may not be able to go against it. The family's expectations of the medical system as well as their fears and hopes for their family member shape their reality and those possibilities that they perceive as possibilities for them, yet the patient can still die regardless of their expectations. The family dwells in the possibilities and attachments that are set up by their connection with the patient and the situation but are also influenced by their past experiences and commitments. Most families do not have the knowledge or previous experience to imagine an alternate trajectory. The family in the exemplar was literally not able to see that the patient was dying. They relied upon the oncologist's opinion that the patient was going to be fine.

In the ED, where time is measured in minutes to hours, we see and experience a snapshot of time in the patient's illness or injury trajectory. In addition, ED clinicians are true generalists who need to possess a moderate to significant amount of knowledge in many different specialties. Although a maximum grip and an embodied realism can be shaped relatively quickly by illnesses and injuries that are commonly or repeatedly seen by clinicians, maximum grip of conditions or scenarios that are completely new or seen less frequently is at risk for not coming into focus, and errors in judgment may ensue.

The family is situated so differently from the healthcare clinicians' perspective. Perhaps my intentional arc of being a clinically empathic nurse coping with the distress of the patient, family, and healthcare team lead me to bring the family to a place of maximum grip of what "doing everything" meant in this case for their mother's body and well-being. This woman's body had become a subjugated docile body reduced to signs and symptoms of disease (Foucault, 1963/1973). After the family saw the violent actions being applied to the docile body of a loved one, the person lying in the bed was transmogrified back from being a "patient" and returned to being their "family member." The family could also see that it was respectful and humane to stop the resuscitation. Before seeing what "everything" meant to the clinicians, the family and ED clinicians lived in two different perceptual worlds.

CONCLUSION

Phronesis, praxis, skillful comportment, and the local ED clinical practice set up the background from which caring practices and virtuous action can be possible. Each individual person uses perception through all senses to attempt to situate him or herself in the right context to attain a maximum grip. Maximum grip is always being refined by new perceptions, understandings, and experiences.

The integration of Aristotle's notions of phronesis and praxis with Merleau-Ponty's ontological notions of intentional arc and maximum grip in the context of the culture and practices of the ED offers a unique view of clinical and ethical practice at the end of life in the emergency setting. The intentional arc of embodied caring for people at the end of life calls us to act virtuously based upon previous experience, meanings, and local practices. The maximum grip of the ultimate particulars of the situation, combined with one's experiential and theoretical knowledge, opens up situated possibilities for the expert clinician.

References

Adams, K., & Corrigan, J. M. (Eds.). (2003). *Priorities for national action: Transforming health care quality.* Washington, DC: National Academies Press.

American Medical Association. (2002). *Code of medical ethics. Current opinions with annotations.* Chicago: AMA Press.

American Medical Association's Council on Scientific Affairs. (1996). Good care of the dying patient. *Journal of the American Medical Association, 275,* 474-78.

American Nurses Association. (1995). *Nursing's Social Policy Statement.* Washington, DC: Publisher.

American Nurses Association. (2001). *Code of ethics for nurses with interpretive statements.* Washington, DC: American Nurses Association.

Benner, P. E. (2000). The roles of embodiment, emotion and lifeworld for rationality and agency in nursing practice. *Nursing Philosophy, 1,* 5-19.

Benner, P. E., Hooper-Kyriakidis, P., & Stannard, D. (1999). *Clinical wisdom and interventions in critical care.* Philadephia: Saunders.

Benner, P. E., Tanner, C. A., & Chesla, C. A. (1996). *Expertise in nursing practice: Caring, clinical judgment, and ethics.* New York: Springer.

Benner, P. E., & Wrubel, J. (1989). *The primacy of caring.* Menlo Park, CA: Addison-Wesley.

Billings, J. A., & Block, S. (1997). Palliative care in undergraduate medical education: Status report and future directions. *Journal of the American Medical Association, 278,* 733-738.

Bourdieu, P. (1992). *The logic of practice.* Stanford University, Stanford, CA.Chan, G. K. (2004). End-of-life care models and emergency department care. *Academic Emergency Medicine, 11,* 79-86.

Chow, E., Harth, T., Hruby, G., Finkelstein, J., Wu, J., & Danjoux, C. (2001). How accurate are physicians' clinical predictions of survival and the available prognostic tools in estimating survival times in terminally ill cancer patients? A systematic review. *Clinical Oncology, 13,* 209-218.

Clarke, E. B., Curtis, J. R., Luce, J. M., Levy, M., Danis, M., Nelson, J., et al. (2003). Quality indicators for end-of-life care in the intensive care unit. *Critical Care Medicine, 31,* 2255-2262.

Corley, M. C. (1995). Moral distress of critical care nurses. *American Journal of Critical Care, 4,* 280-285.

Dreyfus, H. L. (1991). *Being-in-the-world: A commentary on Heidegger's being and time.* Cambridge, MA: The MIT Press.

Dreyfus, H. L., & Dreyfus, S. E. (1999). The challenge of Merleau-Ponty's phenomenology of embodiment for cognitive science. In G. Weiss & H. F. Haber, (Eds.), *Perspective on embodiment: The intersections of nature and culture,* Vol. 2004. New York: Routledge.

Dreyfus, H. L., Dreyfus, S. E., & Benner, P. E. (1996). Implications of the phenomenology of expertise for teaching and learning everyday skillful ethical comportment. In P. E. Benner, C. A. Tanner, & C. A. Chesla (Eds.), *Expertise in nursing practice: Caring, clinical judgment, and ethics* (pp. 258-279). New York: Springer.

Dunne, J. (1997). *Back to the rough ground. Practical judgment and the lure of technique.* Notre Dame: University of Notre Dame Press.

Emanuel, L., von Gunten, C., & Ferris, F. (Eds.) (1999). *The Education for Physicians on End-of-life Care (EPEC) curriculum: The EPEC Project.* Princeton, NJ: Robert Wood Johnson Foundation.

Ferrell, B., Virani, R., & Grant, M. (1999). Analysis of end-of-life content in nursing textbooks. *Oncology Nurse Forum, 26,* 869-76.

Ferrell, B., Virani, R., Grant, M., Coyne, P., & Uman, G. (2000). End-of-life care: Nurses speak out. *Nursing2000, 30,* 54-57.

Ferrell, B. R., & Grant, M. (Eds.) (2001). *End-of-Life Nursing Education Consortium (ELNEC) Curriculum. The ELNEC Project.* Washington, DC: American Association of Colleges of Nursing.

Field, M. J., & Cassel, C. K. (1997). Approaching death. Improving care at the end of life. (pp. 437) Washington, DC: Institute of Medicine.

Foucault, M. (1973). *The birth of the clinic: An archaeology of medical perception.* Vintage Books. (Original work published 1963).

Gadamer, H.-G. (1960/1989). *Truth and Method.* The Continuum Publishing Company, New York.

Halpern, J. (2001). *From detached concern to empathy.* New York: Oxford University Press.

Heidegger, M. (1962). *Being and time.* New York: Harper & Row.

Hill, T. P. (1995). Treating the dying patient: The challenge for medical education. *Archives of Internal Medicine, 155,* 1265-1269.

Iserson, K. V. (1996). Withholding and withdrawing medical treatment: an emergency medicine perspective. *Annals of Emergency Medicine, 28,* 51-54.

Jameton, A. (1984). *Nursing practice: The ethical issues.* Englewood Cliffs, NJ: Prentice Hall.

Kaufman, S. R. (1998). Intensive care, old age, and the problem of death in America. *The Gerontologist, 38,* 715-725.

Kaufman, S. R. (2002) A commentary: Hospital experience and meaning at the end of life. *The Gerontologist, 42,* 34-39.

Kierkegaard, S. (1843/1967) Serial number 1030. In H. V. Hong & E. H. Hong (Eds.), *Søren Kierkegaard's journals and papers,* Vol. 1, A-E (p. 450). Bloomington, IN: Indiana University Press.

Lunney, J. R., Foley, K. M., Smith, T. J., & Gelband, H. (Eds.) (2003). *Describing death in America*. Washington, DC: National Academies Press.

Lunney, J. R., Lynn, J., Foley, D. J., Lipson, S., & Guralnik, J. M. (2003). Patterns of functional decline at the end of life. *Journal of the American Medical Association, 289*, 2387-2392.

Malone, R. E. (2003). Distal nursing. *Social Science & Medicine, 56*, 2317-2326.

McCaig, L. F., & Ly, N. (2002). National Hospital Ambulatory Medical Care Survey: 2000 Emergency Department Summary, p. 31. Hyattsville, MD: National Center for Health Statistics.

Meacham, J. A. (1990). The loss of wisdom. In R. J. Sternberg (Ed.), *Wisdom*. New York: Cambridge University Press.

Merleau-Ponty, M. (2001). *Phenomenology of perception*. New York: Routledge. (Original work published 1945).

National Institute of Nursing Research. (2004). *2004 areas for research opportunity, Vol. 2004*. Washington, CD: National Institute of Nursing Research.

Quint, J. C. (1967). *The nurse and the dying patient*. New York: Macmillan.

Rabow, M. W., Hardie, G. E., Fair, J. M., & McPhee, S. J. (2000). End-of-life care content in 50 textbooks from multiple specialties. *Journal of the American Medical Association, 283*, 771-778.

Rubenfeld, G. D., & Randall, C. J. (2001). End-of-life care in the intensive care unit: a research agenda. *Critical Care Medicine, 29*, 2001-06.

Rushton, C. H. (1992). Care-giver suffering in critical care nursing. *Heart & Lung, 21*, 303-306.

SUPPORT Investigators. (1995). A controlled trial to improve care for seriously ill hospitalized patients. The study to understand prognoses and preferences for outcomes and risks of treatments (SUPPORT). The SUPPORT Principal Investigators [see comments] [published erratum appears in JAMA 1996 Apr 24; 275(16):1232]. *Journal of the American Medical Association, 274*, 1591-1608.

Taylor, C. (1979). *Hegel and modern society*. Cambridge, UK: Cambridge University Press.

Taylor, C. (1985). *Philosophy and the human sciences: Philosophical papers 2*. Cambridge, UK: Cambridge University Press.

Timmermans, S. (1999). *Sudden death and the myth of CPR*. Philadelphia: Temple University Press.

Weick, K. E. (1999). That's moving. Theories that matter. *Journal of Management Inquiry, 8*, 134-142.

Weick, K. E. (2001). Positive organizing and the organizational tragedy. In K. E. Weick & K. M. Sutcliffe (Eds.), *Managing the unexpected. Assuring high performance in an age of complexity* (pp. 66-80). San Francisco: Jossey-Bass.

CHAPTER 7

The Living Tradition of Interpretive Phenomenology

KAREN A. BRYKCZYNSKI AND
PATRICIA BENNER

INTRODUCTION

The purpose of this chapter is to describe how interpretive phenomenology (IP) initially developed and continues to evolve as a philosophy and research tradition in nursing, anthropology, and sociology of health and medicine. The IP research methodology has evolved over time through the conduct of articulation research studies, interpretive ethnographies, and studies of human experiences of health and illness. Benner explained that articulation research describes, illustrates, and gives language to "taken-for-granted areas of practical wisdom, skilled know-how, and notions of good practice" (Benner, Hooper-Kyriakidis, & Hooper, 1999, p. 5). The philosophical underpinnings are described in *The Primacy of Caring (POC)* (Benner & Wrubel, 1989) and *Interpretive phenomenology (IP)* (Benner, 1994). Discourses and debates that have arisen over philosophical and methodological issues are discussed. *From Novice to Expert: Excellence and Power in Clinical Nursing Practice (FNE)* (1984; 2000a) and *POC* (1989) are the foci of much of the discussion since *FNE* was the initial interpretive phenomenological research study and *POC* was the initial description of the philosophical background.

PHILOSOPHICAL BACKGROUND

Interpretive phenomenology as a philosophy and a qualitative research methodology has its origins in the work of several philosophers listed here in approximate order of influence: Heidegger (1927/1962), Kierkegaard, (1848/1962; 1843/1985), Gadamer (1960/1995), Merleau-Ponty (1945/1962), Dreyfus (1991), Taylor (1971; 1985a; 1985b; 1985c; 1993), Geertz (1973; 1987), Benner (1984; 1994), van Manen (1990), and Packer and Addison (1989). While initially referred to as Heideggerian hermeneutic phenomenology (HHP), the term interpretive phenomenology (IP) has become more widely accepted and used in recognition of the multiple philosophical origins of this research tradition. Interpretive phenomenology has been particularly significant in the health care professions. This chapter will focus on the interpretive phenomenological research and philosophy developed from Benner and colleagues.

The starting point of IP is a deconstruction of a Cartesian theoretical and epistemological understanding of the human world and the commonalities of human experience. But an oppositional stance against the Cartesian perspective is avoided. Instead, Benner and Wrubel (1989) maintained that a Cartesian science and epistemology are valuable; and that like all human perspectives, are finite and thrown, and therefore systematically leave out other aspects of human experience and common humanity.

DEVELOPMENT OF INTERPRETIVE PHENOMENOLOGICAL RESEARCH

Benner's landmark book, *FNE* (1984; 2000a), introduced IP as a new qualitative methodology for nursing research. It offered a radically different perspective from the cognitive rationalist quantitative paradigm prevalent during the 1970s and 1980s (Chinn, 1985; Webster, Jacox, & Baldwin, 1981). It constituted an interpretive turn—a movement away from epistemological, linear, analytic, and quantitative methods toward a new direction of ontological, hermeneutic, holistic, and qualitative approaches. This approach has the capacity to uncover, highlight, articulate, and bring recognition to embedded qualitative aspects of practice that are not apparent from a quantitative perspective. Benner noted that this research methodology constitutes a situation-based interpretive approach to describing nursing practice that overcomes some of the problems of reductionism. It also overcomes problems of global and overly general descriptions. It begins with a critique of Cartesian epistemology, and focuses its study on human beings from within their lifeworld and projects, embodiment, and their skilled know-how embedded in practice situations and coping with injuries, acute and chronic illness, and health promotion (Benner, 2000b).

> "Intricate nuanced narrative descriptions are the essence of the IP research approach, which dictates that data be collected through situation-based dialog and observation of actual practice."

Intricate nuanced narrative descriptions are the essence of the IP research approach, which dictates that data be collected through situation-based dialog and observation of actual practice. The fact that *FNE* was written in hermeneutic fashion and read more like literature than a research report may account for some of the misconceptions about the methodology. Although details of this complex project are included in the text of *FNE*, they recede into the background in the face of the more engaging clinical narratives. The IP methodology developed over time as Benner conducted several research projects and worked with doctoral students. In describing the tradition and skill of IP, Benner stated that "the interpretive researcher creates a dialog between practical concerns and lived experience through engaged reasoning and imaginative dwelling in the immediacy of the participants' worlds" (1994, p. 99).

There is no stepwise formula to follow in conducting an interpretive phenomenological study. However, certain research practices typical of this approach can be stated as follows:

- Participant observations and interviews are employed for data collection.

- Interviews provide narrative access to the person's particular experience, capture the temporal progression of situations, and elicit stories in everyday language (Chesla, 1995).

- Identification of paradigm cases, exemplars, and thematic analysis are three interrelated interpretive strategies used for analyzing the narrative and observation data.

- A research team is involved in interpreting the data.

The appendix in *Expertise in Nursing Practice: Caring, Clinical Judgment, and Ethics* (Benner, Tanner, & Chesla, 1996) provides a clear and succinct delineation of the IP method.

The particular form of small group interviews and first-person, experience-near accounts of real practice experiences used in IP differ from participant reports of opinions or generalizations about practice. *Experience-near* narratives require the story teller to dwell in the story as experienced, including thoughts and concerns, providing accounts of actual events, including dialog, all with as much detail as possible. The interviewers and other participants listen carefully to the story without interrupting unless understanding of the story breaks down and requires clarification or to fill in any parts of the story or sequence of events or understanding that they did not achieve in listening to the story. The philosophical underpinning for narrative accounts is that the person's perceptions and meanings—or at the very least, how the world presents itself to the storyteller in practice—is uncovered.

This narrative approach comes from Kierkegaard's (1843/1985) insights on how indirect discourse from within a particular world shows up what counts and what presents itself in the lived experience of narrator in the situation. First-person experience accounts give windows into what the story teller notices, how his concerns organize the story, and a sense of the storyteller's sense of salience about the situation. Geertz (1973) also made extensive observations about the distinctions between first-person experience-near accounts and opinions and generalizations, or even lists of events.

Reasoning across transitions both in the agent's understanding of the situation and the situation itself are very different than what Taylor (1993) calls the snap-shot formal criterial reasoning of a scientific experiment. *Snap-shot* reasoning attempts to capture all relevant criteria and essential characteristics at a particular point in time. It freezes situations in time, abstracts them, and judges them according to the same fixed formal criteria. Both practical reasoning and scientific judgments are useful in different contexts for different purposes. Practical reasoning tries for optimal solutions to problems as they unfold.

Dreyfus notes that IP seeks to overcome Cartesian epistemology that holds to a representational view of the mind and a mind-body dualism. An interpretive phenomenological understanding of the human being is distinct from the Cartesian private subject standing over against or apart from an objective, separate world (1991). The human being is embodied, situated, finite, and thrown into a particular culture, time, and place. This situated, social, sentient person dwells in a world of common meanings, habits, practices, meanings, and skills that are socially prior to the individual human existence and that are also socially disclosed or encountered.

These socially situated meanings, habits, practices, and skills from within the person's lifeworld are the foci of IP. IP relies upon socially shared, common, taken-for-granted background meanings that generate disclosive social spaces or "clearings" constituted by shared social practices, embodied intentionality, habits, rituals, practices, and everyday life. Disclosive shared spaces or clearings allow common, taken-for-granted meanings and social practices to show up: that is, become visible and intelligible. A specific nursing unit in a hospital or the nursing staff at a particular hospital are examples of shared disclosive spaces. This is important for understanding why the original domains and competencies of nursing practice described in FNE (1984) were not simply applied widely as formal frameworks for practice. Instead, the domains and competencies need to be adapted for use in each institution through the study of clinical practice at each specific locale because of the socially embedded, relational, and dialogical nature of clinical knowledge (Benner & Benner, 1999). A social disclosive space, or a culturally constituted "clearing," is defined as social level of shared taken-for-granted meanings that are available in a culture, sub-culture, or particular lifeworld. Human beings and their socially created situations together make some shared meanings accessible and visible. For example a culture focused on hunting wild animals for food will have many practices, symbols, and shared social understandings about what it means to hunt. In the hospital a nurse who forms effective interpersonal caring relationships will create different disclosive spaces for patients than will nurses who are rushed, efficient in their manner, and who do not get to know the patient as a person.

DISCOURSES AND DEBATES

The living tradition of IP continues to evolve through the engagement of a community of scholars in research studies, communication of research findings in publications, and philosophical discourses and debates using the skills of analysis, synthesis, criticism, and understanding to convey meaning and clarify thinking. "The commentary and articulation of IP are similar to the kind of reasoning in transitions that occurs in particular practices such as nursing, medicine, practical moral reasoning and law" (Benner, 1994, p. xiv). Philosophical discourses and debates have arisen over suggested ambiguities, misinterpreted assumptions, perceived inconsistencies, unidentified distinctions, and/or misunderstood conclusions. These debates have typically developed from lack of clarity about the researcher's philosophical background and/or incommensurability between different philosophical traditions.

> "The commentary and articulation of IP are similar to the kind of reasoning in transitions that occurs in particular practices such as nursing, medicine, practical moral reasoning and law."

FNE: RECEPTION BY THE NURSING COMMUNITY

Although *FNE* was enthusiastically received by clinical nurses, nurse administrators, and nurse educators around the world, it was initially interpreted by some academicians and administrators as promoting traditionalism and devaluing education and theory for nursing practice (Cash, 1995; Christman, 1985). Benner believes that the scope and complexity of nursing practice are too extensive to rely upon idealized, decontextualized theoretical views of practice alone. Formal mechanistic theories of nursing set up an "ideal" view of practice and "real" practice, rendering practice as a mere technical application of theory that more or less fits the "real" world of actual practice. These abstract theories view practice as a pale or distorted shadow of theory and ignore the socially embedded knowledge and skilled know-how in practice. According to this perspective, abstract theoretical knowledge is considered superior to experiential knowledge and there is no awareness of the knowledge that develops in clinical practice. Gordon (1984) cautioned that formal models are sometimes misused when they are applied without judgment as maps that direct care and produce conformity.

Benner stated "The platonic quest to get to the general so that we can get beyond the vagaries of experience was a misguided turn. ... We can redeem the turn if we subject our theories to our unedited, concrete, moral experience and acknowledge that skillful ethical comportment calls us not to be beyond experience but be tempered and taught by it" (Benner, 1992, p. 19). This is a call for a more interpretive dialogical stance between theory and practice. It is not a valorization of one and a denigration of either theory or practice, but rather an open dialogical stance to both.

The fact that there have been varied interpretations and critiques of *FNE* is not surprising given its innovative and qualitative nature, the evolution of the IP philosophy and the new methodology it introduced over time, and its widespread influence (Benner, 1984; 1994; Brykczynski, 2010; Cash, 1995; Christman, 1985; Darbyshire, 1994; Edwards, 2001; Benner & Wrubel, 2001; English, 1993; Padgett, 2000; Paley, 1996; Rudge, 1992; Thompson, 1990, 2000). Critiques from Cash (1995), Paley (1996), and Padgett (2000) are from a stance of Cartesian epistemology that does not address the reasons for critiquing Cartesian epistemology in order to study the person in the situation. An IP stance starts with assumptions of common experiences of human existence: embodiment, the intertwining of mind, body, and world; finitude and temporality experienced as throwness into the future; and historical facticity. For example, a woman born in the 21st century in the West has very different possibilities and self-understandings than her counterpart in the 18th century.

FNE: INTERPRETATIONS OF EXPERTISE

FNE is an example of articulation research wherein understanding develops through dialog with a social tradition or practice, observations, and conversation (Benner, 1984). This kind of research gives us a way of recognizing experiential aspects of practice that are relational, contextual, basic, and pervasive that elude formal mechanistic and epistemological theoretical approaches. This approach gives voice to knowledge and notions of the good embedded in clinical nursing practice. Benner's approach is phenomenological and not cognitive, yet an ongoing debate has developed over cognitive interpretations of Benner's concepts of expertise and intuition. The phenomenological perspective creates controversy among quantitative researchers, analytical philosophers, and cognitive rationalists who seek precision, control, and fully articulated theories that can be supported or refuted definitively (Gobet & Chassy, 2008).

FNE radically changed descriptions of skill acquisition, skilled know-how, and expertise. The nurse with the most degrees, published articles, presentations, and funding, as well as the highest position, was not necessarily an example of an expert in nursing practice. The studies of nursing expertise defined and described nursing practice expertise by the actual practice of nurses who provided the most accurate, insightful, and innovative nursing care. This perspective created controversy in academic nursing circles because formal degrees and administrative or faculty positions are valued there as the primary criteria and evidence for expertise. Academics also generally value formal and quantified decision-making strategies over practical reasoning, skill acquisition, or situated cognition (Lave & Wenger 1991; Sullivan & Rosin, 2008). According to the Dreyfus model of skill acquisition (Dreyfus & Dreyfus, 1986) and Benner's use of it in nursing practice, the term expert refers to *situated*, skilled know-how. It is not a trait or a talent model. Therefore, an expert can be expected to perform at lower skill levels when entering new situations or positions.

According to the Dreyfus model, expertise develops over time through direct personal encounters that alter preconceptions and prior understanding. Each expert nurse develops a repertoire of experiences that involve holistic pattern recognition and deep situational understanding of situations common to nursing practice. *FNE* claims that skills, perceptual acuity, and awareness are acquired through clinical experience. For example, fuzzy emotional recognition and gestalts of a situation enable the clinician to sense patient changes over time and/or impending complications prior to the surfacing of more-concrete objective signs and symptoms of clinical deterioration. Fuzzy recognition refers to the ability to detect patterns from ambiguous, indistinct, unstructured situations (Benner & Tanner, 1987). A specific example is the ability to notice family resemblances among several family members of different generations whose objective features may be quite different.

Clinical narratives and direct observations in practice with informal situated interviews about that practice reported by nurses illustrated that novice and expert nurses differed in their clinical judgment skills as well as their commitment and involvement in situations. There were many examples of formative experiences of learning how to be more effective in their practice. For example, nurses claimed in their clinical narratives that if they failed to get an appropriate quick medical response to an accurate early warning of an impending patient crisis, they were more insistent and effective in future early warning situations. Nurses also noted how difficult it was to effectively communicate and support their patients emotionally during a critical event early in their practice because they were so caught up in doing all the interventions required. They explained that they had worked to improve their availability, communication, and support to patients; and over time, had improved their patient support as they increased their technical and communication skills.

By and large, *FNE* was both a critical and affirmative inquiry that articulated the significance of nursing practice and then uncovered and made public the complex lifesaving work done by nurses in their daily practice. However, it was not just a laudatory project, but was also a critical project in the sense of identifying and revealing the cultural crisis inherent in failing to promote and reward the diagnostic, skilled interventions and skillful lifesaving caring practices in today's high-tech world of health care dominated by cost consciousness.

Expertise, according to this model, is *embodied*. Our bodies have intelligence and are capable of knowing, and it is this perceptual acuity and skilled know-how that can be further examined by our rational minds (Dreyfus, 1979). This idea is based upon an integrated holistic view of mind and body. It is perhaps the least-understood aspect of this model because at the time of this early work, the dominant societal perspective was cognitivism, which used the computer as a representational model of the mind/brain. By being an embodied human in situations, being present in the situation, and performing skills, a nurse develops knowledge in her hands—and all senses—so that the nurse acts from a deep background understanding or sense of salience of most clinical situations. In addition, nurses learn to make temporal, situated, or context-dependent qualitative distinctions: for example, between a normal pulse and a thready pulse; or between psychological withdrawal and withdrawal linked with increased intracranial pressure.

This concept of embodied intelligence derives from the Aristotelian tradition and maintains that the body is essential for intelligent behavior (Benner & Benner, 1999; Benner & Wrubel, 1989). This is a radical turn away from the Platonic tradition so widely held in nursing that underlies cognitive notions that intellectual, reflective activity is computational and representational and therefore higher on the hierarchy of human capacities than skilled activity. It is also a turn away from the notion that rational thought is possible without embodied emotional engagement in the world.

> To say that expertise is embodied is to say that through experience skilled performance is transformed from the halting, stepwise performance of the beginner—whose whole being is focused on and absorbed in the skilled practice at hand—to the smooth, intuitive performance of the expert who performs so deftly and effortlessly that the rational mind, feelings and perceptions are available to interact with the patient and others in the situation and to perceive salient aspects of the situational context. (Brykczynski, 1998, p. 352)

FNE: INTERPRETATIONS OF INTUITION

During the 1960s and 1970s, when nursing began striving for recognition as a scientific discipline (Watson, 1981), intuition became a forbidden word that was considered too subjective, feminine, mysterious, and unscientific for use by nurse scientists (McCain, 1965). *FNE* brought new meaning to the term "intuition" (Benner, 1984; 2000a). It became respectable again because, according to the Dreyfus model and Benner's use of it in nursing practice, intuition is a complex skill based upon experience and education. This concept of intuition involves embodied skills put forth by Dreyfus (1979) and Merleau-Ponty (1945/1962), which enable emotional attunement and fuzzy recognition of problems. *FNE* illustrated that intuition signifies experience-based situation recognition, which can lead to early warnings of impending complications and can sometimes be lifesaving. Clinical nurses felt relieved, validated, and liberated by this new perspective on intuition that empowered them to again openly share what they often called their "gut feelings"—the gestalt of the situation—and learning they acquired from working alongside more experienced nurses (Brykczynski, 2003). Intuition has become an important topic for nursing research investigation and has been identified as a characteristic of expert performance in many fields (Lave, 1988; Sudenow, 1978).

DEVELOPING CLINICAL PRACTICE COMPETENCIES

FNE led to redefinition of the terms "competence" and "competency." In nursing service, the idea of developing clinical competencies from actual practice, provided an alternative to the objective measurement-oriented approaches of expert consensus and job analyses so popular in competency-based testing in the early 1980s (Benner, 1982). During the 1960s and 1970s in education, the press to specify all that was known or could be known as behavioral objectives became so pervasive that nurse educators and nurse clinicians were told that if something could not be stated as a behavioral objective, then it was not important to include in curriculum planning—and, for all intents and purposes, did not exist (Lenburg, 1976). These objective approaches were so enthusiastically promoted because they were capable of consistently measuring clearly defined skills and behaviors (Mager, 1962; Popham & Baker, 1970) and conveying an atmosphere of certainty. However, they had serious limitations in terms of assessing relational or contextual skills, and their relevance for complex, dynamic, real-world nursing situations was questionable at best. Styles' (1975) plea for broadening the perspective on objectives to encompass unpredictable and qualitative aspects that occur serendipitously was welcomed by some clinical educators as a more balanced approach (see also Dunne, 1993).

FNE introduced the idea of developing competencies from practice that were based on the intent, functions, and meanings of the activity. Such an approach produces competencies that can be judged as reasonable, appropriate, and meaningful in a given context, thereby offering an alternative to context-stripping measurement approaches that were claimed to be generalizable. This dialogical, relational, and contextual approach to describing competencies has been critiqued as too relativistic to be useful (Cash, 1995). However, Benner and her colleagues argued that agreement can be reached by those who share common background practices and that understanding of a diagnosis or clinical state changes over time as confirmatory and nonconfirmatory data accumulate and are understood in a nonreversible and nonrelativistic way (Benner et al., 1991, 1996, 1999; Taylor, 1993).

RESPONSES TO COGNITIVE CRITIQUES

Darbyshire (1994) clarified several fundamental differences between cognitive and phenomenological understanding in his response to the critique of Benner's application of the novice to expert model published by a master's student in Scotland (English, 1993). English expressed concern that the model had been accepted and applied widely in nursing without being tested or objectively validated. Darbyshire noted that English's major criticism was that Benner's research is not described in positivistic and cognitive terms; in fact, he adds that English apparently did not recognize that her work actually critiques that dominant worldview (Allen, Benner, & Diekelmann, 1986; Benner, 1985). Darbyshire found English's complaint that Benner failed "to seek further clarification of exactly what is entailed in gaining expertise" (p. 389) as completely unfounded given her years of researching and reporting understanding of skilled nursing practice (Benner, 1991; Benner et al. 1991; Benner, Tanner, & Chesla, 1992; Benner & Wrubel, 1989). Darbyshire clarified that while English bemoaned objective, detached criteria for expertise, Benner's research instead maintained that expertise develops in an alternative manner through the nurse's involved, engaged caring stance; and after the event, reflection upon what took place.

In responding to Cash's (1995) critique of her work as a retreat into validation of practice by authority and tradition, Benner (1996) noted that Cash failed to distinguish between the living tradition of any practice *and traditionalism*. Benner locates her articulation research project in "the Feminist tradition of consciousness raising that seeks to name silences and to bring into public discourse poorly articulated areas of knowledge, skill and self-interpretations in clinical nursing practice" (p. 670). She noted that Cash misrepresented and erroneously read cognitive assumptions into the philosophical background for Benner's work when she mentioned the following:

- Polanyi's (1958/1962) example of bicycle riding as being based on theory rather than being prior to any theory of bicycle riding;

- Classifying the Dreyfuses' (Dreyfus & Dreyfus, 1986) description of a repertoire of contextualized examples as *templates* (Cash's notion of templates represents a cognitivist computer model of the mind); and

- Referring to Heidegger's (1927/1962) three modes of engagement as "categories of explicit understanding" (Cash, p. 528) instead of level of engagement, skill, and functioning of different persons or equipment in the situation.

In response to Cash's question about how expert coders can be determined in using this work, Benner explained that interpretive data are not coded by using formal criteria. She also pointed out that Cash did not take into account the fact that Benner's articulation research involved small group interviews, observations of practice, and consensual validation with nurse participants and nurse readers in addition to the research team, which included two nurses and an anthropologist.

PHILOSOPHICAL AND METHODOLOGICAL DEBATES

Gobet and Chassy's (2008) critique of Benner's work is quite similar to Cash's earlier critique. They presented a cognitivist alternative to the Dreyfus Model of Skill Acquisition (Dreyfus & Dreyfus, 1986). There are empirical similarities between the phenomenological and cognitivist accounts of skill acquisition and expertise, but an incommensurable difference between the two paradigms at the level of explaining how the brain, mind, body, and world work together. The major empirical debate raised by Gobet and Chassy (2008) has to do with methodology, as if the two philosophical paradigms could and should share the same methods. Gobet and Chassy assumed that a theory-method split is possible, also ignoring the ways that method influence the data collected and how it is interpreted.

Gobet and Chassy (2008) did not make the ontological stances of cognitivism and phenomenology explicit, assuming that similarities in empirical findings have the same implications, while overlooking the differences in the assumptions about the way the mind works between the two paradigms on how the mind and embodied skilled know-how work together. Gobet and Chassy also overlooked the extensive participant observations and informal interviews in the practice context that are central to all Benner and colleagues' studies of nursing practice. Because Benner and colleagues (Benner, 1984; 2000a; 2000b; 2000c; Benner, Tanner, & Chesla, 2009; Benner et al. 1999) do not think that practitioners can or do remember all the details of their practical know-how, observation with informal clarifying interview questions are essential and always used in the research.

Gobet and Chassy (2008) offered a dated artificial intelligence (AI) version of cognitivism to replace the Dreyfus Model of Skill Acquisition (Dreyfus & Dreyfus, 1986), and Benner's work on intuition and expertise in nursing in particular. Most AI cognitive theorists have moved beyond earlier versions of AI that use an old-fashioned Turing Machine model of the computer, but not Gobet and Chassy. Drawing on Gobet and Simon's (2000), work they develop the Template Theory (TempT) of expertise modeled on a representational and computational view of the mind:

- TempT suggests a different approach: while it acknowledges the importance of understanding a patient as a whole, it also proposes that this whole is decomposable into parts and their relations. Thus, in principle, instructional methods can be developed for teaching these components incrementally (Gobet & Chassy, 2008).

- A related implication is that TempT proposes—unlike Benner's theory—that human knowledge can be approximated as chunks and templates, and that instructional methods can be developed to foster the acquisition of these knowledge structures (Gobet & Wood, 1999).

- Another implication is that analysis can identify efficient ways in which these elements can be taught in the curriculum. The use of patient narratives, which is seen as essential in Benner's approach, does not play such an important role within the framework of TempT; narratives may offer valuable cases studies, but may be replaced by other methods less based on phenomenology. Thus, while agreeing that "expertise takes time to develop," we disagree that "it is neither cost-effective nor practical to try to 'teach' it in formal educational programs" (Gobet and Chassy refer to Benner, 1984, p. 184) (Gobet & Chassy, 2008, p.133).

Gobet and Chassy (2008) questioned whether all (analytical) thinking is ruled out and never used by the expert in the Benner research, but no such claim is made. Indeed, analytical thinking is always required in novel and breakdown practice situations, just as it is required in the novice stages of learning a new practice. Instead, what Benner and colleagues (Benner et al., 1999) found so different between the novice and the expert is the difference between the working background knowledge and skilled know-how and perceptual acuity between the novice and expert. The difference in background-situated knowledge and understanding changes what can be noticed by the novice and expert nurse. What is in the background of the novice and expert's attention and grasp of the situation is quite different based upon the expert's experientially learned perceptual and skilled know-how from gaining situated knowledge and a sense of salience in the real world of practice.

Merleau-Ponty (1945/1962) noted the gulf between what can be externalized and made explicit by Cartesian accounts of a representational mind, and the measureable physiological, biochemical activities of the mechanistic Cartesian brain-body. Practical reasoning, or getting around in the real and already meaningful world, is also such an in-between term not articulated in a Cartesian account of the body (Dreyfus 1991; Merleau-Ponty, 1945/1962). In the Dreyfus and Dreyfus (1986) account of skill acquisition, the expert engages in action in an engaged, ready-to-hand way. Each new situation can shift and reshape experiential learning. The kind of experiential learning required for expertise or wisdom is quite different from elemental technical learning about things that can be standardized across situations.

Bourdieu (1990) pointed out that at the heart of practical reasoning lies a grasp of the nature of the situation. This holistic grasp is also highlighted by Merleau-Ponty (1945/1962) and Dreyfus (1979; 1991). Engaged reasoning is described as "embedded thinking" by AI workers and as the "intentional arc" by Merleau-Ponty (1945/1962), meaning that the agent is solicited by the meaningfulness of the situation. As Dreyfus (2007) states:

For Heidegger, the ready-to-hand is not a fixed function, encountered in a predefined type of situation that triggers a predetermined response that either succeeds or fails. Rather, as we have begun to see and will soon see further, readiness-to-hand is experienced as a *solicitation* that calls forth a *flexible response* to the *significance* of the current situation—a response which is experienced as either improving one's situation or making it worse (p. 1144).

Dreyfus explained that in perceiving the nature of a situation, one learns to perceive what is salient; and, on the basis of that sense of salience, what must be done to accomplish what needs to be done for the sake of some concern or change in the situation. In a world of underdetermined, illness-shaped situations, the nurse usually enters the situation with a purpose; however, after the nurse is proficient or expert, he can be easily solicited by the situation itself, noticing what needs to be addressed and what needs to be attended to (Benner, Tanner, Chesla, 2009; Benner et al., 1999). To act in an expert manner, the practitioner has to have a maximum grasp of the situation (Chan, see Chapter 6 of this book). When the grasp of the situation turns out to be wrong, the practitioner has to allow disconfirming evidence to alter her/his understanding of the situation. Defining the situation as ill-structured or well-structured, as Hammond and colleagues have (Hammond, Hamm, Grassia, & Pearson,

1987), is a step in the right direction but not so useful in professional education because the crucial teaching and learning concerns, not techne or well-structured problems, but underdetermined, complex, unfolding problems that yield, at best to fuzzy logic, or to the recognition of family resemblances, or even anecdotal narrative comparisons based upon a deep background understanding of similar and dissimilar real clinical situations. To quote Dreyfus (2007) on Merleau-Ponty again:

> According to Merleau-Ponty, as an agent acquires skills, those skills are "stored," not as representations in the agent's mind, but as the solicitations of situations in the world. What the learner acquires through experience is not represented at all but is presented to the learner as more and more finely discriminated situations. If the situation does not clearly solicit a single response or if the response does not produce a satisfactory result, the learner is led to further refine his discriminations, which, in turn, solicit ever more refined responses. For example, what we have learned from our experience of finding our way around in a city is "sedimented" in how that city looks to us. Merleau-Ponty calls this feedback loop between the embodied coper and the perceptual world the intentional arc (p. 1144).

This is why clinical nursing faculty find it necessary to coach novice students in their grasp of the clinical situation, often enriching the novice's understanding of what they need to notice (Benner, Sutphen, Leonard-Kahn, & Day, 2009).

Chess has been used as the major exemplar in debates over AI and expert systems (Dreyfus, 1979; Dreyfus & Dreyfus, 1986). Gobet and Chassy (2008) and Benner and colleagues agree that chess and nursing practice are quite different. Nursing is far more open-ended, underdetermined, and relational than chess. It is curious that Gobet and Chassy emphasized the role of emotion in memory retrieval and cognition, without noting the role of emotion in perception. For example, emotions are triggered when nurses sense that they do not have maximum grasp of a situation just as a patient's trends in signs and symptoms may yield a foreboding or early warning sense on the part of the nurse (Benner et al., 1999; Benner, Tanner & Chesla, 2009). Attunement to the patient's condition (problem attunement) and relational attunement play a central role in the acquisition of expertise. If nurses are too detached and unconnected to their clinical work, they may fail to notice subtle changes in the patient's clinical condition. If nurses are too detached and distant in their relationship with the patient as a person, they may not notice subtle cues, and the patient may not disclose their complaints or fears to the nurse.

Emotions are central to perception and rationality because emotions signal preference, danger, attractiveness, and so on (Benner, 1994; Damasio, 1999; Sherman, 1997). Damasio ascribed the six so-called primary emotions of happiness, sadness, fear, anger, surprise, or disgust to the person, while he ascribed the so-called secondary or social emotions of embarrassment, jealousy, guilt, or pride to the social realm. However, private and social distinctions do not hold up because all emotions—including happiness, sadness, fear, anger, surprise, or disgust—are always about something, and in relationship to something. It is hard to imagine any emotional state that is not social in the sense of having some access or interaction with one's experienced world and relational connections with other.

Damasio (1999) also called attention to background emotions—such as well-being or malaise, calm or tension—and summoned empirical evidence for the capacity of people to read facial expressions and emotional states. Damasio noted that contrary to Descartes' assumption that mind and emotions are private, unknowable, and individual possessions, people can become astute in reading background emotions. Even background emotions that are not specific emotional responses to current events are evident and embodied in feelings, postures, gestures, and facial expressions. These background emotions give persons access to the world. Emotions are formed in response to notions of good practice, of signals of danger or warning, possibility, harm and so on.

The Dreyfus Model of Skill Acquisition (Dreyfus & Dreyfus, 1986) is not a trait or template matching model of skill acquisition. Expert skilled know-how and knowledge use are situated and acquired through experiential learning in social contexts over time. Although the amount of time required for professionals to graduate from school as experts (because in order to become experts they would have to have extensive in-depth experience with all the relevant major patient populations such as patient with cardiovascular disease, or care of the woman in labor and so on would be too long), graduates from all professional schools could be much further along and much better prepared for situated experiential learning if both teachers and learners shifted their understanding of teaching and learning a practice from formal decision-making models, such as the Template Model (See discussion above on the Gobet and Chassy template model (Gobet & Chassy, 2008), to include knowledge use as well as knowledge acquisition (Eraut, 1994) and to situated thinking-in-action based upon learning communities (Benner, Sutphen, Leonard-Kahn, & Day, 2009; Lave & Wenger, 1999; Sullivan & Rosin, 2008).

Finally, because medical and nursing practices are science-using practices that contain the requirement of teamwork and the justification of one's action through well-stated rationales and clinical arguments, Benner and colleagues concluded that medical and nursing educators need to attend to the narrative structure of clinical nursing and medicine, particularly the narrative structuring of reasoning through transitions in the patient's condition, and/or changes in the patient's condition (Benner et al., 1999; Montgomery, 2005).

UNDERSTANDING AND ARTICULATING THE BODY-MIND-WORLD INTERCONNECTION

John Paley's critiques (1996; 2000; 2002) did not attempt to articulate the philosophical stance of the authors he critiques, nor his own, but he writes from assumptions of British Empiricism, and hence a Cartesian view of the mind. Paley (2000) criticized Benner's research for differing from this view while making little or no attempt to articulate or understand distinctions and differing assumptions between British Empiricism and the philosophical stance of IP. For example, in critiquing the Benner, Janson-Bjerklie, Ferketich, and Becker (1994) study of autonomy, responsibility, and the limits of control in the cultural and lived meaning of coping with asthma, Paley assumed that Benner and colleagues are taking an oppositional stance that asthma is either all in the mind or all in the body (lungs). This is a puzzling misguided interpretation because the explicit stated aims of the research study reject this oppositional dualistic stance toward coping with asthma, or any other disease. Paley's critiques (1996; 2000; 2002) of these works primarily stem from his *misreading* the research he critiqued.

Benner et al. (1994) studied the body-mind-world and lived experience of people living and coping with asthma. The participants were interviewed three times about coping with actual, recent, and pivotal illness experiences with asthma episodes. The research study described informal understandings of asthma as an illness with social-cultural meanings, and resultant self-understandings. The larger study described how participants engage in self-care that includes medical and health-promotion strategies (such as diet, exercise, rest, stress management) and complementary therapies. The study findings focused on how constitutive shared cultural meanings and social constructions of an illness influence persons' self-care. The authors did not hold up implicitly or explicitly a compliance/noncompliance model. Instead, they uncovered the participants' struggles with when to use medical interventions, self-care, health promotion, and alternative strategies.

Paley constructed his critique on imagined formal philosophical arguments or propositions about mind-body relationships rather than descriptive data presenting the participants' encounter with common cultural beliefs that asthma is considered "psycho-somatic" or "all in the mind." Benner (2000d) disagreed with Paley's point that all arguments are reduced to the broad term "Cartesianism." The following quote from the chapter makes Benner and colleagues' stance clear:

> Unrealistic expectations for personal control that confuse the healthy are even more confusing and troubling for the chronically ill. The quest to transcend the body and overcome frailty and suffering was led early in the [Western] tradition by Socrates' oppositional view of mind, spirit and body. Rawlinson (1986) describes Western moral links to suffering as a disruption to the project of producing an autonomous subject. In this project suffering must have a sense, or particular meanings related to control and responsibility, in order for the autonomous subject to maintain that he or she owns the power to control his or her own ends: [quote from Rawlinson, 1986, is omitted here]. . . . Indeed, senseless suffering assaults a sense of meaning and justice in Western philosophy beginning with Plato and extending through Kant and Christian Platonism. (Benner et al, 1994, p.226)

This is indeed a broad framing of Western meanings of illness and suffering, mind and body. However, such a framing is compatible with the participants' descriptions and does not intend, nor does it import, formal philosophical arguments and claims because the focus is on the cultural level of interpretations and commonly held folk views of asthma as illustrated in the following interview excerpt from a participant who struggles to refute and reject a psychosomatic cultural view of asthma. The participant, Sara, is a 47-year-old, single Caucasian woman who has had asthma for 30 years:

> Asthma has always been in my experience a disease that is not considered a true disease. It is a personality defect that takes a physical form, and so I think that's one reason I never even talked about having asthma . . . I never told anyone. If it had anything do with breathing, or with any kind of physical weakness, it was a moral, character weakness, defect, and asthma was in part of that. It just wasn't like a broken leg or something. (Benner et al, 1994, p.226)

Sara's interview is particularly informative for health care professionals who have ambivalent attitudes toward chronic illness:

> When I have worked with people, medical people or people in the alternative health field, when they first see me, they are enthusiastic and then they discover that I'm not going to get well and then they get depressed and disturbed and a little hostile, and I don't like that. . . . Why am I such a terrible

> person in my very core? I've always been sick and never been well and no matter what I do, I don't get better. . . . I think my fear has always been that I'm sick because there's something sort of basically corrupt about me, and my mind, my brain, tells me this isn't true, but there is a primitive part of me that's very afraid. . . . (Benner et al., 1994, p. 245)

Paley (2000) drew the conclusion that persons considered "acceptors" are painted as persons who must adopt the medical model and not embrace any supplemental methods. This is contrary to the data and research as reported. Those persons who described themselves as "coming to terms with" or "accepting their asthma" also described a larger range of strategies for managing their asthma, stress reduction, rest, nutrition, prudent use of medication, avoidance of triggers, and so on. They talked of acceptance not as a passive resignation, the way that "acceptance" in illness has typically been defined in the literature. Rather, "coming to terms" with their illness included a clearer understanding of triggers, asthma management, and stress reduction.

It is true that the participants, for the most part, were not accepting moral responsibility or blame for their illness. Most often, they were railing against the socially ascribed and stigmatized interpretation of asthma that they considered to be erroneous and left over from "psycho-somatic" interpretations of the illness. Benner and colleagues' interpretation did not imply that the participants embraced the social attributions of blame and responsibility that they encountered from others. Most often, they defended against it. The point was to describe this social stigmatization and burden, as the participants described it. However, the folk theory that "asthma is all in the mind" (psychological determinism or psychosomatic theory of the disease) can lead to self-doubt and unwarranted shame for some participants, especially on the part of those who actively "rejected" the illness.

Those participants who rejected the cultural Cartesian folk suggestions that illness alternated between extreme positions of the illness being "in their mind or thinking" or "externally caused" complained and struggled to counteract these erroneous stigmatizing views. We suggest that such informal models of asthma as an illness mirror the folk psychology of a psychosomatic cause of the illness that most of the participants encountered from social interactions in their everyday life. This folk description of psychosomatic causation places the cause of the illness in the body—most often when physical determinants and cures can be found—and in the mind when no physical causality or cures can be identified. Participants tell stories of being "falsely accused" of not having a "real" physical illness that can appropriate absolution accorded by conceptually placing the root causes of diseases in the mechanical/biochemical body.

A clearer definition of the term "mentalism," which Paley left broad and unarticulated, might shed some light on his interpretation and prevent the untenable position of having either the mind or body disappear. A nondualistic choice is that asthma or any other chronic illness is never just in the mind or just in the body, or just in the "germ" or world. As soon as persons respond emotionally to the sensations of their illness, those very responses can alter the physical functioning (Janson-Bjerklie et al. 1986). The mind responds to chronic illness sensation and experiences, however these responses are not consistent over time, even within the person (Janson-Bjerklie et al. 1986).

Paley (2000) asked how "anti-dualism" can lead to such a dogmatic rejection of the idea that states of the body are clinically influenced by states of mind." But nowhere do Benner and her colleagues ever declare that states of the body are un-influenced by the mind just as they assert that the body is also influenced by the mind. This is where Paley's erroneous reading of Benner and colleagues' research report creates confusion, and can lead only to a restatement of what the article actually claimed rather than Paley's misinterpretation. Nowhere does the research report make such a dogmatic rejection of either the mind influencing the body, or the body and world influencing the mind. The Benner, Janson-Bjerklie, Ferketich & Becker (1994) chapter addresses the social meanings of responsibility for causing and managing the illness that the participants actually encountered. Both participants and current theories of asthma etiology point to a multifactorial model of causation of asthma that is broader than just "mind" or "mentalism." In addition to a hereditary tendency to have hyper-reactive airways that constrict in response to physical irritants—cold air, laughing, exercise, inhaled irritants (such as allergens and environmental pollutants), infections, and inflammatory reactions—the research report explicitly points to the person's symptom perception, self-care, and emotional responses to the illness episodes as well. Paley alluded to a range of mental states (but failed to include a person's habits and social practices, as shown in the research) that might be incorporated in crediting mental powers for influencing comfort, health, and well-being.

Just as the disease cannot be located fully in the mind, the body, or the world, neither can it be assumed that the mental influence on the body is always good, or that the body does not influence the mind. It is precisely in the area of "mentalism" that more articulation is needed in order to avoid misattributing moral responsibility or unrealistic visions of personal control over the illness to persons with asthma and other chronic illnesses (Benner, 2000d).

UNDERSTANDING THE DISCOURSE OF PHENOMENOLOGY: MAKING LIFEWORLD AND EMBODIED INTENTIONALITY AND LIVED EXPERIENCE VISIBLE

From Descartes and Kant, we have inherited rich, descriptive language for the physiological, mechanical, biochemical body and the transcendental intentionality of the mind, will, thought, attitudes, and beliefs. We have little or no language to describe the lived body that skillfully inhabits and comports itself in lifeworlds. Merleau-Ponty (1945/1962) described aspects of the social and skillful habitual body as "middle terms" between pure intentionality (mind as pure intentional and conceptual thought) and the physiological, biochemical body. He suggested that investigating these middle terms more fully could help us better understand mind-body-world relationships. Benner's work has focused on the person's lived sentient body in the lifeworld and physical world.

The goal in *POC* (Benner & Wrubel, 1989) is to expand the terms for mind-body-world relationships so that stress and coping, complementary healing practices, and everyday nurturing and care of the body can be given full conceptual and practical space. Contrary to Paley (2000, 2002) and others' misunderstanding (Gobet & Chassy, 2008; Horrocks, 2000), Benner and colleagues' work argued against a single-factor, representational view of the mind that carries with it a narrow representational view of the mind or "mentalism." Mentalism, so defined, attributes "pure or deliberate, clear intentionality to the mind in controlling the body." Such a view accords the person "full access" or "control" of body, mind, or world. Our intertwining view of mind-body-world based upon the work of Merleau-Ponty (1945/1962) does not imply a dogmatic rejection of the influence of the mind and does not preclude forms of control that Paley describes.

In *POC*, Benner & Wrubel (1989) sought to give fuller conceptual space to feelings and to thinking about feelings. For example, one can learn new thought and habit patterns and emotional responses that can influence lung functioning, well-being, and healing. And certainly this draws on mental powers, but tacit knowledge and relaxation strategies play a more direct role on influencing bodily states than direct deliberate willed control of the mind over the body. Presumably, when thought patterns become habituated, they function differently than when they are fully conscious and deliberate. However, this doesn't mean that a unidirectional or analysis of variance model of causality is the only explanatory system possible or that all mental responses are cognitive and deliberate. Benner and Wrubel (1989) rejected a "pure intentionality" or a representational view of thought or "mental" activity. It is a major conceptual lacuna that Western epistemology does not have adequate language for the "nonmentalistic" yet personal, embodied skills of dwelling in relationships, responding skillfully to everyday circumstances, or experiencing different states of mind through visualizations or emotional responses to circumstances or physical sensations. Alternative therapies, such as biofeedback and the Alexander Technique (a method for improving ease and freedom of movement, balance, support, and coordination), illustrate this by demonstrating that engaging the deliberate, intentional mind does not work as well as engaging the embodied, quasi-emotional skills of imaginatively dwelling in another state or situation.

In *POC*, Benner and Wrubel (1989) made claims for an anti-dualistic view of the person based on Merleau-Ponty's (1945/1962) writings on the body. They argued for replacing a dualistic mind/body view, by a notion of the embodied person engaged in the world through habits, thoughts, and practices. Such a view augments visions of "pure intentionality" or "pure mentalism," where the person is envisioned as having direct conscious control of bodily responses. This position does not dogmatically reject the influence of thought or the mind. It does, though, reject a dualistic either/or view of the relationship between mind and body. And it also rejects a representational view of the mind's powers. In *POC*, Benner and Wrubel (1989) created a richer language and understanding of healing practices that do not also entail unrealistic visions of mental control over illnesses, or underestimate the power of bodily sensation and experience to influence the mind. Both of these extreme versions of mentalism or bodily separatism are too easily linked to failure or shame. This is the way that moral responsibility is embedded in the Cartesian view of an executive mind and a mechanistic body: a view now regarded as inaccurate (Benner, 2000b; Damasio, 1994; Lakoff & Johnson, 1999). Benner and colleagues explored ways that habits of thought, skillful comportment, social relationships, practices, and lifeworld are implicated in living with chronic illness—and this is highly relevant to nursing practice.

Benner and Wrubel (1989) claimed that it is impossible to give an adequate account of complementary therapies or the healing practices without a richer language of the socially constituted embodied person. Human beings are engaged in particular socially shared lifeworlds (i.e., worlds that also influence the mind, and indeed, set up the conditions of possibility for imagining and participating in any healing practices). This engagement includes mind, body, (person) lifeworld, and environment. The philosophical task is not to switch oppositional terms in mind-body dualism, giving the mind more or less credit than the body, but rather to reconceptualize mind-body-world relationships. Such a project entails developing a new account of human agency and possibility that is not limited to either Descartes' or Kant's views of the person. The following quote from *POC* clearly incorporates a view of the influence of habits, thought, skills and practices on illness, and corrects Paley's mistaken view that we have dogmatically rejected the mind's influence in illness experience:

> We have much to learn from expert patients who have developed habitual, skilled bodies in response to a chronic illness. A respect for the habitual, skilled body of the patient with a chronic illness causes the clinician to respect the patient's knowledge and develop lines of clinical inquiry that go beyond a mere mapping of symptoms onto pre-existing explanations. The patient's learning about his or her own illness becomes a source of clinical discovery and inquiry in its own right (p.74).

We applaud Paley's thought project of trying to accord conceptual space for the role of the mind in healing, and encourage him to also include the social, sentient body and world in order to break new ground in thinking about health, illness, disease, healing, and recovery. Paley's misattributions of Benner and Wrubel and other colleagues' work point to crucial philosophical work to be done in conducting research on the possibilities of complementary medicine. If the mind is brought back into an integrated nondualistic vision of mind-body-world relationships, the concept of "mind" has to be more than "pure consciousness," "pure intentionality," or purely "representational." Likewise, a richer account of embodiment (not just the physiological, genomic, biochemical body) has to be conceptualized. Switching back and forth between physicalism and mentalism stays within dualistic oppositional metaphors, limiting inquiry and explanation, and limits analysis methods to search only for the direction or source of influence, rather than how mutual influence occurs—or, more importantly, how to facilitate beneficial mutual influences between the mind, body, and world of the person.

QUESTIONING THE LEGITIMACY OF NURSES' UNDERSTANDING AND USING PHENOMENOLOGY

Horrocks (2000) disagreed with Dreyfus' interpretation of Heidegger, and infers that Benner has used only secondary sources for interpreting Heidegger. It is correct to say that Benner follows Dreyfus' interpretation of Heidegger, and that she has been highly influenced by his widely accepted and illuminating interpretations of Heidegger. However, Benner has also read most of the original English translations of Heidegger. Benner chose to inform her own reading with her mentor and widely acknowledged authority on Heidegger (namely, H. L. Dreyfus), and the interpretation of Kierkegaard by Jane Rubin (1984), who was also mentored by Dreyfus. Dreyfus (1991; 2007) covers more than 50 years of scholarship. Direct and clear scholarly debate between Horrocks and Dreyfus regarding their interpretations of Heidegger would be welcome but has not yet happened.

Horrocks (2002) took an elitist philosophical stance about the work of Heidegger (1926/1962), Kierkegaard (1843/1985), and Merleau-Ponty (1945/1962). We agree with Horrocks that the technical and often-obtuse philosophical language of Heidegger limits access and use of his texts to all audiences. Yet Heidegger's work to critique and deconstruct Cartesian mind-body-world and examine the structures and concerns of care that ontologically constitute being in the world is indeed enlightening (Benner, 2000b, 2000c). Heidegger believed in the primacy of practices and everyday comportment in the world. Heidegger provided extensive dialogs about medical care, and often used examples from a carpenter's workshop to illustrate skillful expert practice and the impact of lack of skill or some other practice breakdown to alter the way the person engaged with the practice of carpentry while hammering. Horrocks (2002) departed from Heidegger's stance when he stated

> . . . if one attempts to explain the ideas at the philosophical level (and in the case of Heidegger very complex ideas) is this appropriate for a general readership of nurses? If it is not appropriate then that means that there is the potential for nurse academics not to fully explain the philosophy that they are using (even if they understand it), and use the arguments at the nursing level to obscure the arguments at the philosophical level (p. 37).

Horrocks (2002) seemed to think that discourse, in order to be "philosophical," must stick to a technical, specialized philosophical language, and that such a language is inappropriate for a general nurse readership. We disagree with these assumptions, and the patronizing tone in relation to nurses' capacities for understanding philosophical issues. We believe that everyday practical understandings can illuminate philosophy, and that philosophy translated and made relevant to practical concerns can become clearer and more relevant. Indeed, this was Heidegger's approach as well. We resist the notion that philosophy should be left only to technical philosophical language and thus only accessible to philosophers who know how to read the technical "code" words. Instead, we try to articulate and make the "code words" more accessible to everyone's understanding. Benner and Wrubel (1989) asserted that because of the nature of meeting people in health and illness, where the impact of one's existentiell (those culturally given understandings of self and world) understandings of existence are often disclosed, nurses have enriched preontological understandings of being. *POC* has been accessible to many nurses and phenomenologically oriented philosophers.

At the time of writing *POC*, there were fewer philosophical works in nursing. Now, there are many more philosophical works in nursing, including the journal *Nursing Philosophy*. For the past 28 years, nursing doctoral students at the University of California, San Francisco have successfully taken courses in Heidegger, Kierkegaard, and Merleau-Ponty taught by Dr.

Bert Dreyfus at the University of California, Berkeley. Nurses have taken these philosophy courses based on their interest and rich preontological understandings of world, embodiment, and engagement in skilled practices. Their research topics have focused on illness experience, coping, recovery, skilled know-how, and caring practices. These topics evolved directly from the nursing doctoral students' own existential dwelling in the world of nursing as evidenced in the researcher's studies in this work.

The goal of *POC* is to make the nature of human existence in the *world* visible in relation to the experience of stress (e.g., anxiety, depression, fear, foreboding) and other forms of challenge or breakdown in meanings and self-understandings in a person's world due to illness or injury. Ontological structures of care enable human beings to dwell in a meaningful human world and respond appropriately to meaningful situations of enjoyment, fear, challenge, danger, worry, happiness, and so on.

CONCLUSION

This chapter provides a general overview of the development of the philosophy and methodology of interpretive phenomenology. Then, the dialogs created by various critiques of Benner and colleagues' work are presented from an interpretive phenomenological perspective along with commentary. Theory and method are intertwined interpretations in this work. In other words, methodological approaches create an interpretive screen just as theory does. An interpretive phenomenological perspective focuses on persons in social situations and lifeworlds, in some mode of involvement or concerns. Articulation of habits, practices, taken-for-granted shared background meanings, tacit knowledge, skilled know-how, everyday coping, and knowledge and self-understandings embedded within a social context or lifeworld is a primary aim in order to understand common human experiences and concerns. It is assumed that existence in the world is so taken for granted, ubiquitous and largely in the background of attention, that articulation creates new understandings and knowledge. Articulation occurs at both the ontological and ontic levels. IP researchers encourage a dialog between Cartesian accounts of mind and body with a phenomenological account of the lived body experience of dwelling in a lifeworld, and experiencing health and illness.

IP claims that pluralistic approaches to human knowledge and existence are essential to study human beings, rather than a unified science that attempts to cover all aspects and realms of human experience and activity. Most of the critiques of Benner and colleagues' work have come from a unified view of rational/empirical science methods and a unified Cartesian theory of the nature of human beings. There have been few internal critiques, or even critiques that start with an understanding of an IP stance toward human science. Misinterpretations of Heidegger by Horrocks (2002) have led to confusing arguments that provide little insight into the usefulness of articulating the ontological nature of being human and dwelling in a lifeworld in relation to the human experience of illness, injury, and finitude, nor do they shed light on ("ontic") caring practices designed with an understanding of the ontological nature of care. Nevertheless, the dialog is evocative, and sheds light on the contestations and disagreements over what it means to be human within nursing. The studies in this book demonstrate what can be revealed, noticed, and articulated when stepping outside a decontextualized stance toward human beings and toward more situated embodied engaged studies of being human in a lifeworld with all the concerns and potential hazards of dwelling in human lifeworlds.

References

Allen, D., Benner, P., & Diekelmann, N. (1986). Three paradigms for nursing research: methodological implications. In P. L. Chinn, (Ed). *Nursing research methodology: Issues and implementation*. Rockville, MD: Aspen.

Benner, P. (1982). Issues in competency-based training. *Nursing Outlook, 20*(5), 303-309.

Benner, P. (1984). *From novice to expert. Excellence and power in clinical nursing practice*. Menlo Park, CA: Addison-Wesley.

Benner, P. (1985). Quality of life: A phenomenological perspective on explanation, prediction, and understanding in nursing science. *Advances in Nursing Science, 8*(1), 1-14.

Benner, P. (1992). The role of experience, narrative, and community in skilled ethical comportment. *Advances in Nursing Science, 14*(2), 1-21.

Benner, P. (1994). The tradition and skill of interpretive phenomenology in studying health, illness, and caring practices. In P. Benner (Ed.), *Interpretive phenomenology: Embodiment, caring, and ethics in health and illness* (pp. 99-126). Thousand Oaks, CA: Sage.

Benner, P. (1996). [A commentary on the article Benner and expertise in nursing: A critique by K. Cash]. *International Journal of Nursing Studies, 33*, 669-674.

Benner, P. (2000a). *From novice to expert. Excellence and power in clinical nursing practice* (2nd ed.). Saddleback, NJ: Prentice-Hall (Addison-Wesley).

Benner, P. (2000b). The roles of embodiment, emotion and lifeworld for rationality and agency in nursing practice. *Nursing Philosophy, 1*(1) 5-19.

Benner, P. (2000c). "The quest for control and the possibilities of care." In M Wrathall & J. Malpas (Eds.), *Heidegger, coping and cognitive science: Essays in honor of Hubert L. Dreyfus Vol. 2* (pp. 293-383. Cambridge, MA: The MIT Press.

Benner, P. (2000d). Response to asthma and dualism by John Paley. *Journal of Advanced Nursing, 31*(6), 1300-1303.

Benner, P. (2008). Interpretive phenomenology. In L. Given (Ed.), *Sage encyclopedia of qualitative methods* (pp. 461-464). Thousand Oaks, CA: Sage.

Benner, P, & Benner, R. V. (1999). The clinical practice development model: Making the clinical judgment, caring, and collaborative work of nurses visible. In B. Haag-Heitman (Ed.). *Clinical practice development: Using novice to expert theory* (pp. 17-42). Gaithersburg, MD: Aspen.

Benner P., Hooper-Kyriakidis P., & Stannard D. (1999). *Clinical wisdom and interventions, in critical care: A thinking-in-action approach.* Philadelphia: Saunders.

Benner, P., Janson-Bjerklie, S., Ferketich, F., & Becker, G. (1994). Moral dimensions of living with a chronic illness: Autonomy, responsibility and limits of control. In P. Benner (Ed.), *Interpretative phenomenology: Embodiment, caring and ethics* (pp. 225-254). Thousand Oaks, CA: Sage.

Benner P, Sutphen M, Leonard-Kahn V, Day L. (2009). *Educating nurses.* A call for radical transformation. San Francisco: Jossey-Bass Publishers.

Benner, P., & Tanner, C. (1987). Clinical judgment: How expert nurses use intuition. *American Journal of Nursing, 87*(1), 23-31.

Benner, P., Tanner, C. A., & Chesla, C. (1991). The nature of clinical expertise in intensive care nursing units. *Anthropology and Work Review, 11*(3), 16-19.

Benner, P., Tanner, C. A., & Chesla, C. (1992). From beginner to expert: Gaining a differentiated clinical world in critical care nursing. *Advances in Nursing Science, 14*(3), 13-28.

Benner, P., Tanner, C. A., & Chesla, C. A. (1996). *Expertise in nursing practice: Caring, clinical judgment, and ethics.* New York: Springer.

Benner, P., Tanner, C. A., & Chesla, C. A. (2009). *Expertise in nursing practice: Caring, clinical judgment, and ethics* (2nd ed.). New York: Springer.

Benner, P., & Wrubel, J. (1989). *The primacy of caring: Stress and coping in health and illness.* Menlo Park, CA: Addison-Wesley.

Benner, P., & Wrubel, J. (2001). Response to: Edwards S. D. (2001) Benner and Wrubel on caring in nursing. *Journal of Advanced Nursing 33*(2), 167-171. Blackwell Science Ltd, *Journal of Advanced Nursing, 33*(2), 172-174.

Brykczynski, K.A. (1998). Clinical exemplars describing expert staff nursing practices. *Journal of Nursing Management, 6,* 351-359.

Brykczynski, K, (2003, September). *The impact of "Novice to Expert."* Presented as a Benner Novice to Expert Celebration Panelist, Charting the Course: The Power of Expert Nurses to Define the Future, Boston, Mass.

Brykczynski, K.A. (2010). Patricia Benner: Caring, clinical wisdom and ethics in nursing practice. In M. Alligood & A. Marriner-Tomey (Eds.). *Nursing theorists and their work* (7^{h} ed., pp. 137-164). St. Louis, MO: Mosby.

Bourdieu, P. (1990). *The logic of practice.* (R. Nice, Trans.). Stanford: Stanford University Press. Brykczynski, K. A. (1998). Clinical exemplars describing expert staff nursing practices. *Journal of Nursing Management, 6,* 351-359.

Cash, K. (1995). Benner and expertise in nursing: A critique. *International Journal of Nursing Studies, 32,* 527-534.

Chesla, C. A. (1995). Hermeneutic phenomenology: An approach to understanding families. *Journal of Family Nursing, 1,* 68-78.

Chinn, P. L. (1985). Debunking myths in nursing theory and research. *Image: The Journal of Nursing Scholarship, 18*(2), 45-49.

Christman, L. (1985). [Review of the book *From novice to expert*]. *Nursing Administration Quarterly, 9*(4), 87-89.

Damasio, A. (1994). *Descartes' error: Emotion, reason, and the human brain.* New York: Putnam.

Damasio, A. (1999) *The feeling of what happens: Body and emotion in the making of consciousness.* New York: Harcourt Inc.

Darbyshire, P. (1994). *Skilled expert practice: Is it all in the mind?* [A response to English's critique of Benner's novice to expert model]. *Journal of Advanced Nursing, 19,* 755-761.

Dreyfus, H. L. (1979). *What computers can't do: The limits of artificial intelligence* (revised ed.). New York: Harper & Row.

Dreyfus, H. L. (1991). *Being-in-the-world. A commentary on Heidegger's being and time (Division I)*. Cambridge, MA: The MIT Press.

Dreyfus, H. L. (2007). Why Heideggerian AI failed and how fixing it would require making it more Heideggerian. *Philosophical Psychology*, (Routledge) Vol. 20, No. 2, 247-268. (April 2007). Reprinted in *Artificial Intelligence*, (Elsevier), Vol. 171, issue 18, (December 2007), 1137-1160 Special Review Issue. http://dx.doi.org/10.1016/j.artint.2007.10.012. Reprinted in *The mechanical mind in history*, Husbands, P., Holland, O., & Wheeler, M. (Eds.). Cambridge, MA: The MIT Press) 2008.

Dreyfus, H. L., & Dreyfus, S. E. (1986). *Mind over machine. The power of human intuition and expertise in the era of the computer*. New York: Free Press.

Dunne, J. (1993). *Back to the rough ground, Practical judgment and the lure of technique*. Notre Dame, IN: University of Notre Dame Press.

Edwards, S. D. (2001). Benner and Wrubel on caring in nursing. *Journal of Advanced Nursing, 33*(2), 167-171.

English, I. (1993). Intuition as a function of the expert nurse: A critique of Benner's novice to expert model. *Journal of Advanced Nursing, 18*, 387-393.

Eraut, M. (1994). *Developing professional knowledge and competence*. Philadelphia: Falmer Press, Taylor and Francis.

Gadamer, H. G. (1995). *Truth and method*. (2nd revised ed.). (J. Weinsheimer & D. G. Marshall Trans.). New York: The Continuum Publishing Company. (Original work published 1960).

Geertz, C. (1973). *The interpretation of culture*. New York: Basic Books.

Geertz, C. (1987). Deep play: Notes on the Balinese cockfight. In P. Rabinow & W. Sullivan (Eds.), *Interpretive social science: A second look* (pp. 195-240). Berkeley, CA: University of California Press.

Gobet. F., & Chassy, P. (2008). Towards an alternative to Benner's theory of expert intuition in nursing: A discussion paper. *International Journal of Nursing Studies 2008 Jan; 45*(1):129-139. Epub 2007 Mar 2.

Gobet, F., & Simon, H.A. (2000). Five seconds or sixty? Presentation time in expert memory. *Cognitive Science, 24*, 651-682.

Gobet, F., & Wood, D. J. (1999). Expertise models of learning and computer-based tutoring. *Computers and Education, 33*, 189-207.

Gordon, D. R. (1984). Research application: Identifying the use and misuse of formal models in nursing practice. In P. Benner (Ed.). *From novice to expert. Excellence and power in clinical nursing practice* (pp. 225-243). Menlo Park, CA: Addison-Wesley.

Hammond, K. R., Hamm, R. M., Grassia, J., & Pearson, T. (1987). Direct comparison of the efficacy of intuitive and analytical cognition in expert judgment. *IEEE Transactions on Systems Man and Cybernetics, 17*, 753-770.

Heidegger, M. (1962). *Being and time*. (J. MacQuarrie & E. Robinson, Trans.). New York: Harper & Row. (Original work published 1927).

Heidegger, M. (1993). The question concerning technology. In D. F. Krell (Trans.), (revised ed.), *Basic writings*. San Francisco: Harper. (Original work published 1953.)

Horrocks, S. (2000). Hunting for Heidegger: questioning the sources in the Benner/Cash debate. *International Journal of Nursing Studies, 37*(3), 237-243.

Horrocks, S. (2002). Edwards, Benner and Wrubel on caring. *Journal of Advanced Nursing, 40*(1), 36-41.

Janson-Bjerklie S, Boushey H.A., Carrieri, V.K., & Lindsey, A.M. (1986) Emotionally triggered asthma as a predictor of airway response to suggestion. *Research in Nursing and Health*. 1986 June;9(2):163-70.

Kierkegaard, S. (1962). *The present age*. (A. Dru, Trans.). New York: Harper & Row. (Original work published 1848).

Kierkegaard, S. (1985). *Fear and trembling*. (A. Hanney, Trans.). New York: Penguin. (Original work published 1843).

Lakoff G., & Johnson M. (1999). *Philosophy in the flesh, the embodied mind and its challenge to western thought*. New York: Basic Books.

Lave, J. (1988). *Cognition in practice: mind, mathematics and culture in everyday life (learning in doing S.)* Cambridge, UK: Cambridge University Press.

Lave, J., & Wenger, E. (1991). *Situated learning: Legitimate peripheral participation.* New York: Cambridge University Press.

Lenburg, C. B. (1976). *Criteria for developing clinical performance evaluation.* New York: National League for Nursing (23-1634).

McCain, R. F. (1965). Nursing by assessment—not intuition. *American Journal of Nursing, 65,* 82-84.

Mager, R. T. (1962). *Preparing educational objectives.* Palo Alto, CA: Fearon.

Merleau-Ponty, M. (1962). *Phenomenology of perception.* (C. Smith, Trans.) London: Routledge & Kegan Paul. (Original work published 1945.)

Montgomery, K. (2005). *How doctors think: Clinical judgment and the practice of medicine.* New York: Oxford University Press.

Packer, M. J., & Addison, R. B. (1989). *Entering the circle. Hermeneutic investigation in psychology.* Albany, NY: SUNY Press.

Padgett, S. M. (2000). Benner and the critics: Promoting scholarly dialogue. *Scholarly Inquiry for Nursing Practice: An International Journal, 14,* 249-266.

Paley, J. (1996). Intuition and expertise: Comments on the Benner debate. *Journal of Advanced Nursing, 23,* 665-671.

Paley, J. (2000). Asthma and dualism. *Journal of Advanced Nursing, 31*(6), 1293-1299.

Paley, J. (2002). Benner's remnants: culture, tradition and everyday understanding. *Journal of Advanced Nursing, 38*(6), 566-573.

Polanyi, M. (1962). *Personal knowledge: Towards a post-critical philosophy.* New York: Harper and Row. (Original work published 1958).

Popham, W. J., & Baker, E. L. (1970). *Systematic instruction.* Englewood Cliffs, NJ, Prentice-Hall.

Rawlinson, M. C. (1986) "The sense of suffering." Journal of Medicine and Philosophy. 11 39-72.

Rubin, J. (1984). *Too much of nothing: Modern culture, the self and salvation in Kierkegaard's thought.* Unpublished doctoral dissertation, University of California, Berkeley.

Rudge, T. (1992). Reflections on Benner: a critical perspective. *Contemporary Nurse, 1*(2), 84-88.

Styles, G. M. (1975). Serendipity and objectivity. *Nursing Outlook, 23,* 311-313.

Sherman N. (1997). *Making a necessity of virtue: Aristotle and Kant on virtue.* Cambridge, MA: Cambridge University Press.

Sudenow, D. (1978). *Ways of the hand: the organization of improvised conduct.* Cambridge, MA: Harvard University Press.

Sullivan, W. M., & Rosin, M. S. (2008). *A new agenda for higher education: Shaping a life of the mind for practice.* San Francisco: Jossey-Bass.

Taylor, C. (1971). Interpretation and the sciences of man. *The Review of Metaphysics, 25*(1), 3-34, 45-51.

Taylor, C. (1985a). *Philosophical papers* (Vols. I & II). Cambridge, UK: Cambridge University Press.

Taylor C. (1985b). Theories of meaning. In *Philosophical papers* (Vol. I, pp. 248-292). Cambridge, UK: Cambridge University Press.

Taylor, C. (1985c). What is human agency? In C Taylor (Ed.), *Philosophical papers* (Vol. I, pp. 15-44). Cambridge, UK: Cambridge University Press.

Taylor, C. (1993). Explanation and practical reason. In M. Nussbaum & A. Sen (Eds.), *The quality of life* (pp.208-31). Oxford: Clarendon.

Thompson, J. L. (1990). Hermeneutic inquiry. In L. E. Moody (Ed.), *Advancing nursing science through research* (Vol. 2, pp. 223-280). Newbury Park: Sage.

Thompson, J. L. (2000). [Commentary on the article *Benner and the critics: Promoting scholarly dialogue by S. M. Padgett*]. *Scholarly Inquiry for Nursing Practice: An International Journal, 14,* 267-271.

van Manen, M. (1990). *Researching lived experience. Human science for an action sensitive pedagogy.* Albany, NY: SUNY Press.

Watson, J. (1981). Nursing's scientific quest. *Nursing Outlook, 29,* 413-416.

Webster, G., Jacox, A., & Baldwin, B. (1981). Nursing theory and the ghost of the Received View. In J. C. McCloskey & H. K. Grace (Eds.), *Current issues in nursing* (pp. 26-35). Boston: Blackwell Scientific.

PART II

Interpretive Phenomenological Studies

8 Articulating, Preserving, and Promoting Holistic Aspects of Nurse Practitioner Practice 145

9 Sustaining Purpose and Motivation: Weaving Caring and Self-Care Together in Nursing Practice 169

10 Sustaining Family Life and Health Through Rituals, Routines, and Practices in Well Families with School-Age Children. 195

11 Listening with Care to Teen Mothers and Their Families 217

12 Life-Course Considerations for Adolescents Born with Spina Bifida: Toward Authentic Care and Transparency of the Other 243

13 Our Patients: Heretics, Believers, Agnostics, and Ecumenists. 259

14 Dwelling in the World: Realms of Meaningful Involvement in Late Life 287

15 Patients' and Family Members' Experiences of Hospital End-of-Life Care 313

16 End of Living: Maintaining a Lifeworld During Terminal Illness 337

CHAPTER 8

Articulating, Preserving, and Promoting Holistic Aspects of Nurse Practitioner Practice

KAREN A. BRYKCZYNSKI

INTRODUCTION

The purpose of this chapter is to explore how interpretive phenomenology (IP) can enhance understanding of the nature of nurse practitioner (NP) practice. The philosophical debate about the nature of advanced nursing practice has developed from the longstanding controversy in nursing about the degree to which the NP role embodies fundamental nursing tenets and practices (Fawcett, Newman, & McAllister, 2004; Mauksch, 1975; Rogers, 1975; Watson, 1995; Weston, 1975) and does not simply mimic medical practice. In this chapter, I discuss how Benner's (Benner, 1984; Benner, Tanner, & Chesla, 1996; Benner, Hooper-Kyriakidis, & Stannard, 1999) articulation research with nurses has informed my interpretive phenomenological investigation of NP practice. I will continue the dialog about the nursing dimensions of NP practice through historical ruminations and discussion of interpretive phenomenological studies of NPs. Following Benner's (2000) interpretation of Heidegger (1953/1993), I explore the relationship between theory and practice with regard to advanced practice nursing, and I suggest directions for future research to further clarify these issues.

> *"The philosophical debate about the nature of advanced nursing practice has developed from the longstanding controversy in nursing about the degree to which the NP role embodies fundamental nursing tenets and practices."*

BACKGROUND OF THE NATURE OF NP PRACTICE ISSUE

The dominant discourse in health care has been focused on economics and technology with little attention to care and humanistic aspects (Benner, 2000; Rashotte, 2005). This is of concern because when economic issues are paramount, caring practices may be devalued, and the holistic healing dimensions of nursing care may be marginalized and silenced (Weiss, Malone, Merighi, & Benner, 2002). These more qualitative aspects of care are covered over and risk being lost if they are not recognized, promoted, preserved, and rewarded. Rashotte argued that the primarily economic and instrumental perspective of the majority of NP research to date has failed to capture the nature of what it means to be a NP and has reinforced the idea that NP practice is no more than what can be readily observed and measured. Rashotte (2005) called for dialogical research approaches "to evoke the richness and depth of what it means to be a NP" (p. 60).

Bullough (1992) claimed that a collaborative model forms the basis of practice for NPs, nurse midwives, nurse anesthetists, and mental health clinical nurse specialists (CNSs), and a nursing model constitutes the practice foundation for other CNSs. I believe all nurses practice according to a collaborative model to some extent. There is a postmodern blending of nursing and medical knowledge and skills in NP practice reflecting an "and" rather than a dichotomous "either-or" perspective (Brykczynski, 1999; Johnson, 1993). Fawcett et al. (2004) challenged NPs to clarify what a blending of nursing and medical knowledge signifies and to articulate the nursing dimensions of advanced practice nursing. In a dialog with Fawcett, McAllister (Fawcett et al. 2004) stated the belief that "much of what we do in advanced practice nursing is on an unconscious or intuitive level of awareness" (p. 138). Interpretive phenomenology can uncover taken-for-granted, intuitive, and other unrecognized aspects of care (such as contextual and relational aspects) that are embedded in practice so they can be recognized and valued.

> *"Historical evidence suggests that what we call the expanded role today was common nursing practice yesterday"*

Over time, health professional roles have evolved and continue to evolve in response to changing needs of society. "Historical evidence suggests that what we call the expanded role today was common nursing practice yesterday" (DeMaio, 1979, p. 272). Examples of NP precursors developed during the early 1900s include infant hygiene nurses, school nurses, and Frontier Nursing Service nurses (DeMaio, 1979; Kalisch & Kalisch, 1978). This historical perspective suggests that there was actually a decrease in the scope of nursing practice as medicine came to dominate the health care field with its model of research-based scientific practice, developed following the Flexner report in 1910 (Aaronson, 1989; Kalisch & Kalisch, 1978).

Flexner, a sociologist, was sponsored by the Carnegie Foundation to conduct a study of all the medical schools in the U.S. and Canada. He found that there was a profusion of schools with inadequate standards. As a result of his report, many medical schools closed and medical education was organized exclusively at the graduate level in university-affiliated schools. A request for Carnegie funding to conduct a similar study of nursing education was denied, yet they did sponsor studies of dental, legal, and teacher education (Kalisch & Kalisch, 1978). Rather than abandoning nursing and moving into the medical realm, NPs might be portrayed more accurately historically as reclaiming aspects of nursing practice that they were excluded from by more politically powerful physicians and nursing's own efforts to formalize clear distinctions between nursing and medicine (American Nurses Association, 1955; Levy, 1968; Safriet, 1992).

An example of organized medicine limiting nursing's scope of practice occurred when the American Academy of Pediatrics was established during the 1930s and pediatricians claimed well-child care as the practice of medicine (Ford, 1992). An example of organized nursing limiting the scope of nursing practice was the so-called "model definition" of nursing practice developed by the American Nurses Association (ANA) in 1955, which specifically restricted nurses from diagnosing and prescribing. Bullough (1984) observed, "The fascinating thing about the disclaimer [regarding diagnosis and prescription] is that it was made not by the American Medical Association, but the American Nurses Association. . . . In effect, organized nursing surrendered without any battle over boundaries" (p. 374). In reference to the impact of the model ANA definition, Safreit (1992) stated, "Even at the time the ANA's model definition was issued . . . it was unduly restrictive when measured by then current nursing practice" (p. 417). Keeling and Bigbee (2005) claimed that the model ANA definition limited expansion of the scope of advanced nursing practice for the rest of the 20th century while the nursing "profession struggled with the dichotomy of 'care versus cure' and the legalities of 'medical' versus 'nursing' diagnosis" (p. 20).

Assertions that NPs have abandoned nursing and become "junior doctors" derive from the fundamental belief that nursing practice can and should be precisely distinguished from medical practice. However, this perspective is simply not consonant with reality. The boundaries between nursing and medicine have changed over time, expanding and contracting in response to the economic, social, and political climate (Allen, 1997). During the early 1900s, there was a great deal of overlap and competition; after the Flexner report in 1910, the boundaries became more distinct; and then during the 1960s, with the development of coronary care units and the birth of the NP role, the boundaries became more indeterminate again (Brykczynski, 2000; Edwards, 1997; Kalisch & Kalisch, 1978; Keeling, 2004). Recently, with perceived economic and political threats to physician power and control over health care in the U. S., there have been increasing attempts by some state and national medical societies to restrict the practice of advanced practice nurses (APNs) (Whitcomb, 2006); solidify the practice boundaries of medicine; and legally protect use of the MD title (Bupert, 2007).

In describing the overlap between nursing and medicine, the early NP leader Ingeborg Mauksch (1981) explained:

> Historically, nurses have taken over tasks originally done only by physicians, such as taking temperatures and blood pressures, and so it is now with physical assessment. Yet, these tasks have never been the main component of nursing care. The primary functions of nursing fall into two other realms: First, the emphasis on health maintenance and health and self care education and second, the care of the ill and the dying. (p. 4)

A double standard exists with regard to the performance of given tasks by physicians versus nurses. This is a long-standing issue that has not been acknowledged and therefore has not been addressed openly and adequately (Brykczynski, 2000). Over time, the scope of nursing practice has expanded in isolated rural areas and poor sections of major cities in the U. S. while contracting in affluent urban medical centers. In similar fashion, hospital nurses have commonly been able to perform functions and provide services on nights, weekends, and holidays that were reserved for physicians only during normal working hours (Brykczynski, 2000). Most importantly, underlying the notion of a double standard is the false belief that physician provided care is superior to the same care provided by a nurse. In fact, research comparing care provided by MDs and NPs has demonstrated that NPs provide care of equal and in some cases better quality than physicians (Freund & Fox, 1999; Gearon, 2005; Mundinger, et al., 2000). In essence, as Safreit (1992) has pointed out, the claim that care provided by a physician is superior, is more a restraint of trade issue than an issue of quality of care. A highly trained physician specialist is not the most appropriate provider for the majority of clinical problems encountered in primary health care settings; and in the face of escalating health care costs, it is unreasonable to pay for primary care at specialist prices (Mundinger, 1994).

With the initiator of the NP role, Loretta Ford (1996), I maintain that the nature of nursing is "timeless and enduring," and I agree with Mauksch (1981) that nursing is "a health-oriented and restorative discipline" (p. 11). I believe that the colloquial phrases "to nurse a drink" and "to doctor a drink" contain aspects of practical wisdom that reflect fundamental differences in the meaning of nursing practice and medical practice. "Nursing a drink" suggests spending time with it: holding it, savoring all aspects of it, and making it last as long as possible. "Doctoring a drink," on the other hand, conveys the idea of adding various ingredients to make it better. These common phrases shed light on the subtle, yet fundamental, differences between nursing and medicine, and suggest the possibility of articulating qualitative distinctions between them.

Moore and Komras (1993) offered the following description of patient-centered care, which highlights the nursing perspective:

> The essence of patient-centered care is reflected in the subtle difference between curing and healing. Largely, the American health care system is focused on curing.... Healing, however, makes one whole or well. It implies an integration of body, mind, and spirit. Whereas curing focuses on the disease or injury, healing focuses on the person experiencing the disease or injury.... When healing is the goal, the definition of success is expanded to include what the patient has learned and how well the patient is able to cope even though complete curing may not be possible. Healing implies that patient care operates on several levels: mental, emotional, and spiritual, as well as physical. It implies that patients are provided with the information and resources they need in order to use their experience of illness as an opportunity to learn about themselves and to move toward a sense of well-being. (p. 53)

Although the disciplines of nursing and medicine overlap, each has its particular history, traditions, philosophies, concepts and theories, practices and ways of being with patients and families. Nursing practice is distinguished by an orientation to holistic care, a philosophy of collaboration with patients and their families and other health professionals, a tradition of care and concern, a rich and varied history, and an ever-growing body of knowledge. Advancing understanding of clinical nursing practice requires articulation of the knowledge that develops as nurses expand their scope of practice and incorporate new knowledge and skill into their repertoire (Benner, 1985).

Advocacy for quality patient care has long been a basic component of nursing practice for all nurses. Because of nursing's holistic perspective, nursing advocacy extends to all aspects of patient care (whether dietary, medical, rehabilitation, preparation for surgery, peaceful death, or discharge) and occurs in all settings (whether hospital, home, extended care facility, or community agency). Perhaps Aaronson's (2007) perspective that rather than defining nursing as a single, discrete discipline, it might be more accurately conceptualized as an interdiscipline integrating knowledge from many disciplines, including biology, biomedicine, philosophy, psychology, sociology, and so on.

> *"Nursing's focus on people, its blend of medical, behavioral, and social science expertise, and its commitment to caring, teaching, counseling, and supporting patients are the characteristics of nursing that make nurses so uniquely qualified to provide advanced practice and primary health care services to the public."*

Benner and colleagues (1996) found that "experienced nurses feel enormous responsibility for what might ordinarily be viewed as medical practice" (p. 305). In their study of expertise in nursing practice, they found that nurses felt personally responsible for persuading physicians to change treatment plans when they perceived that a patient was not benefiting from them. Their research described the collaborative skills that nurses develop when making a case for a change in the medical treatment plan. Allen (1997) lent support to this view, noting that a number of studies have shown that nurses often influence patient care and medical decision-making. These observations help make the case that all nursing practice is collaborative with medicine—not just NP practice.

In 1981, Fagin claimed primary care as nursing's academic discipline and visualized it as an integral component of nursing in all its aspects. She reaffirmed that perspective in 1999 with the observation that primary care had been brought into mainstream nursing education beginning at the undergraduate level, with graduate education expected for NPs. "Assessing, monitoring, coordinating, and managing the health status of patients over time: Being a primary care provider" was identified as a central competency of NPs in the domain *Management of Patient Health/Illness Status* in my dissertation research (Brykczynski, 1989/1999, p. 153). This broad competency has now been differentiated into 25 competencies in the latest revision of the National Organization of Nurse Practitioner Faculties (NONPF) (2006) Domains and Core Competencies of NP practice. Baer (1999) observed that "nursing's focus on people, its blend of medical, behavioral, and social science expertise, and its commitment to caring, teaching, counseling, and supporting patients are the characteristics of nursing that make nurses so uniquely qualified to provide advanced practice and primary health care services to the public" (p. 87). Mundinger (2002) claimed that it is the health perspective of nurses and their recognition of the whole person that distinguishes the care they provide not only in primary care settings, but in any setting.

PHILOSOPHICAL, CONCEPTUAL, AND THEORETICAL PERSPECTIVES

Principles, concepts, models, and theories from nursing, biological, behavioral, medical, and sociocultural disciplines provide a broad foundation for nurses to understand and interpret complex health and illness situations (Aronson, 2007; Kenny, 2006). Efforts to incorporate advanced practice nursing into philosophical, conceptual, and theoretical nursing literature have been taking place for some time (Cody, 2006; Nicoteri & Andrews, 2003). For example, Smith (1995) stated that: "The core of advanced practice nursing lies within nursing's disciplinary perspective on human-environment and caring interrelationships that facilitate health and healing. This core is delineated specifically in the philosophic and theoretic foundations of nursing" (p. 3).

Heidegger's phenomenology can be helpful for expanding our understanding of the relationship between theory and practice in nursing. Nursing practice entails more than simple application of theory. Conceptual knowledge, although essential, is not sufficient. As Benner observed, "In order to make good clinical judgments, the nurse must be skillful in moral and clinical perception" (Benner, 2003, p. 494).

Benner (2000) described nursing practice as "a socially embedded way of knowing and revealing," and she described the relationship between theory and practice as "a dynamic dialogue in which understanding is refined, refuted, altered, and enhanced" (p. 308). Fawcett (1997) put forth an unnecessarily linear and static perspective in claiming that the hallmark of professional nursing was the use of conceptual models and theories of nursing to guide practice. Kenny (2006) incorporated this linear approach in her description of the application of theory-based nursing practice, which follows the nursing process and involves the consideration of relevant models and theories during the initial assessment phase. This perspective may be helpful for teaching beginning nursing students. However, after experience is acquired in actual practice, the sequential steps of the nursing process are replaced by the dynamic thinking-in-action and response-based practice described by Benner and colleagues (Benner, 1984; Benner et al., 1996; 1999).

Nursing practice is centered in human experiences of health and illness in the context of the nurse/patient relationship and the holistic situation. In teaching NP students how to understand their practice in terms of their personal knowledge and moral agency as clinicians, it can be helpful for them to engage in interpretation of narratives from their own practice (Benner, 2003). Through study of their own clinical narratives (see Benner, 1993, for clinical narrative format), they can come to recognize and understand the taken for granted knowledge that becomes embedded in their practice over time.

A major assignment in the master's level theory course that I teach is for NP students to describe three clinical situations from their own experiences and then analyze and reflect upon them to uncover the beliefs, values, and practices that have central meaning for them. After completing this initial reflective activity, NP students join with others in their specialty area and share their clinical narratives, philosophies, and practice models to develop a shared practice model. This aspect of the assignment encourages students to engage in dialog about their practice and facilitates the development of shared communities of practice. It is hoped that this experience will initiate a continuing dialog with colleagues about shared practices and meanings of relevant concepts, theories, philosophies, and research that they find most relevant for the health concerns of their patients.

The disconnection often experienced by students when trying to understand their practice in terms of more abstract theoretical concepts can be clarified by consideration of the differences between practical and theoretical knowledge. Benner distinguished between these two types of knowledge based on the work of Kuhn (1970) and Polanyi (1958), and explained that both types of knowledge are required in clinical nursing practice. Theoretical knowledge can be acquired through reading or observing in a decontextualized fashion, whereas the development of practical knowledge necessitates actual involvement in situations because it is contextual and transactional. Understanding of the distinctions between *techne* or technique—as described by Plato and Aristotle's idea of praxis (or practice) that requires phronesis (or practical judgment) and entails development of character, practical reasoning, skilled know-how and comportment—can help clarify why the lived experiences of practice cannot be fully captured in precise, abstract theoretical terms (Benner, 2003).

In addition to the inherent clinical uncertainty arising from incomplete mastery of available knowledge and unknowns, there are questions regarding the best choice of action in a given situation. According to Benner (1994), an interpretive process is involved in learning to develop the best account of a clinical situation and to make the best clinical judgment under the circumstances of uncertainty associated with clinical situations. Ethical dilemmas over fetal, genetic, and death and dying issues have contributed to the transition from the certain, law-like, factual world of biomedical science to the more uncertain, complex life-world, which demands dialog and active participation of patients and their families along with input from health care professionals from many disciplines. Thus, a uniquely human model, such as the Dreyfus model of skill acquisition (Dreyfus & Dreyfus, 1986), which Benner applied to clinical nursing practice, is appropriate for understanding the complexities of real world practice in which technical and relational skills are intricately interwoven.

INTERPRETIVE PHENOMENOLOGICAL RESEARCH WITH NPS

Early research findings from study of primary-care NP practice demonstrated the incorporation of the following central aspects of nursing practice:

- Family orientation
- Collaboration
- Long-term association with patients over time
- Person-centeredness
- Comprehensive care inclusive of health maintenance and promotion, and illness detection, treatment, and prevention (Hochheiser, 1974)

My dissertation research (Brykczynski, 1985) was conducted during the 1980s when there was a perceived division in NP programs into two different types: those that followed a nursing model, and those that followed a medical model. This division arose from the initial establishment of NP programs outside of academic nursing because of opposition to the NP role from major nursing organizations (Ford, 1982) and nurse academicians (Rogers, 1975). This dichotomous classification of NP programs was based upon the ANA's (1955) previously mentioned attempt to formally differentiate nursing practice from medical practice and reflects the positivistic philosophy prevalent in nursing at that time (Watson, 1981; Webster, Jacox, & Baldwin, 1981).

> *"The most fundamental and powerful change brought about by the NP role was that NPs were allotted time alone with patients in an office with the door closed."*

My preparation as a NP was post-masters following eight years as a medical-surgical staff nurse, preparation as a cardiovascular CNS, and four years teaching nursing at the baccalaureate level. My participation as a baccalaureate faculty member in a project funded by Kellogg to prepare nursing faculty for teaching primary care, and later as a Robert Wood Johnson Foundation nurse faculty fellow in primary care, helped me realize that providing comprehensive care over time and establishing ongoing collaborative relationships or partnerships with patients and families was congruent with and fully utilized the skills and knowledge of nurses. As a result of these experiences, I developed a broad understanding of primary health care, and the rigid distinctions between what was considered nursing and what was considered medicine piqued my interest to study the question: "Whither the nurse in nurse practitioner?" (Weston, 1975).

I believe that the NP role opens a window of opportunity to further our understanding of nursing's unique contribution to care. I disagree with the claim, first asserted by Rogers (1975), that NPs have abandoned the discipline of nursing and sold themselves out to medicine to practice as "junior doctors." Instead, I maintain with Lynaugh (1999) that the most fundamental and powerful change brought about by the NP role was that NPs were allotted time alone with patients in an office with the door closed. This development is significant because of the increased distancing of nurses from patients brought about by organizational restructuring in the name of increased efficiency and cost effectiveness, which disrupts opportunities for nurses to establish caring relationships with patients (Malone, 2003).

The NP role puts the nurse in a situation where what happens between nurses and patients can unfold and develop freely. That is, with the introduction of the primary care NP role, a major spatial-structural change occurred whereby the NP had a designated private room in which to interview and examine the patient. This spatial-structural change gave the NP private time alone with the patient and was accompanied by the major functional change of having responsibility for diagnosing and treating the patient's health and illness concerns. Designated private time with the patient, along with responsibility for diagnosis and treatment, enabled the NP to establish a caring and healing relationship and also allowed for maintaining continuity by scheduling follow-up visits with patients over time as their primary care provider.

The twofold purpose of my dissertation research was to describe the clinical judgment of NPs and to describe commonalities and distinctions between NP practice in particular and nursing practice in general. Discussion of selected findings will be organized here using the four major components of the clinical encounter:

1. The agenda establishes and clarifies the reason for the visit.

2. The history entails systematic collection of details of the patient's health and current concern from the patient's verbal responses and written reports of previous visits.

3. The physical exam consists of systematic collection of objective data using standardized techniques.

4. The plan involves four components: ordering diagnostic and laboratory tests, pharmacological and nonpharmacological treatments, followup, and patient education.

The Agenda

Here is an example of the NP partnering with the patient for joint establishment of the agenda and collaborative care:

> An NP's careful assessment of a 32-year-old man resulted in a diagnosis of glioma. His brain tumor was found to be inoperable, yet he found this terminal prognosis more acceptable than the turmoil he had been through during the uncertain diagnostic phase when he went from provider to provider trying repeatedly to find someone who would take his symptoms seriously and figure out what was wrong with him.

The details illustrating the NP's assessment expertise in this situation are described elsewhere (Brykczynski, 1989/1999). Following the diagnostic period, the patient's major concern was to be able to see his son as much as possible before his death. The NP provided support and encouragement to him and his mother as he negotiated with his estranged wife for opportunities to visit his son. The NP also collaborated with other health professionals in coordinating his care. This situation conveys the NP's attention to broader concerns beyond direct disease-focused care.

The History

During the history phase, the NPs studied attended to patients' life experiences, were alert to subtle cues, and acted as sounding boards. Here is an example:

> An NP assessed a 38-year-old man who was seeing the NP for the first time and was complaining of chest pain and shortness of breath. The NP related that his history did not fit any clear picture; and she observed that while she was collecting his history, he kept referring to his wife. She felt a connection there and asked, "How is your wife?" It turned out that his wife was diabetic and had recently given birth to their sixth still-born baby. He exclaimed, "I just can't take it anymore!" The NP also learned that this man had been married before and that his only child died in a car accident while he was away in the military service. After uncovering these tragic circumstances, the NP and the patient sat together in shared sadness (both holding their heads in their hands), and she said to herself, "He doesn't have heart disease" (cardiac)—"He has heart disease" (heartache)—thereby signifying that she understood his problem to be more functional and emotional rather than structural and physical. The NP recommended family counseling for this couple.

This situation illustrates assessment expertise, which involved spending time with patients, focused listening, and recognizing subtle contextual and relational aspects. In this situation, the NP demonstrated her ability to perceive the clinical situation accurately and to make qualitative distinctions with regard to heart disease. Even though she had not seen this patient before, she was able to recognize that his history did not fit the typical picture of chest pain; she noticed his repeated statements about his wife; and she made him feel comfortable enough to tell her about his anguish. This situation highlights that there is more to NP practice than just identification of diseases and that the context in primary care is the patient's life.

The Physical Exam

During the physical exam component, the NPs attended to both the patient's physical and psychological comfort and interspersed teaching into the exam process. For example, one NP began teaching about ear hygiene while examining a patient's ears, and another checked whether the patient was becoming short of breath while she was auscultating her lung fields. Then during the plan component (the following step), the NPs maximized teachable moments and personalized interventions for patients. Here is an example:

> An employee-health NP noticed that an employee (a ward clerk) who complained of back pain was quite short in stature. The NP recommended a cushion for her chair; and after assessing her activity level, incorporated teaching about back exercises to give her a more active role in her care.

A more medically focused scenario for back pain in employee health would be for the provider to order an analgesic for pain relief and a muscle relaxant. Throughout the study, it was apparent that NPs incorporated teaching into any and all components of the encounter as a topic arose or the opportunity presented itself.

The Plan

The following situation illustrates the significance of continuity of care.

> Several NPs in the study staffed a coagulation clinic, which was set up specifically for follow-up and management of patients discharged from the hospital on long-term anticoagulant therapy. These NPs described clinical situations that illustrated not only the importance of careful attention to various medications ordered by other providers that could alter patients' prothrombin

times, but also the importance of adequate instruction about proper precautions to take and necessary diet and lifestyle modifications.

Their approach enabled patients to take a more active role in monitoring their health status, which was especially important when they saw various providers for different problems who might not be so cognizant of anticoagulant interactions with other drugs. These NPs related that it was common for their anticoagulant clinic patients to stop by their clinic after an appointment with another provider to find out from them whether it was okay to take their newly prescribed medications before they had the prescriptions filled.

This careful attention to follow-up is highlighted by the maxim, "Follow-up is everything."

Attention to continuity of care, a central aspect of NP practice, accounts for their being sought out not only for primary care, but for in-patient acute care as well, where follow-up is a challenge because of medical staff rotation.

The findings from direct observations of NP practice and narrative clinical situation interviews indicated many continuities in nursing and nurse practitioner practice. All the domains of nursing practice identified and described by Benner (1984) were illustrated in the observations and clinical narratives of the NPs. The only major change was the consolidation of the two domains—*the diagnostic and patient monitoring function* and *administering and monitoring therapeutic regimens*—into a single domain more typical of primary health care: specifically *management of patient health/illness in ambulatory care settings* (Brykczynski, 1989/1999).

Later, in response to interest in blending the NP and CNS roles during the early 1990s, Fenton and Brykczynski (1993) conducted secondary analyses of findings from studies of CNS (Fenton, 1985) and NP (Brykczynski, 1985) practice. All of Benner's initial domains were evident in CNS practice, also, and Fenton identified an additional domain: the Consulting Role of the Nurse for CNSs. Both studies had incorporated Benner's domains of nursing practice as interpretive frameworks, so secondary analysis of the data enabled comparing and contrasting CNS and NP practice qualitatively.

This comparative analysis of actual practice situations gathered through observations and clinical narrative interviews indicated that CNSs and NPs shared a core of advanced practice competencies, but also pointed to distinct differences in role expression in each of the domains of nursing practice. NP practice was typically oriented to both health and illness concerns and primarily involved direct provision of care to individual patients and their families. CNS practice was generally more focused on illness and encompassed broader aspects such as teaching staff, providing consultation, and acting as change agents and role models.

In an interpretive study of clinical decision making in family primary care, family nurse practitioners (FNPs) and family physicians (FPs) appeared to take the uncertainty that pervaded clinical situations in stride (Brykczynski, 1991). Four types of uncertainty were illustrated in the observations and were interpreted to be typical of the open, unstructured nature of clinical judgment in primary health care settings.

- Informational
- Diagnostic
- Treatment
- Patient response

The providers were not observed to be perplexed, mystified, or immobilized by the uncertainty; instead, they were pragmatic in their collection of subjective and objective data, assessment of complex patient situations, and development of plans for intervention and follow-up. They relied upon past experience (a stock of personal knowledge; Atkinson, 1984), collaboration, consultation, referral, and follow-up to function as primary care providers. Here is an example:

> An FNP, who was also a certified nurse midwife (CNM), relied upon her past experience with women who had developed rashes during pregnancy as well as her intuitive understanding of the particular situation when working with a pregnant woman who presented with a pruritic rash during her third trimester.
>
> In caring for this woman, the FNP checked published literature and followed protocol by ruling out the worst-possible scenarios (such as syphilis or rubella), but she did so on the background of the primary care maxim, "Common things occur commonly." She continued to assess the situation during follow-up visits and instituted empirical trials of corticosteroid cream and penicillin, both of which were subsequently discontinued because of lack of effectiveness. She also consulted with her collaborating physician regarding

management of the rash, and they concluded that a "wait and see" approach with close monitoring and encouragement to continue using the calamine lotion that alleviated her itching somewhat was most appropriate in this situation.

The FNP was aware that the woman was experiencing a great deal of stress about her impending delivery because of her husband's insistence that she deliver at an unfamiliar hospital because of dissatisfaction with past treatment at the nearby hospital where she (the FNP) had hospital privileges. As the date of the delivery approached, the FNP met with the couple to clarify and finalize the plans for the delivery. The FNP reported after the study was completed that the woman's rash resolved spontaneously following the baby's birth.

This situation, which exemplified smooth functioning in the face of the complexity and pervasive uncertainty of family primary care, can be understood by reference to the previously mentioned research on human expertise and intuition (Dreyfus & Dreyfus, 1986). The Dreyfus brothers claimed, "When things are proceeding normally, experts don't solve problems and don't make decisions, they do what normally works" (Dreyfus & Dreyfus, 1986, pp. 30-31). Thus, as clinicians accrue experience, they build up a repertoire of past whole situations that constitute the background for managing current situations, and they seem to be able to "go with the flow." This is similar to what McCallister was referring to by her comment that much of advanced nursing practice takes place on an intuitive level (Fawcett et al. 2004).

"Healing begins with listening" was a maxim identified in an interpretive phenomenological study of the healing role of NPs (Lewis & Brykczynski, 1994, p. 207). One of the NPs related her understanding of healing as follows:

> Healing is different things to different people. Sometimes it's just listening to this person and letting him talk. There may not be a thing I can do about it but listen.... They kind of go through a catharsis and it makes them feel better to talk about it. I guess listening is the main thing to me... The climate of healing is set more by being attentive and by sitting down and actually facing the patient and not reading the chart or anything while you are with them. (Lewis & Brykczynski, 1994, p. 209)

Another NP stated

> I give them lots of information. I serve as an advisor to them. I see myself as a resource person. My agenda is to wake up inside of them what is left that is still their strengths. I try to motivate them for what they want in order to empower them and to give them back a sense of control that they have lost. This woman and I had a relationship for 9 or 10 months. I would anticipate things for her and prepare her for what to expect. I kept in touch with her as a person. (Lewis & Brykczynski, 1994, p. 212)

These excerpts illustrate the interpersonal relationship skills of the NPs and convey the meaning that healing signifies self healing. The NP serves as a facilitator and resource person who provides anticipatory guidance, emotional support, information, and education to enable patients to better care for themselves.

Secondary analysis of data from my dissertation and the Lewis study (1994) was undertaken by using Benner's competency "establishing a healing relationship" as an interpretive framework. Examples replicated here illustrated NPs being present—"being with" patients in their lived world and trying out ways to participate with them in making decisions and learning to live with their particular health and illness situations (Brykczynski & Lewis, 1997). In the following excerpt (Brykczynski & Lewis, 1997, pp. 521-522), an NP describes how she mobilizes hope for herself in a long-term, complex, multiproblem patient situation:

> I've always liked her and despite the fact that she's been real destructive in her life, she's done some very positive things in her life too. I mean she's raised a family; she still takes care of her grandchildren. Her kids are really crazy about her. She has a husband who's an alcoholic, as she is, and she constantly talks about leaving him, but they've been together for many years and I suspect that she'll continue to talk about him and how she is going to leave him and maybe she won't. So, I don't know, I mean maybe I don't have any expectations as such, except to just sort of be there—you know to provide a service. Maybe if I set low expectations then I can't be disappointed. . . . But also, I guess her behavior at this point is less destructive than it has been in the past. I mean the alcohol is not good, but it's better than IV heroin and she seems to have a certain stability in her life that makes her functional.

The NP's ability to interpret "stability" as positive for this patient enables her to remain hopeful about this woman's future possibilities for maintaining and improving her health and affirms the NP's commitment to caring for her over time.

The observation that patient involvement was actively promoted by the NPs in the aforementioned studies takes on increased significance in view of more recent attention to the second half of the patient visit (Elwyn, Edwards, & Kinnersley, 1999; Lazare, Putnam, & Lipkin, 1995). Further investigation of this aspect of the NP-patient relationship may increase understanding of why NP patient visits have been reported to last longer than visits to physicians (Brown & Grimes, 1993). Lazare and colleagues (1995) noted that of the three functions of the medical interview

1. Determining and monitoring the nature of the problem

2. Establishing, maintaining, and concluding the therapeutic relationship

3. Patient education and implementation of treatment plans

the third has been "most overlooked and inadequately performed" (p. 14).

Elwyn et al. (1999) commented in their discussion of the neglected second half of the patient encounter that data have repeatedly indicated that there is minimal sharing of information about the identified problems, discussion of treatment options, or decisions about preferred future management plans. Yet, it is well known that standardized treatment guidelines are based on pooled data that may be difficult to individualize to a particular patient. The practice of personalizing or individualizing care, which involves developing a shared understanding of how to proceed in specific patient care situations, has been a longstanding component of nursing care (Benner, 1984; Peplau, 1952), and it was evident in the clinical situations described here.

> *"The nurse-patient relationship sets up the conditions of possibility for the patient to disclose their concerns, fears and discomforts."*

Findings from the interpretive phenomenological studies of NP practice described here consistently portray NP practice as holistic, collaborative, and patient-centered as well as focused on continuity and coordination of care. However, as Benner (2003) commented:

> The nurse-patient relationship sets up the conditions of possibility for the patient to disclose their concerns, fears and discomforts. If the nurse is too hurried, or too task oriented to notice the patient's and family's experience, then the level of disclosure on the part of the patient/family will be constrained. (p. 492)

In the face of pressures to be more cost-effective, NPs are faced with increasing caseloads. Therefore, they need to be familiar with research findings highlighting the value-added dimensions of nursing care so that they can be articulate in advocating for the allocation of sufficient time for patient visits. They also need to document their impact on patient outcomes by collecting ongoing comprehensive follow-up data.

Recently, Nicoteri and Andrews (2003) commented that, "Although the education includes learning the essentials of nursing theory and of the NP role and how to incorporate nursing theory into clinical practice, the major thrust of NP education is learning medical language, physical assessment and diagnostic evaluations pertaining to disease, pathophysiology, and pharmacology" (pp. 495-496). Yet, they also noted that:

> Since the inception of the role . . . the emphasis is holistic in nature—that is, diagnosing and treating human responses to illness and life changes in collaboration with the patient and utilizing preventive measures as the key elements, not just treatment of the disease state. The NP maintains nursing skills while adding the necessary medical skills to be an advanced practice nurse. (p. 495)

We cannot expect NP students to blend nursing and medical aspects into an integrated holistic practice without clinicians to emulate and without specific emphasis and guidance from faculty. Basic nursing knowledge and skills that students bring with them to NP programs need to be further developed during their NP program (Hanson & Hamric, 2003). This is especially true today, as more graduate students are admitted to NP programs with little or no prior nursing experience.

Hagedorn (2004) pointed out that in the face of organizational and policy initiatives, increasing technology, focus on evidence-based treatment, and emphasis on health care costs, NPs are expected to find faster, simpler ways to provide care. She challenged NPs to envision how attention to holistic, caring practices might alter the relationship between the patient and the NP and the way care is provided. She stated that viewing the NP as a "junior doctor" or physician-extender limits the possibilities for caring to emerge in clinical NP/patient relationships. The question about whether the nature of NP practice is too focused on medical aspects to the exclusion of nursing aspects has recently resurfaced given the increased emphasis on cost containment and technological capabilities.

Additional studies focused on articulating holistic aspects of NP practice are needed to honor the significance of these more qualitative aspects of practice so they can be recognized, taught, emulated, and practiced by clinicians regardless of their discipline. There is an urgent need for collaborative interdisciplinary practice to address the health care crisis in the U. S. today (Institute of Medicine (IOM), 2001; Professions Education Workforce (PEW, 1995). The IOM reported in 2001 that while biomedical science and technology continue to make major rapid advances, the health care–delivery system has been unable to consistently provide high quality care to all Americans. The U. S. spends more on health care than any other industrialized nation, yet the life expectancy and overall health of our citizens is below that of some Third World countries, and millions of Americans have no health insurance (Abramson, 2004). Three areas identified by the IOM (2001) for emphasis in health professional education are:

- Basic skills for patient-centered care
- Evidence-based practice
- Multidisciplinary training

Nursing can make major contributions in all three of these areas.

CONCLUSION

This chapter expands the usual historical context for understanding the development of the NP role and discusses findings of IP research studies to advance the dialog about the nature of advanced practice nursing for NPs. It claimed that NPs are nurses first and also have much in common with all nurses. NPs are in a position to play a major role in collaborative interdisciplinary practice to meet national health care needs. There is an opportunity for nurses to serve as leaders in healing our ailing health care system. For effective leadership, we need to recognize that all nursing practice is collaborative and interdisciplinary, and we need to promote peer supportive rather than peer critical interactions and dialog.

References

Aaronson, L. S. (1989). A challenge for nursing: Re-Viewing a historic competition. *Nursing Outlook, 37*(6), 274-279.

Aaronson, L. S. (2007). *Translational research: Bridge or destination?* Keynote address for the 21st Annual Conference of the Southern Nursing Research Society, February 22, Galveston, TX.

Abramson, J. (2004). *Overdo$ed America. The broken promise of American medicine*. New York: HarperCollins.

Allen, D. (1997). The nursing-medical boundary: A negotiated order? *Sociology of Health & Illness, 19*(4), 498-520.

American Nurses Association. (1955). ANA board approves a definition of nursing practice. *American Journal of Nursing, 5*, 1474.

Atkinson, P. (1984). Training for certainty. *Social Science in Medicine, 19*(9), 949-956.

Baer, E. D. (1999). Philosophical and historical bases of advanced practice nursing roles. In M. D. Mezey & D. O. McGivern (Eds.), *Nurses, nurse practitioners: Evolution to advanced practice* (pp. 72-91). New York: Springer.

Benner, P. (1984). *From novice to expert. Excellence and power in clinical nursing practice.* Menlo Park, CA: Addison-Wesley.

Benner, P. (1985). The oncology clinical nurse specialist: An expert coach. *Oncology Nurse Forum, 12*(2), 40-44.

Benner, P. (1993). Clinical narrative accounts that illustrate nursing practice. Retrieved March 10, 2007 from, http://www.bennerassociates.com

Benner, P. (1994). The tradition and skill of Interpretive Phenomenology in studying health, illness, and caring practice. In *Interpretive phenomenology: Embodiment, caring, and ethics in health and illness* (pp. 99-127). Thousand Oaks, CA: Sage.

Benner, P. (2000). The quest for control and the possibilities of care. In M. A. Wrathall & J. Malpas (Eds.), *Heidegger, coping, and cognitive science. Essays in honor of Hubert L. Dreyfus* (Vol. 2, pp. 293-309). Cambridge, MA: The MIT Press.

Benner, P. (2003). Clinical reasoning: Articulating experiential learning in nursing practice. In L. Basford & O. Slevin (Eds.), *Theory and practice of nursing. An integrated approach to caring practice* (2nd ed., pp. 492-503). Cheltenham, UK: Nelson Thornes.

Benner, P., Hooper-Kyriakidis, P., & Stannard, D. (1999). *Clinical wisdom in critical care: A thinking-in-action approach.* Philadelphia: Saunders.

Benner, P., Tanner, C. A., & Chesla, C. A. (1996). *Expertise in nursing practice caring, clinical judgment, and ethics.* New York: Springer.

Brown, S. A., & Grimes, D. E. (1993). *A meta-analysis of process of care, clinical outcomes and cost effectiveness of nurses in primary care roles: Nurse practitioners and certified nurse midwives.* Washington, DC: American Nurses Association.

Brykczynski, K. A. (1985). Exploring the clinical practice of nurse practitioners. (Doctoral dissertation, University of California, San Francisco). *Dissertation Abstracts International, 46,* 3789-B. (University Microfilms No. DA8600592).

Brykczynski, K. A. (1991). Judgment strategies for coping with ambiguous clinical situations encountered in family primary health care. *Journal of the Academy of Nurse Practitioners, 3*(2), 79-84.

Brykczynski, K. A. (1999). An interpretive study describing the clinical judgment of nurse practitioners. *Scholarly Inquiry for Nursing Practice: An International Journal, 13*(2), 141-166. (Original work published 1989).

Brykczynski, K. A. (1999). Reflections on clinical judgment of nurse practitioners. *Scholarly Inquiry for Nursing Practice: An International Journal, 13*(2), 175-184.

Brykczynski, K. A. (2000). Role of the nurse practitioner in primary health care. In P. Meredith, & N. M. Horan (Eds.), *Adult primary care* (pp. 3-25). Philadelphia: Saunders.

Brykczynski, K. A., & Lewis, P. H. (1997). Interpretive research exploring the healing practices of nurse practitioners. In P. Kritek (Ed.), *Reflections on healing* (pp. 518-535). New York: NLN Press.

Bullough, B. (1984). The current phase of the development of nurse practice acts. *St Louis Law Journal, 28,* 365-395.

Bullough, B. (1992). Alternative models for specialty nursing practice. *Nursing and health care, 13,* 254-259.

Bupert, C. (2007). Congressman tries to protect medical doctors. *The Journal for Nurse Practitioners, 3*(1), 12-13.

Cody, W. K. (2006). The nursing discipline and the development of nursing knowledge. In W. K. Cody (Ed.), *Philosophical and theoretical perspectives for advanced nursing practice* (4th ed., pp. 2-3). Boston: Jones and Bartlett Publishers.

DeMaio, D. (1979). The born-again nurse. *Nursing Outlook, 27*(4), 272-273.

Dreyfus, H., & Dreyfus, S. E. (1986). *Mind over machine. The power of human intuition and expertise in the era of the computer.* New York: Free Press.

Edwards, J. B. (1997). Collaboration between medicine and nursing education in community-based settings. In J. C. McClosky & H. K. Grace (Eds.), *Current issues in nursing* (5th ed., pp. 537-544). St. Louis, MO: Mosby.

Elwyn, G., Edwards, A., & Kinnersley, P. (1999). Shared decision-making in primary care: The neglected second half of the consultation. *British Journal of General Practice, 49*, 477-482.

Fagin, C. M. (1981). Primary care as an academic discipline. *Primary care. A contemporary nursing perspective* (pp. 13-30). New York: Grune & Stratton.

Fagin, C. M. (1999). Primary care as an academic discipline. In M. D. Mezey & D. O. McGivern (Eds.), *Nurses, nurse practitioners: Evolution to advanced practice* (pp. 95-109). New York: Springer.

Fawcett, J. (1997). Conceptual models of nursing, nursing theories, and nursing practice: Focus on the future. In M. R. Alligood & A. Marriner-Tomey (Eds), *Nursing theory: Utilization & application* (pp. 211-221). St. Louis, MO: Mosby.

Fawcett, J., Newman, D. M. L., & McAllister, M. (2004). Advanced practice nursing and conceptual models of nursing. *Nursing Science Quarterly, 17*(2), 135-138.

Fenton, M. V. (1985). Identifying competencies of clinical nurse specialists. *Journal of Nursing Administration, 15*(2), 31-37.

Fenton, M. V., & Brykczynski, K. A. (1993). Qualitative distinctions and similarities in the practice of clinical nurse specialists and nurse practitioners. *Journal of Professional Nursing, 9*, 313-326.

Ford, L. C. (1982). Nurse practitioners: History of new idea and predictions for the future. In L. H. Aiken (Ed.), *Nursing in the 1980s: Crises, opportunities, challenges* (pp. 231-247). Philadelphia: Lippincott.

Ford, L. C. (1992). Advanced nursing practice: Future of the nurse practitioner. In L. H. Aiken, C. Fagin (Eds.), *Charting nursing's future agenda for the 1990s* (pp. 287-299). Philadelphia: Lippincott.

Ford, L. C. (1996). Personal communication cited in Komnenich, P. (1998). The evolution of advanced practice in nursing. In C. M. Sheehy & M. McCarthy (Eds.), *Advanced practice nursing: Emphasizing common roles* (pp. 8-46). Philadelphia: F. A. Davis.

Freund, C. M., & Fox, J. A. (1999). Research in support of nurse practitioners. In M. D. Mezey & D. O. McGivern (Eds.), *Nurses, nurse practitioners: Evolution to advanced practice* (3rd ed., pp. 32-71). New York: Springer.

Gearon, C. J. (2005). Medicine's turf wars. *U.S. News & World Report.* Retrieved April 1, 2007 from http://www.usnews.com/usnews/health/articles/50131/31turf_2.htm

Hagedorn, M. I. (2004). Caring practices in the 21st century: The emerging role of nurse practitioners. *Topics in Advanced Practice Nursing eJournal, 4*(4).

Hanson, C. M., & Hamric, A. B. (2003). Reflections on the continuing evolution of advanced practice nursing. *Nursing Outlook, 51*, 203-211.

Heidegger, M. (1993). The question concerning technology. In D. F. Krell (Trans.), *Basic writings* (revised ed.,). San Francisco: Harper. (Original work published 1953).

Hochheiser, L. (1974). Summary. In L. Hochheiser, J. Lewis, & H. Bailit (Eds.). *Proceedings of the nurse practitioner research conference* (pp. 80-89). University of Connecticut. Rockville, MD: National Institutes of Health Center for Nursing Research, Division of Nursing, Bureau of Health Professions, Health Resources and Services Administration (HRSA).

Institute of Medicine. (2001). Committee on Health Care in America. *Crossing the quality chasm: A new health system for the 21st century.* Washington, D.C.: National Academy Press.

Johnson, R. (1993). Nurse practitioner-patient discourse: Uncovering the voice of nursing in primary care practice. *Scholarly Inquiry for Nursing Practice: An International Journal, 7*(3), 143-157.

Kalisch, P. A., & Kalisch, B. J. (1978). *The advance of American nursing*. Boston: Little, Brown and Company.

Keeling, A. W. (2004). Blurring the boundaries between medicine and nursing: Coronary care nursing, circa the 1960s. *Nursing History Review, 12*, 139-164.

Keeling, A. W., & Bigbee, J. L. (2005). The history of advanced practice nursing in the United States. In A. B. Hamric, J. A. Spross, & C. M. Hanson (Eds.), *Advanced nursing practice. An integrative approach* (3rd ed., pp. 3-45). St. Louis, MO: Elsevier Saunders.

Kenney, J. W. (2006) Theory-based advanced nursing practice. In W. K. Cody (Ed.), *Philosophical and theoretical perspectives for advanced nursing practice* (4th ed., pp. 295-310). Boston: Jones and Bartlett.

Kuhn, T. (1970). *The structure of scientific revolutions* (2nd ed.). Chicago: University of Chicago Press.

Lazare, A., Putnam, S. M., & Lipkin, M. (1995). Three functions of the medical interview. In M. Lipkin, Jr., S.M. Putnam, & A. Lazare (Eds.), *The medical interview. Clinical care, education, and research* (pp. 3-19). New York: Springer-Verlag.

Levy, J. (1968). The maternal and infant mortality in midwifery practice in Newark. *American Journal of Obstetrics and Gynecology, 77*, 42.

Lewis, P. H., & Brykczynski, K. A. (1994). Practical knowledge and competencies of the healing role of the nurse practitioner. *Journal of the Academy of Nurse Practitioners, 6*(5), 207-213.

Lynaugh, J. E. (1999). The interaction between nurse practitioner and patient: A paradigm for care. In M. D. Mezey & D. O. McGivern (Eds.), *Nurses, nurse practitioners: Evolution to advanced practice* (pp. 110-120). New York: Springer.

Malone, R. E. (2003). Distal nursing. *Social Science and Medicine, 56*, 2317-2326.

Mauksch, I. G. (1975).Nursing is coming of age . . . through the nurse practitioner movement. Pro. *American Journal of Nursing, 75*, 1834-1843.

Mauksch, I. G. (1981). Introduction. *Primary care. A contemporary nursing perspective* (pp. 1-11). New York: Grune & Stratton.

Moore, N., & Komras, H. (1993). *Patient-focused healing. Integrating caring and curing in health care*. San Francisco: Jossey-Bass.

Mundinger, M. O. (1994). Advanced practice nursing—Good medicine for physicians? *New England Journal of Medicine, 330*(3), 211-214.

Mundinger, M. O. (2002). Twenty-first-century primary care: New partnerships between nurses and doctors. *Academic Medicine, 77*(8), 776-780.

Mundinger, M. O., Kane, R. L., Lenz, E. R., Totten, A. M., Tsai, W., Cleary, P. D., . . . Shelanski, M. L. (2000). Primary care outcomes in patients treated by nurse practitioners or physicians. A randomized trial. *Journal of the American Medical Association, 283*(1), 59-68.

National Organization of Nurse Practitioner Faculites (NONPF). (2006). *Domains and core competencies of nurse practitioner practice*. Washington, D.C.: NONPF. Retrieved November 14, 2009 from http//:www.nonpf.com

Nicoteri, J., & Andrews, C. (2003). The discovery of unique nurse practitioner theory in the literature: Seeking evidence using an integrative review approach. *Journal of Academy of Nurse Practitioners, 15*(11), 494-500.

Peplau, H. E. (1952). *Interpersonal relations in nursing*. New York: Putnam.

PEW Health Commission. (1995). *Critical challenges: Revitalizing the health profession for the twenty-first century*. San Francisco: Center for Health Professions.

Polanyi, M. (1958). *Personal knowledge*. Chicago: University of Chicago Press.

Rashotte, J. (2005). Knowing the nurse practitioner: Dominant discourses shaping our horizons. *Nursing Philosophy, 6*, 51-62.

Rogers, M. E. (1975). Nursing is coming of age . . . through the practitioner movement. *American Journal of Nursing, 75*, 1834-1843.

Safriet, B. J. (1992). Health care dollars and regulatory sense: The role of advanced practice nursing. *Yale Journal on Regulation, 9*, 417-488.

Smith, M. C. (1995). The core of advanced practice nursing. *Nursing Science Quarterly, 8*, 2-3.

Watson, J. (1981). Nursing's scientific quest. *Nursing Outlook, 29*, 413-416.

Watson, J. (1995). Advanced nursing practice . . . and what might be. *Nursing and Health Care: Perspectives on Community, 16*, 78-83.

Webster, G., Jacox, A., & Baldwin, B. (1981). Nursing theory and the ghost of the received view. In J. C. McCloskey & H. K. Grace (Eds.), *Current issues in nursing* (pp. 26-35). Boston: Blackwell Scientific.

Weiss, S. M., Malone, R. E., Merighi, J. R., & Benner, P. (2002). Economism, efficiency, and the moral ecology of good nursing practice. *Canadian Journal of Nursing Research, 34*(2), 95-119.

Weston, J. L. (1975). Whither the "nurse" in nurse practitioner? *Nursing Outlook, 23*, 148-152.

Whitcomb, M. E. (2006). The shortage of physicians and the future role of nurses. *Academic Medicine, 81*(9), 779-780.

CHAPTER 9

Sustaining Purpose and Motivation: Weaving Caring and Self-Care Together in Nursing Practice

BONNIE RAINGRUBER AND CAROL ROBINSON

Benner and colleagues (Benner, Tanner, & Chesla, 1996; Benner & Wrubel, 1989) eloquently addressed the pivotal nature of caring in the nursing profession by describing how letting situations, relationships, and patients matter shapes our practice and understanding. Heidegger's (1926/1962) work provided the foundation for this understanding by detailing how caring allows us to open ourselves, notice possibilities, see how history influences us, and recognize significance in daily life. In effect, by caring for others and the world around us, we create a *clearing (a kind of understanding that comes from shared practices and traditions that allow us to make sense of our community, culture, and world)*. We find purpose and meaning in life—or, rather, it finds and surrounds us in an effortless, engaged way.

Heidegger (1926/1962) spoke of this way of being in the world as being richly woven with the in-order-to's, the for-the-sake-of's, the to-those-ends. Meaning and purpose are tied to caring about others and one's own situation. Intertwined with this world of caring about others is caring about self: noticing one's own possibilities, being aware of one's own history, and letting self matter. Self-care is not selfish. Rather, self-care creates its own clearing in the same way that caring for others does. In this clearing, nurses find a renewed sense of motivation and purpose, which enriches their practice.

Situation is one of the commonly explored lines of inquiry within interpretive phenomenology (IP). Attending to situation includes an examination of the constraints and resources of a given place, culture, or context. The reality that the context in which something happens shapes the nature of the experience is central to interpretative inquiry (Benner, 1994). One example of the importance of place is seen in the explanation of Benner et al. (1996) regarding how "skill acquisition and the development of clinical expertise are dependent on the social ecology of the unit" and on the existence of a sense of trust and possibility within any given nursing unit (p. 230). This same sense of trust and possibility in life is also needed to grow as an individual.

Interpretive phenomenology (IP) allows us to explore our lived world, embodied understandings, everyday concerns, and commitments as well as those of others. IP and reflective healing practices such as meditation, yoga, tai chi, and Reiki allow us to shed light on the meaning of being and interpret expressions of the inner life of human beings (Palmer, 1969). Like reflective healing practices (RHP), the interpretive process has no clear end. Both RHP and IP are circular endeavors in which one develops understanding a bit at the time after dwelling, reflecting, revisiting, and experiencing.

This chapter focuses on the interrelatedness of self-care and caring for others. Narratives from a study of a meditation, yoga, tai chi, and Reiki retreats (reflective healing practices) will be presented and interpreted to illustrate nurses' views of how reflective healing practices (RHP) improved their own health and strengthened their ability to care for patients.

THE INTERRELATEDNESS OF SELF-CARE AND OTHER-CARE

Koloroutis (2004) agreed that the essence of care is found in developing relationships and moments of connection with patients. She suggested that relationship-based care consists of

- A nurse's relationship with patients and families
- A nurse's relationship with self
- A nurse's relationship with colleagues

Koloroutis (2004) also spoke of the relationship nurses that have with themselves as being fundamental to being a productive member of an organization. She explained that this relationship with self is grounded in both self-knowledge and self-care. Koloroutis (2004) stressed that hospitals need to encourage self-care for nurses, teach ways to manage stress, and create a space for nurses to balance demands within the profession with their own physical and emotional health and well-being.

Although numerous scholars within nursing (Benner & Wrubel, 1989; Peplau, 1952; Watson, 1988) have argued that relationship and caring are the most fundamental and healing aspect of nursing, this philosophy has not been fully operationalized in the daily workings of most hospitals. In agreeing with the recommendation of the Pew Health Professions Commission Task Force on reinvigorating health care, Koloroutis (2004) emphasized that relationship-centered care is the way to bring health back into health care for patients, families, and health care professionals as well.

The values of nurturing and protecting patients, fostering their growth, and promoting patient health have long been central to nursing practice (Benner, 2000). The history of nursing has been one of self-sacrifice and other-focused caring (Benner & Wrubel, 1989). Moreover, the structure of nursing practice today—with back-to-back 12-hour shifts, complex patient assignments, and rotating days off—actually undermines a nurse's opportunity for self-care and reinforces this self-sacrificing stance. Echoing this view, Brathovde (2006) pointed out that self-care practices are neither typically encouraged by hospitals today nor routinely taught within nursing school.

However, caretaking must be woven with and by self-care if nurses are to sustain their practice (Benner et al., 1996). We live in a world where we care for others and expect in turn to be cared for (Benner & Wrubel, 1989). Genuine caring is not duty-based nor self-sacrificing: It is nurturing and sustaining to both the patient and the nurse (Benner & Wrubel, 1989). Weaving self-care practices into the fabric of hospital culture enables nurses to take note of their own bodily responses, foster the sense of purpose and motivation in their practice, and create a way to sustain caring practices.

Benner and Wrubel (1989) have argued that the best cure for burnout is to create a community of connected and sustaining relationships. To be truly healthy, it is necessary to have a sustaining relationship with one's patients, colleagues, and self. Self-care practices allow nurses to reconnect with their own bodies; their history and life experiences; and their hopes and vision of the profession, peers, and patients. Extending one's own possibilities, attending to one's own growth, and honoring one's own health is also part of what it means to be a nurse. In our hectic, fast-paced world, it is as vital to have a relationship with oneself as it is necessary to have sustaining relationships with others.

USING REFLECTIVE PRACTICES AS SELF-CARE

A number of researchers have argued that reflective healing practices such as tai chi, yoga, meditation, and Reiki healing provide a way for nurses to avoid stress, decrease burnout, and cope with the complex challenges of working with acutely ill patients (Brathovde, 2006; Cohen-Katz et al. 2005; Gold & Thornton, 2001; Mackenzie, Poulin, & Seidman-Carlson,

2006; Oman, Hedberg, & Thoresen, 2006; Tsai & Crockett, 1993; Whelan & Wishnia, 2003). Watson (1988) stressed that nurses who are self-aware and able to find balance between mind, body, and spirit are more accessible to and present with their patients. She further suggested that meditation, yoga, and other such practices help nurses shift their focus when it is time to move from working with one patient or family to another or from managing one crisis to the next.

Schwartz (1990) explained that stress contributes to diminished health and burnout when individuals are so overwhelmed by stimuli that they cannot attend to cognitive, emotional, bodily, or psychological feedback and use it to regulate their activities. Becoming overrun and overwhelmed by stimuli during a busy shift caring for several complex patients is a common occurrence in most hospitals. Schwartz suggested that interventions that encourage individuals to attend to subtle physical, emotional, and cognitive impressions such as tai chi, yoga, meditation, and Reiki healing offer great promise as a way to decrease stress and promote health. (Reiki is discussed in depth later in this chapter.) It is in the learning to listen to subtle feedback and embodied feelings obtained during reflective healing practices that nurses learn to honor their body and provide the best patient care possible.

SIMILARITIES BETWEEN RHP AND NURSING PRACTICE

Expert nurses are highly skilled at noticing subtle distinctions and listening to embodied impressions that alert them to assess further or intervene in a way that matches patient need. At advanced levels of skilled nursing practice, nurses attend to emotions, listen to fuzzy resemblances (immediate recognition based on integration of observed patterns and past experience), and notice subtle patterns that help them take action on behalf of their patients (Benner, 1994). Likewise, repeated practice with tai chi, yoga, meditation and Reiki helps nurses attend to embodied emotions, fuzzy resemblances, and subtle feelings that allow them to notice patterns in their own life and ways of being. By listening to their own body and what it is telling them, nurses increase their understanding of how clinical and life situations affect them.

> *"Attending to emotion offers the possibility of bringing a past interpretation of a situation into the present where past history can be reinterpreted and reconstituted."*

In nursing practice, emotions provide a way to compare similar and dissimilar patient situations and intervene in an attuned, effective manner (Benner & Wrubel, 1989). "Attending to emotion offers the possibility of bringing a past interpretation of a situation into the present where past history can be reinterpreted and reconstituted" (Benner & Wrubel, 1989, p. 97). This "...emotional attunement is essential to effective coping" (Benner & Wrubel, 1989, p. 97) in clinical practice.

In a similar way, emotional attunement attained through reflective healing practice allows a nurse to compare similar and dissimilar personal narratives, emotional responses, and even clinical experiences. Reflective healing practices "… provide a way of allowing feelings to instruct, heal and create a sense of well-being" (Benner & Wrubel, 1989, p. 171). Reflection is a highly effective way of coping with the stress of nursing practice.

Being totally present with a patient (Benner et al., 1996) helps a nurse pick up on subtle clinical nuances. Likewise, being totally present in the moment during reflective healing practices helps nurses notice what their body, their intuition, and their history have to say. Being present in the moment brings a sense of meaning and purpose to everyday experience. Self-care healing practices encourage nurses to reinterpret their past and create a future replete with new possibilities through the use of visualization, letting go, and reflection.

The feelings, images, and impressions that derive from reflective healing practices are not merely individualistic musings. Images common to a given culture, a particular way of being, or a given professional heritage arise on a regular basis in meditation, yoga, tai chi, and Reiki practice as they do in dream work or narratives of nursing practice. The experiences that show up in reflective healing practices tell a story of a shared world of experience common to life within Western society and tradition. They help a nurse recognize and understand her place and uniqueness within this shared world.

Benner and Wrubel (1989) commented that the skilled body is a major coping resource in clinical practice. Reflective healing practices enable nurses to enhance physical and emotional strength during stressful times and are excellent ways to enhance coping. Habitual meanings and ways of being in the world are "...taken up by our bodily postures and sets to action.... Learning new bodily postures through relaxation exercises or yoga opens up new bodily meanings" (Benner & Wrubel, 1989, p. 173-174). The habitual body learns to adopt a new way of being, "a more fluid, relaxed, or confident stance" (Benner & Wrubel, 1989, p. 174). This new way of being then influences the nurse's interactions with patients and co-workers.

A STUDY OF REFLECTIVE HEALING PRACTICES OFFERED DURING A SELF-CARE RETREAT

What type of reflective healing practice is most effective with which nurse in what setting has not been determined. Factors such as age, level of physical ability, personal interest, availability of the classes, and administrative support are key factors to consider when designing a self-care program to decrease stress among registered nurses working in inpatient settings (Detert, Derosia, Caravella, & Duquette, 2006).

In this context, the question arose regarding whether reflective healing practices learned in a group setting, capable of supporting a strong unit-based culture, might encourage self-care, mentorship, and collaboration among nurses. For that reason, a pilot study was undertaken to examine the effectiveness of offering a self-care retreat for nurses.

The study was funded as a small portion of a three-year Health Resources and Services Administration residency program created to retain nurses. The first author was the primary investigator of that grant. She created the retreat schedule, attended the event, arranged for the self care classes, and analyzed nurses' evaluations with the assistance of the second author. Nurses who attended were volunteers who were not paid for their time or travel. Nurses' rooms, their food, and the classes that were included in the retreat were provided without cost. Asilomar, a state park alongside the Pacific Ocean, was selected as the location for the two-day, weekend self-care retreat. Asilomar was chosen for its intentional lack of telephones and televisions in the bedrooms, along with the spaciousness of the ocean setting. Moreover, Asilomar is proximal to Sacramento, where the hospital employing the participating *mentees* (new nurses or nurses transferring to a new unit) and their mentors was located. The purpose of the research was to identify which experiences and perceptions the nurses considered to be meaningful during the course of the self-care retreat.

Retreat Self-Care Options

Four self-care practices were included in the retreat at Asilomar. Meditation, yoga, tai chi, and Reiki healings were offered to 56 nurses (mentees and mentors) who volunteered to attend the retreat. Everyone attended a class in which each of these reflective self-care classes was offered. Reiki is a Japanese form of hands-on-healing in which the practitioner places his or her hands on or near the head, throat, chest, abdomen, hands, knees, and feet of an individual to redistribute energy.

For this retreat, Reiki sessions were one-half hour in length, during which nurses rested on a massage table fully clothed as soft music played in the background. Each nurse participated in one Reiki healing session.

Tai chi, yoga, and meditation classes were one hour in length. Each of these three classes was offered twice during the two-day retreat. Tai chi, based on the Yang short form, consisted of a series of gentle movements and walking meditations designed to stretch the body, enhance concentration, and improve body alignment. Yoga classes consisted of an introduction to breathing techniques and poses that included sweeps, downward dog position, and gentle spinal twists accompanied by soft music. At the end of the yoga session, nurses lay on the floor in the corpse position as the teacher led a five-minute guided meditation. The meditation teacher led a guided relaxation exercise that included instruction in grounding, breathing, and work with colors to assist nurses to let go of stressful feelings and images.

Retreat Qualitative Phenomenological Approach

Nurses were given a written self-care journal and asked to reflect a number of questions and prompts. Those questions and prompts included

1. What were the least-/most-helpful components of the self-care retreat at Asilomar?

2. Describe any sensations or feelings you noticed in your body during the course of the retreat.

3. Talk about why it is important for nurses to take good care of themselves.

4. What are the advantages and disadvantages of having self-care options offered in a retreat setting away from the hospital?

The journal was distributed at noon on Saturday after informed consent to participate in the study had been obtained. Nurses returned the journal at the end of the day on Sunday.

The purpose of the research was to identify which experiences and perceptions the nurses considered to be meaningful during the course of the self-care retreat. Heideggerian phenomenology (1926/1962) was used because this approach allows for accessing the meaning and significance of lived experience. In this approach, participants are asked to share both their lived experience and reflective understandings (Caelli, 2000).

Journal entries were compared one with another as parts of each journal were examined and contrasted with the overall sum of all entries to identify unifying, repeated concerns

(Benner, 1994). As the researchers looked for similarities and contrasts within the journals and dwelled in the text, exemplars were found that illustrated commonalities inherent in the nurses' narratives. Independently visiting and revisiting the text allowed the researchers to identify common themes. When wording used to describe these common themes differed, both researchers revisited the journals to find quotes that accurately captured the nurses' understandings. Consensus regarding findings was achieved by using this approach.

The results of phenomenological studies are most applicable to other populations that are similar to those for which the data was collected who also have a similar background of understanding and experience (Heidegger, 1926/1962; Sandelowski, 1986). It is the job of the reader to compare the group studied with demographic profiles in his or her setting and determine whether the findings have relevance for other hospitals or institutions. In the following tables are descriptions of the participants in this study. Table 9-1 lists participant demographics, Table 9-2 lists self-rated indicators, and Table 9-3 lists nurses' evaluation of the self-care options. Of the 56 in attendance, 2 nurses attended the retreat but did not attend all self-care classes and did not return their journals. Thus, detailed responses are used of the 54 nurses who did attend the self-care classes and return their journals.

Table 9-1 Participant Demographics

Age, years		**Marital Status**	
Average	43	Single	17
Range	25-61	Married	33
		Divorced	4
Experience, years			
As an RN	16	**Level of educational attainment**	
Range	1-35	Diploma	1
At current hospital	12	ADN	8
Of current hospital experience	1-35	BSN	40
		MSN	5
Sex		**Race**	
Female	50	Asian	15
Male	4	East Indian	3
		Hispanic	3
		Caucasian	33

Table 9-2 Self-Rated Indicators

	Quite a bit below average	Below average	Average	Above average	Quite a bit above average
Weight	0	3	26	17	8
Stress at home	0	5	25	21	3
Stress at work	0	3	13	26	12
Problems sleeping	14	7	18	12	3
How often I call in sick	31	7	9	4	3
Amount of daily caffeine use	9	8	17	18	2
Amount of weekly exercise	11	19	16	7	1
Amount of smoking	None = 54	0	0	0	0

Past experience with:
  Tai chi = 3
  Yoga = 8
  Meditation = 3
  Reiki = 4
  None = 36					

Table 9-3 Nurses' Evaluation of the Self-Care Options

Self-Care Option	Very helpful	Helpful	Undecided	Somewhat helpful	Not helpful
Tai chi	12	17	11	9	5
Yoga	41	9	1	3	0
Reiki	40	11	3	0	0
Meditation	22	16	9	7	0
Entire retreat	47	7	0	0	0

It is important to note that the tai chi class was held outside and that it started to mist and then rain. This sudden change in weather may have affected nurse's evaluations of the tai chi class as it was the only one that was offered outside. Also, a number of moves in the Yang style tai chi classes were covered during a one-hour period. When comments by participants were less than optimal, nurses mentioned the pace of the tai chi class was faster than they could follow in a one-hour class session.

Retreat Results

Nurses described three main themes in their written journals. These themes included that

- Self-care and caring are intertwined.
- The retreat setting helped clear a space to relax, gain perspective, and connect with peers.
- Feeling embodied sensations made the self-care experience memorable and motivating.

Exemplars from the journals are presented here illustrating each of these themes. Because the quotes often contained statements that illustrated more than one of the themes, they were organized under the most prevalent theme present within the quote. The reader is invited to participate in consensual validation of the results and review the quotes presented to determine whether the comments convey the suggested interpretations (Sandelowski, 1986). As Lincoln and Guba (1985) explained, descriptions of human experience are credible if readers recognize the experience presented as something they have encountered after having read the participant's words. Numerous quotes are included to articulate the taken-for-granted meanings and to give voice to the nurse's experiences and understandings.

SELF-CARE AND CARING ARE INTERTWINED

Nurses wrote in their diaries that self-care and caring are intertwined. They explained that nurses need to take care of themselves to be able to care for patients and get along with their co-workers. Nurses attending the retreat commented that taking time for self-care helped them notice insights about their life and career. They felt that by making time for self-care they created a feeling of effortless progress.

Taking Care of Yourself as a Nurse

In exemplars 1, 2, and 3, nurses described that you have to take care of yourself as a nurse if you expect patients to pay attention to the health-related teaching you are doing in your practice. To have patients truly hear what you have to say about health, you have to be a believable role model. Self-care improves your own health. It also bolsters the authenticity of your patient teaching and ability to care for others.

Exemplar 1

Setting aside your work responsibilities helps you remember that you have a responsibility to take care of yourself, too. You can't take care of others if you can't take care of yourself. Somehow, patients can feel you are being disingenuous if they can sense you don't take care of yourself when you're telling them how to eat, or exercise, or rest. When you're stressed out, as a nurse patients feel your tension. The yoga class helped me listen to my body and relax. Just focusing on breathing helped me. I felt gentle and peaceful afterward. The retreat has given me tools to take better care of myself. That will help me to be the most compassionate, caring, and giving nurse that I can be. A gift to myself is really a gift to my patients.

Exemplar 2

Patients don't believe you if you are teaching them about being healthy or relaxing, and you clearly aren't relaxed or healthy. Patients read body language and emotions, too, just like nurses do. You have to walk the walk, or no one really hears the patient teaching you are doing.

Exemplar 3

I liked the hands-on-healing session the best. When I went back to my room afterward, my face actually looked different. I was visibly more relaxed. I had rosy cheeks. You can't teach other people how to take care of themselves if you don't take care of yourself. The retreat reminded me that I'm going to slow down my daily life. I'm also going to take one of the self-care classes at the hospital when I get back home. I realized the classes are run by really good instructors. You need an introduction to the classes like this retreat provided to know you want to take them on a weekly basis. As a nurse, you have to use your body and your soul every day, so it's important to take the time to take care of them.

The Interconnectivity of Caring for Others and Self-Care

In exemplars 4–8, nurses described the interconnected nature of caring for others and self-care. As Benner (2000) commented, we "…do not spring from the womb as autonomous and educated, nor do we go to our graves without requiring care, support and sustenance" (p.

307). Needing care and taking time for self-care are just as much a part of the human condition and the nursing profession as is caretaking.

Self-care and caring are woven together like fine silk. The warp and weave of both these threads must be delicately balanced within nursing practice. Neither can be drawn too tight or ignored, or the fabric will become distorted. Vulnerability and strength, caring and self-care lace together whether it be to fashion a nurse's cap, a set of scrubs, or a well-balanced life.

A benefit of the retreat mentioned by the nurses was the time it provided for co-workers to bond and get to know one another better. Nurses described they felt more connected with their peers and more supportive of them after the retreat. Because nursing decisions and interventions are often a team effort, this sense of connection is vital. Nurses talked about the importance of caring for their peers as part of what it means to be a nurse. Exemplars are detailed here that speak to this theme.

Feeling Connected To Self and Co-Workers

Exemplar 4

> *The yoga class helped me clear my mind and focus on me. The time away from the normal everyday hassles was wonderful. There was nothing to worry about: not commuting, not dinner, not children, not work. After the retreat, I felt very connected with my co-workers and myself. I was also amazed that I have never done anything like this for myself before. I'll return a better nurse, more energized and better able to care for my patients and their families. I plan to take some time each day for myself because I feel it's critical to maintain the vitality needed to advocate for your patients each and every day. I didn't sign up for the weekly self-care classes at the hospital before the retreat because I felt like I didn't have any time to spare. Now I know taking some time for myself will be good for my body, my family, my patients, my practice, and my peers.*

Exemplar 5

> *The Reiki healing session was my favorite activity. It felt like someone was taking care of me instead of me always taking care of others. Even though I like taking care*

of patients, sometimes it just gets to be too much. That's when you have to take care of you too. Just sitting by the fire in the lodge made me feel connected with other nurses and thankful for my job. I've made a silent pack with me to take better care of my body. I know that will help me be a better nurse.

In exemplars 6–8, the nurses reflected on contrary cases—what their life and their nursing practice is like when they don't take the time for self-care.

Exemplar 6

My life is always busy down to each and every minute. It has been so busy and hectic I suddenly realized how much I've forgotten about taking care of me. The retreat reminded me of a time in my life when I did take care of me, and I felt softer and kinder as a nurse. Recently, it seems there is never enough time to do what I need to do. My mind is always racing to get things done or move on to the next task on my to-do list. Walking along the beach, I realized life's design is bigger than just my to-do list. The little things I never get to don't really matter in the grand design. I was drawn to the water and calmed by its vastness and constant movement. The breathing activity in the yoga class helped me to remember this moment is for me, and there is nowhere else I need to be. It was fun to be part of a group all focusing on the same task at the same time. That is something I've missed about nursing recently. Our unit floor plan is a bit isolating. It was nice to be at the retreat with my peers and get to know a different side of each person. The retreat was like a dedication for me: a way out of the pattern of being swamped at work and at home. I can't mentor anyone well until I have found my self, my energy, and my resources again. I can't be a good nurse unless I take care of me.

Exemplar 7

I felt warmth in my feet during the Reiki session. The touch was gentle and barely palatable. In the yoga class, I felt connected with my pose buddy. By the end of the yoga class, it was like I was melting into the mat. Nurses who take care of themselves are better caregivers. If I don't do that, I get squirrelly and resentful. That doesn't help me be a good nurse. I liked having time to just talk with the other nurses I work with on a regular basis. I'll remember the time we shared at Asilomar.

Exemplar 8

> *For nurses, our own health is usually the lowest thing on the priority list. This retreat reminded me it needs to be first. I liked spending time with my peers away from TVs, computers, and work just talking and getting to know each other. Relationship-building helps when it's busy at work. The retreat reminded me how difficult it is to do nothing. Nurses are always planning or doing. Taking time out of a 12-hour shift for yourself isn't the norm. The irony is that clinical ideas pop into your head if you carve out the time to be quiet and take care of yourself. You can do a better job of taking care of others when you have a moment of quiet to take care of yourself.*

The interwoven nature of caring and self-care described in these exemplars provided the nurses with a sense of authenticity, vitality, and motivation. Nurses described that caring and self-care both derive from a place of quiet knowing. Within expert practice, there is a space of quiet, effortless knowing that develops from experience with familiar patterns that take you by the hand and guide you toward effective interventions (Benner et al., 1996). Reflective practices such as tai chi, yoga, meditation, and Reiki healing are much the same. At first, it's hard to sit still and just be. The clatter of 100 thoughts and projects distract you like a list of tasks that must be completed before the end of a nursing shift. It's hard to remember six tai chi moves, let alone which is your right or left hand. You are a beginner, just learning. But with practice, you step into a place of quiet knowing where you notice subtle things about your life, your relationships, and your nursing career. This quiet space isn't a place of effort, but rather a place of insight and joy. The garment of health created in this quiet space is woven one strand, one step at a time with repeated practice just as is expertise in nursing practice.

Benjamin (1988) spoke of the tension between individuation, focus on self, and connecting with others. She used the analogy of Escher's birds "in which the figure and ground are constantly changing in their relation even as their outlines remain clearly distinct…. appearing to fly in both directions…. so that the drawing asks us to look two ways simultaneously" (p. 26). Self-understanding, self-focus, and connection with others are fluid and reciprocal processes that support one another. To sustain oneself as a nurse caring and connecting with others as well as caring for and connecting with oneself are necessary.

HOW THE RETREAT SETTING HELPED CLEAR A SPACE

Nurses talked about how the retreat setting and being away from the hospital helped them clear a space to relax, gain perspective, and connect with peers. Nurses live and work in communities. Each hospital, health care agency, unit, shift, and team has its own culture (Benner et al., 1996). Place and situation matter. Not only does a caring connection with patients shape one's practice as a nurse, but one's place within a unit, a hospital, and an agency also opens possibilities and defines what it means to be a nurse. How we see ourselves as team members and the extent to which we are at home in our environment matters.

To really gain understanding of one's typical environment, getting away can be helpful. Group retreats help nurses learn what sustains and unites them. Group retreats help nurses get to know one another and reflect on their daily practice. It's easier to get a sense of how to create a healing environment in the hospital, on the unit and shift where you work, after a time away and a bit of perspective. In the next two exemplars, nurses described how the lack of distractions at the retreat helped them develop a new perspective regarding nursing practice.

Creating a Space to Gain Perspective

Exemplars 9 and 10 illustrate a shift that occurred for nurses as the retreat progressed. The retreat allowed them to relax, gain perspective, and connect with their peers and their inner self.

Exemplar 9

> *Being at a retreat and not having to make any decisions, even about what to eat or when to do what was really nice. You get to leave your worries behind. The meditation class and focusing on my body helped me to be very aware of my surroundings throughout the retreat. Being away from the hospital felt like a total break—a gift really. I loved being surrounded by the sound and smell of the ocean. It was serene. I liked being away from TVs, traffic, and phones. I also liked spending time with some of the people I share my job with on a daily basis. It was great to get to know them in a different setting. At the end of the retreat I just felt an overwhelming wave of gratitude. Everyone was friendly and positive. What I took away was that's it's important to focus on the positive at work rather than dwelling on the things that are stressful that I can't change. That was a shift in perspective*

for me. If the retreat had been held in a conference room at the hospital, I wouldn't have experienced that feeling of gratitude or come up with the goal of looking for the positives in each day.

Exemplar 10

I just moved so being at home is stressful. There's always something to do even on my days off. At a retreat you have no choice but to relax. During the healing, I felt warmth in my feet and forehead. I also felt like I was rocking from side to side. It was very relaxing. I felt like a kid being away from work and having that be something my manager supported. It was nice to have a retreat where you didn't need to worry about when you had to be somewhere else or what the traffic might be like. Being away from being a mom and a wife and a nurse and walking on the beach helped me realize how blessed I am to be healthy, to have a good job, great friends, and a family. Life felt clearer. I liked being able to socialize and mingle with co-workers and connect with my inner self.

Distance and the Focus on Self-Care

In exemplars 11, 12, and 13, the nurses described how being away from the distractions of everyday hospital life helped them focus on and learn to be open to the new self-care practices. The retreat setting reinforced the message of the classes—to stay in the moment and listen to your body.

Exemplar 11

It was helpful to slow down and forget about life outside Asilomar. There weren't all the distractions here. There was no Vocera [communication device], no phone, no overhead page, no IV beeping, no emergencies. Concentrating in the yoga class on when to inhale and exhale was very soothing to me. That's something I want to bring back into each 12-hour shift that I work. The ocean and the peaceful surroundings enhanced everything the teachers talked about in the classes. The free time brought everything together. The slow, calm, positive attitude of the teachers was relaxing to me. I liked being away from Sacramento and being cared for in an encouraging, gentle way. It was like a group vacation and being pampered but more. It was active and doing, and learning to be good to yourself. Being with a group of people you work with, who you know put their needs on the back burner to care for others all the time and feeling that focusing on yourself is OK was great. I enjoyed the variety of activities and instructors and the sense of connection with fellow nurses. I look forward to running into nurses from other units and sharing a knowing smile about the Asilomar retreat.

Exemplar 12

When I'm stressed out at work, I plan to stop for a moment, breathe, stretch, and use the skills I learned in this retreat. I'll be a more efficient nurse if I take a minute to calm down and take care of myself while I take care of my patients. The retreat also helped me figure out which self-care classes I'm most interested in taking once we get back. Being at the ocean helped me to learn the concepts presented. I'm easily distracted by the sound of overhead pages. Being away from computers, phones, TV, and traffic was a great way to learn self-care. I was open to what the teachers were saying here. I was open to spending with my peers and to getting to know each of them as a person.

Exemplar 13

I feel work is never about what you love doing but who you work with and how you connect with them. You can have a crummy job (although I don't), and it is still fun if you are with positive people. There were positive people everywhere here—my co-workers, the teachers, and the people who worked at Asilomar. I enjoyed connecting with everyone. The change of scenery was nice because it makes you more open to trying new things. I learned a lot of new practices. I felt cared for and appreciated. At the hospital, there would have been constant distractions and interruptions during a weekend retreat. Being away from the noise and busyness of the hospital helped you to realize the importance of building quiet into each day.

Distance from Family; the Importance of Setting

In exemplars 14, 15, and 16, the nurses explained that the beauty of the setting reinforced a feeling that the hospital valued their nursing practice and wanted to retain them. Additionally, the nurses described that scheduling a weekend away from family responsibilities was a practical and workable option for them.

Exemplar 14

We all have very busy schedules, deadlines, projects to complete and a laundry list of things to do on the weekends. I made a decision to set aside this time for me. That was a big step for me because I have young children. After the yoga class, everything just fell into place for me. My body relaxed and my shoulder tension went away. Being close to nature brings a calm, centered feeling that lasts. Being taught relaxation techniques helps me focus and notice more about my surroundings. Healing the mind and the body is a natural thing. Taking care of ourselves leads to a healthier self and being a better nurse, person, wife/husband, mother/father, and human being. Having the retreat away from the hospital highlighted natural ways to care for yourself. Being in a relaxing setting shows the hospital respects and supports the goals of the retreat, and respects and supports nurses.

Exemplar 15

There is little time in my life for self-care and much stress and responsibility in my personal and professional life. I commute and work full time and have a family. The retreat worked great for me. I can steal away for a weekend without too much worry or guilt. It's harder to carve out eight weeks in a row to attend a class before or after a 12-hour shift. During the meditation session, I felt a multicolored energy and calm flow over me. I felt a sense of spirituality during the tai chi class. During the healing session, I felt a fountain of discomfort coming from my umbilical region that went away. I was left with a sense of completeness. Standing 20 feet away from a deer filled me with a sense of awe and peace. I love my job. But the tools I received from this retreat will help me deal with the emotional turmoil and the physical toll of caring for oncology patients. I felt renewed and valued. It was a great thing that the hospital organized this retreat.

Exemplar 16

If the retreat were at the hospital, I would have still been seeing my to-do list with chores and my work schedule floating through my mind. I was far enough away to let go of that, which was great. I felt a warmth in my inner core in the yoga class that is still with me. Nurses work in a stressful environment. We need tools to relax our body and make peace with ourselves. This was a wonderful way for the hospital to show their appreciation for nurses and their desire to retain nurses. It felt special to be away from the hospital.

RETREAT CONCLUSIONS

The retreat setting gave nurses permission to silence their internal to-do list. It allowed them to create a space for relaxation that was far enough away to let go of competing demands on their time. The retreat was a guilt-free escape that was practical given their schedule of working three to four 12-hour days in a row along with family responsibilities. The lack of distraction increased the nurses' receptivity to and ability to learn new self-care practices. Relaxation was mandatory as there were no competing demands or other available activities. The retreat provided a sampler of relaxation skills in a beautiful setting and allowed nurses to select a self-care option that worked for them.

No nurses mentioned a disadvantage of learning self-care practices in a retreat setting although they were invited to address disadvantages in their journal. After the retreat, nurses who went to Asilomar took it upon themselves to create a group e-mail list proc and sent multiple e-mails to one another. These e-mails and the sharing contained within them demonstrated in a very concrete way that the nurses who attended the Asilomar retreat felt connected with and supportive of one another.

It is likely that the fast-paced nature of nursing practice and the constant pull of multiple demands on a daily basis acclimatize nurses to stay busy on a nonstop basis. The pace and heart beat of the hospital is habit forming. The history of self-sacrifice and hard work are woven deeply into the fabric of nursing. Although these qualities alone may no longer sustain nurses, their pull is intense and of course, and in some ways quite positive. Initially, as nurses are learning new self-care skills, it may be necessary to select a retreat-like setting, a place away from the hum and pull of the hospital environment. Otherwise, it may be difficult for nurses to slow their tempo, focus inward, and be quiet enough to hear what their body has to say. Because of the historical traditions that have shaped their practice, nurses may need to learn in a setting that sends a message that self-care is not selfish, but rather a sustaining component of practice. In addition, a retreat-like setting allows nurses to feel valued and supported by their employer, which in turn may promote retention.

Feeling Embodied Sensations Made the Self-Care Experience Memorable and Motivating

In clinical practice, "the narrative memory of concrete events can evoke perceptual or sensory memories that enhance pattern recognition" (Benner et al., 1996, p. 251). Similarly in meditative and reflective practices perceptual and sensory memories shape one's way of looking at, remembering, and responding to the world. Feeling laden memories, fleeting images, and physical sensations that occur during reflective practices stand out as being memorable in the way that exemplars from practice do.

The exemplars in this chapter demonstrate a nurse's understanding of and approach to care. Memories that arise during reflective healing practices help a nurse key into life patterns that are or are not working for them. The vivid nature of these embodied feelings remain with the nurse, often for a period of weeks or months, motivating additional practice. Insights gained from reflective practices can help transform a way of looking at the world, reframe experience, and create new possibilities. This happens because worldviews have an atmosphere or mood surrounding them that shape present and future action and possibility (Heidegger, 1926/1962). When we are aware of that mood, we feel the possibilities and sets to action associated with the experience. As several nurses commented in the following exemplar and others that follow, we value, remember, and are motivated by experiences that are associated with strong physical or emotional sensations.

Exemplar 17

> *During the tai chi class, I could feel energy radiating from my hands. That left me with a feeling of awe and wonder because I'm a really skeptical person. During the healing session, it was strange, but it felt like two people were working on me when actually it was one person. I felt warmth in the area the healer wasn't touching even after he moved to another spot. In the meditation class, I felt a shoulder pain that slowly dissipated over the course of the hour. I'll remember what I learned at this retreat because such strong physical sensations stay with you.*

The Decision to Incorporate Self-care

In the following four exemplars, nurses described being motivated to shift their daily routine or to participate in weekly self-care classes on their return to work because of the retreat experience.

Exemplar 18

During the meditation session, I felt a tingling and sense of electricity. During the hands-on healing, I felt a pulsating energy that was quite pleasant. When I got up off the massage table, the constant tension in my neck was gone, and there was a sense of calm about me. In the yoga class, it felt like I was becoming part of the floor or the earth. That felt relaxing and memorable. This retreat has shown me many different ways to deal with the feelings I have about my job. I love my job but not everything I have to manage. I'll use the grounding and the breathing and the imagery to just let go during the day.

Exemplar 19

I felt encapsulated and safe during the hands-on-healing session. That was a feeling that will stay with me. There was a sense of pulling or release in my lower back area. I'm intense, the hospital is intense, and my job is intense. Being at Asilomar helped me separate and let go. I need to pay more attention to how I'm feeling throughout the day and just breathe when my body tells me to breathe. I'm going to attend the ongoing yoga class when I get back. I felt a sense of peace, vitality, and clarity during the class. I can tell that regular yoga practice will help me be calmer, more precise, and more focused because that's how I feel now. I'm motivated to continue with the yoga classes.

Exemplar 20

I experienced a heightened sense of color and visual clarity following the meditation. During the healing session, I was surprised at how such a gentle touch could produce so much relaxation. A sense of joy went over my body like a wave. It was like a pulse along my back that traveled down my hands and out my fingertips and the soles of my feet. The ache in my hips and back went away. For a time, it felt like someone placing hot rocks on spots all over my body. That's a memory that will stay with me and motivate me to use the tools I've learned to relax at work. Until I arrived, I didn't actually realize the name of the retreat was "self-care for nurses." I thought, "Perfect! That's what I need." I left feeling a sense of self acceptance and joy.

Exemplar 21

The yoga one-nostril breathing exercise opened my sinus, and the twisting poses helped settle my stomach. During the healing session, I felt a lightness all over my body that I won't forget. I was thankful to have this time away from all the stress in my life to think about myself. I'll remember the Asilomar retreat. I started a fire in our lodge and talked to another nurse. In a short time, 15 other nurses joined us and started chatting about where they worked and what they did. It was a nice way to find new friends from work. During stressful times at work, I am going to take 5 minutes for myself and stretch so I can make sure I'm still focused on what is going on with my patients.

LISTENING FOR THE CALL TO ACTION

Nurses described emotions and physical sensations that they experienced during the self-care retreat in much the same way as Vetlesen (1994) who wrote "…emotions and sensations are active in disclosing a situation to us. …they provide …access to and make us aware of the relevance of an experience" (p. 166). In this study, nurses used the strong physical sensations and emotions as a marker, a Geiger counter of meaning (Raingruber & Kent, 2003), something that pointed to a significant experience that was memorable and motivating for them. As Zuk and Wetmore (1993) commented, sensory experiences and memories, whether they are primarily self- or other-directed, help individuals enhance their own narrative understanding.

Martinsen (1996) spoke of the motivating call to action—the need to intervene on behalf of a patient—that follows strong physical sensations in clinical practice. It is interesting in these exemplars that nurses were motivated to take action to improve their own lives based on similar strong physical sensations. Vetlesen (1994, p. 175) explained that sensations and emotions are ways of being moved or affected by a situation—"a gut take on the situation"—which calls for reflection and subsequent action. Being with feelings and sensations at this retreat allowed nurses to experience and feel, to notice their body's response, and to understand something new about themselves in the process. A number of nurses signed up for the weekly self-care classes offered at the hospital after participating in the retreat.

As Saleebey (1992) commented, a clinician's relationship to practice is always mediated by the body. Burnout and alienation result from a lack of access to embodied responses, bodily energies, sensations, and resources. Practices that connect nurses to embodied sensations offer great promise for enhancing nurses' health, reinvigorating their enthusiasm for nursing, motivating growth, reintroducing a sense of purpose in their practice, and promoting longevity among working nurses.

Limitations of the Study

This study began a needed exploration of the effectiveness of self-care retreats in motivating and retaining registered nurses. Analysis of objective measures and long-term evaluations at more than one hospital are also needed to determine the effectiveness of self-care retreats:

- Follow-up evaluations are necessary to determine how long after the retreat the nurses' practice, health, and self-understanding are influenced.

- Studies that compare and contrast the responses of new graduate and experienced nurses are also needed. For example, would a retreat be more motivating to an experienced nurse who needs to feel valued by an institution after 20 years of service or by a new nurse who needs a break from the stress of beginning practice?

- The difference that location has on the impact of the retreat also needs to be determined. Are some settings more effective than others?

- Would results have differed if additional men had participated? This retreat included only 4 male but 50 female nurses.

- Also, the majority of participants (33 of 54) were Caucasian. Would the journal entries have been similar if additional Black, Hispanic, and Southeast Asian nurses had participated? Future studies with larger and more diverse populations are certainly needed.

- Additionally, focus groups need to be conducted to determine whether qualitative interviews and journal entries yield similar findings.

Implications of the Study

Hospitals dedicate significant resources to recruiting, and orienting new nurses. Given that maintaining a stable workforce is becoming more and more challenging as the nursing shortage intensifies (Schullanberger, 2000), additional options need to be considered. The stress associated with working 12-hour shifts, having rotating days off, and caring for increasingly complex patients continues to contribute to turnover and burnout. Substantial numbers of nurses from inpatient settings are leaving the profession prior to retirement age (Aiken et al., 2001). Koloroutis (2004) argued that hospital-based programs and infrastructures must be developed to bring relationship-based care back to life within our contemporary health care system. She stressed hospitals must start to value self-care for nurses as a critical component of this relationship-based care. One way to reintroduce relationship-based care into inpatient settings is to offer self-care retreats for nurses.

If self-care retreats are an effective way to build a sense of teamwork on a unit and promote a nurse's health or the longevity of his/her career, they are worth the financial investment involved. Nurses who feel valued go the extra mile to support their peers and patients. Nurses who are relaxed are more productive. Hospitals need to find ways to encourage nurses to care for themselves while simultaneously caring for their patients. Retreats are an effective way to introduce nurses to weekly self-care practices. At a retreat, a nurse can sample various options and select the self-care practice that works best for him or her. Self-care retreats are an efficient and popular way to reintroduce a heightened sense of purpose, motivation, caring, and self-care into nursing practice.

We live in webs-of-connection and relationship (Keller, 1986): nurse-patient, nurse-family member, nurse-nurse, and nurse-physician. These relationships sustain caring in our practice. But the sense of connection and relationship with oneself called self-care is just as important. Clarity about one's personal history, values, and dreams—as well as the skill of being present in the moment—are vital qualities that help sustain nursing practice. All the strands in the webs of our lives are important in sustaining balance, creating motivation, bringing joy, and maintaining a sense of purpose in our practice. In this era of increasing technology, embracing high-touch alternative therapies helps nurse administrators, managers, and hospitals create a climate that supports self-care and a balanced work life for nurses providing patient care.

ACKNOWLEDGMENTS

This project was supported by funds from the Division of Nursing (DN), Bureau of Health Professions (BHPr), Health Resources and Services Administration (HRSA), Department of Health and Human Services (DHHS) under grant number 1D64HP03099 titled "RN Residencies: Transitioning to Nursing Specialties." The information or content and conclusions are those of the author and should not be construed as the official position or policy of, nor should be any endorsements be inferred by the DN, BHPr, DHHS, or the U.S. Government.

References

Aiken, L. H., Clarke, S. P., Sloane, D. M., Sochalski, J. A., Busse, R., Clarke, H., Giovnetti, P., ... Shamian, J. (2001). Nurses' reports on hospital care in five countries. *Health Affairs, 20*(3), 43-53.

Benjamin, J. (1988). *The bonds of love: Psychoanalysis, feminism, and the problem of domination.* New York: Pantheon Books.

Benner, P. (1994). *Interpretive phenomenology: Embodiment, caring, and ethics in health and illness.* Thousand Oaks, CA: Sage.

Benner, P. (2000). The quest for control and the possibilities of care. In *Heidegger: Coping and cognitive science: Essays in honor of Hubert L. Dreyfus, Vol 2. Wrathall, Mark and Malpas, Jeff (Eds.)* (pp. 293-309). Cambridge, MA: The MIT Press.

Benner, P., Tanner, C., & Chesla, C. (1996). *Expertise in nursing practice: Caring, clinical judgment, and ethics.* New York: Springer.

Benner, P., & Wrubel, J. (1989). The *primacy of caring: Stress and coping in health and illness*. Menlo Park, CA: Addison-Wesley.

Brathovde, A. (2006). A pilot study: Reiki for self-care of nurses and health care providers. *Holistic Nursing Practice, 20*(2), 95-102.

Caelli, K. (2000). The changing face of phenomenological research: Traditional and American phenomenology in nursing. *Qualitative Health Research, 10*(3), 366-377.

Cohen-Katz, J., Wiley, S., Capvano, T., Baker, D., Deitrick, L., & Shapiro, S. (2005). The effects of mindfulness-based stress reduction on nurse stress and burnout. Part III. *Holistic Nursing Practice, 19*(2), 78-87.

Detert, R. A., Derosia, C., Caravella, T., & Duquette, D. (2006). Reducing stress and enhancing the general well being of teachers using T'ai Chi Chih movements: A pilot study. *Californian Journal of Health Promotion, 4*(1), 162-173.

Gold, J., & Thornton, L. (2001). Simple strategies for managing stress. *RN, 64*(12), 65-68.

Heidegger, M. (1926/1962). *Being and time*. (J. Macquarrie & E. Robinson, Trans.). New York: Harper & Row.

Keller, C. (1986). *From a broken web: Separation, sexism, and self.* Boston: Beacon Press.

Koloroutis, M. (2004). Introduction. In M. Koloroutis (Ed.), *Relationship-cased care* (pp. 1-23). Minneapolis: Creative Health Care Management, Inc.

Lincoln, Y. S., & Guba, E.G. (1985). *Naturalistic inquiry.* Thousand Oaks, CA: Sage.

Mackenzie, C. S., Poulin, P. A., & Seidman-Carlson, R. (2006). A brief mindfulness-based stress reduction intervention for nurses and nurse aides. *Applied Nursing Research, 19*(2), 105-109.

Martinsen, K. (1996, October). *Introduction to lecture one*. Paper presented at the University of California at San Francisco, Logstrup Conference, San Francisco.

Oman, D., Hedberg, J., & Thoresen, C. E. (2006). Passage meditation reduces perceived stress in health professionals: A randomized, controlled trial. *Journal of Consulting and Clinical Psychology, 74*(4), 714-719.Palmer, R.E. (1969). Hermeneutics. Evanston: Northwestern University Press.

Peplau, H. E. (1952). *Interpersonal relations in nursing: A conceptual frame of reference for psychoanalytic nursing*. Itasca, IL: Putnam.

Raingruber, B., & Kent, M. (2003). Attending to embodied responses: A way to identify practice-based and human meanings associated with secondary trauma. *Qualitative Health Research, 13*(4), 449-468.

Saleebey, D. (1992). Biology's challenge to social work: Embodying the person-in-environment perspective. *Social Work, 37*(2), 112-118.

Sandelowski, M. (1986). The problem of rigor in qualitative research. *Advances in Nursing Science, 8*(3), 27-37.

Schullanberger, G. (2000). Nurse staffing decisions: An integrative review of the literature. *Nursing Economics, 18*(3), 124-148.

Schwartz, G. E. (1990). Psychobiology of repression and health: A system approach. In Singer, J. (Ed.), *Repression and dissociation: Implications for personality theory, psychopathology, and health* (pp. 337-387). Chicago: University of Chicago Press.

Tsai, S. L., & Crockett, M. S. (1993). Effects of relaxation training, combining imagery, and meditation on the stress level of Chinese nurses working in modern hospitals in Taiwan. *Issues in Mental Health Nursing, 14*(1), 51-66.

Vetlesen, A. J. (1994). *Perception, empathy, and judgment: An inquiry into the preconditions of moral performance.* University Park, PA: Pennsylvania State University Press.

Watson, J. (1988). *Nursing: Human science and human care.* New York: NLN Press.

Whelan, K., & Wishnia, G. S. (2003). Reiki therapy: The benefits to a nurse/Reiki practitioner. *Holistic Nursing Practice, 17*(4), 209-218.

Zuk, R. J., & Wetmore, A. A., (1993). Teaching the incest narrative: Problems and possibilities. *Feminist Teacher, 7*(3), 21-26.

CHAPTER 10

Sustaining Family Life and Health Through Rituals, Routines, and Practices in Well Families with School-Age Children

KAREN A. PLAGER

INTRODUCTION

Contemporary approaches to health and health promotion activities often focus on the individual. This individualization of health tends to splinter these activities from family life, especially by treating health and related activities as consumer commodities and therapeutic interventions. Still, health and health-related activities are an integral part of the family's world. Persons' basic embodied stances and ways of being in their world are first constituted through membership and participation in shared family life, especially in the early years of life. Within the context of family, a young person takes up basic postures, self-understandings, notions, habits, and practices around health and health-related activities that will be a lifelong part of her/his personhood. To detach health from the everyday habits, skills, and practices of work, rest, recreation, social relationships, eating, and exercise that characterize family life is to contribute to an impoverished understanding of health in the family.

In this chapter, I describe families' everyday practices, routines, and rituals—particularly those centered around mealtimes—to understand how these are meaningful for families; how these shape their health skills, activities, and habits; and what it means to the family to be healthy. This chapter constitutes a portion of the findings from a larger interpretive phenomenological study that examines the meanings of health and health promotion practices in well families with school-age children (Plager, 1995).

A previous paper described how family legacy ("living tradition, an aspect of the family's lifeworld reshaped over time in a family's particular situations and influenced by family, culture and society", p. 52) shapes family and family member identity as well as health in the ways that families extend, flee from, and/or reshape their legacy, as well as what that means for family health concerns and activities in daily life (Plager, 1999). Everyday practices, routines, and rituals—like legacy—are part of the rich warp and woof of the fabric of family life; therefore, these may be reciprocally shaped by—and, in turn, shape—family legacy. In this chapter, I continue to uncover aspects of family legacy by exploring the ways that families' practices, routines, and rituals are shaped by stories from their families of origin.

REVIEW OF THE LITERATURE: DEFINING RITUALS, ROUTINES, AND PRACTICES

The notions of routine and ritual in family life in the United States are well described in the family literature, including Bossard and Boll whose seminal work on family rituals still holds relevance for family scientists and family life today (Bossard & Boll, 1950; Boyce, Jensen, James, & Peacock, 1983; Kantor & Lehr, 1975; Reiss, 1981; Wolin & Bennett, 1984). Family rituals convey a sense of the family's shared identity and solidarity, even to the point that during ritual activities, there is a heightened sense of the family group identity over the individual. Reiss (1981) referred to this as an "undifferentiated oneness" (p. 246) that refocuses, establishes, and maintains the family's sense of social reality. From an interpretive phenomenological (IP) perspective, family rituals are constitutive of the family's world. Participation in ritual is a way that family members are absorbed and involved in the world of their shared family life: what concerns them and what is meaningful for them.

Family rituals are patterns of activity in family life that are meaningful for how the family understands and recognizes itself as a group and as members of the family. Ritual activities (Wolin & Bennett, 1984) may include

- Family traditions that constitute special family rites of passage, such as birthdays, anniversaries, bar/bat mitzvahs, or confirmations

- Family celebrations of holidays generally practiced in the culture

- Patterned family interactions that constitute regular activities in the family, such as dinnertime, bedtime, and ways of settling family conflicts

Family routines are repetitive family activities that involve two or more family members and occur on a regular basis in the life of the family. Routines generally serve to provide for needs, wishes, or requirements to sustain family members and/or the family group and to maintain the household. Routines may also have ritual significance when they take on meaning for the family or family members beyond sustenance and maintenance of the family and household (Boyce et al., 1983). For example, in one of this study's participant families with two daughters, ages 2 and 7, dinnertime is significant in how it is constitutive for what makes a "good" teenager. Even at the young age of these children, the parents were concerned about the kind of teenagers their daughters would become.

Practices, according to MacIntyre (1984), are "any coherent and complex form of socially established human activity" with "goods internal" to the activities that achieve "standards of excellence" and seek a common good (p. 187). In this sense, making and sustaining a family and the life of that family falls under the rubric of practice. A practice, as it is interpreted here, may encompass both family routines and rituals; there is considerable overlap of these three areas of activities in the actual lived experience of any family.

Borgmann (1984) described a special category of practice—a *focal practice*. In a world where technology's patterned pervasiveness infiltrates every corner of our lives with commodification Borgmann claimed that the device paradigm forever threatens to make our lives ones of shallow existence. He described the device or technological paradigm as an invisible and pervasive pattern in contemporary life by which we normally orient or understand ourselves. In everyday life, we come to rely upon technological devices to provide us with easily available commodities. The machinery of a device is inconspicuous. The paradigm's implicit promise is to disburden humans of toil, suffering, and poverty; but paradoxically, it can lead to disengagement, distraction, and a loss of meaningful involvement in life. Borgmann suggested that focal practices center us and engage us in life in more meaningful ways. He claimed that "focal practices naturally reside in the family, and the parents are the ones who should initiate and train their children in them" (p.226). A healthy family, he suggested, is centered upon a focal concern, whether it be a sport or a family meal. In this chapter, I point out how certain practices in the lives of these families are significant in the ways that they focus the family and gather them in an engaged and attentive manner, as opposed to a disengaged and distracted manner. It is within such contexts that many health-related activities take place in the family.

Another special area of practices—recognition practices—are intertwined through all the other practices, routines, and rituals of the families. Benjamin (1988) noted that recognition shows up in many invisible and taken-for-granted ways in our lives because it is so central to human being. This is what Heidegger (1927/1962) meant when he referred to humans as the kind of beings that allow other beings to show up.

Recognition practices constitute the social spaces in the family for individual members to show up and be "known" in the family. One's identity begins to be formed in the family through these practices. Taylor (1991, 1994) pointed out that recognition practices have always existed for human beings. In premodern times, these were largely derived from a preordained social station in society and corresponding roles and activities. Modern ideals of authenticity have undermined the taken-for-grantedness of this premodern way of being socially identified. Now we must depend upon recognition and identity that transpires through an overt and internalized dialog with others. These subtle—and, sometimes, not so subtle—dialogs are the recognition practices that occur and are constitutive of self and other in families. I point to these as I move through this discussion of family routines, rituals, and practices.

A final point merits emphasizing. A family's understanding of the activities that constitute the practices, rituals, and routines in their particular family depends upon a shared background understanding in the culture and society (Heidegger, 1927/1962). No family invents its meanings from whole cloth; rather, it tailors the culturally available meanings according to the particular family needs, wants, desires, and possibilities. This tailoring may occur in invisible and taken-for-granted ways, or it may occur through a conscious effort of the family to orchestrate some sort of change for the family or its members.

Three practices in the lives of the families are common themes in which health concerns of the families show up:

- Gathering practicesw
- Play practices
- Protection practices

This chapter focuses on gathering practices, particularly family dinnertime. Play practices and protection practices are explicated elsewhere (Plager, 1995).

STUDY METHODOLOGY AND DESIGN

The findings in this chapter emerged from a larger study of family health and well-being. Interpretive phenomenology was employed to understand everyday skills, practices, and experiences; and to disclose the meanings and knowledge embedded in these. Using thick description and interpretation, the researcher is challenged to uncover and understand the meanings in the activities and stories of the study participants within the context and temporality of their situations (Benner, 1985, 1994; Chesla, 1988).

Study participants included six well, middle-class, Caucasian, two-parent families with at least one school-age child between 7 and 11 years old. Table 10-1 summarizes the demographics of the participating families.

Table 10-1 Demographics of Participant Families

Ethnicity	All Caucasian
Average age of parents	38.7 years
Age range of parents	35 to 42 years
Education	All college
Employment status:	
One parent working outside the home	4 families
Two parents working outside the home	2 families
Average number of children per family	2.33
Average age of children	7.5 years
Average age of 7- to 11-year-old participants	9 years
Age range of children	2 to 11 years

Note: N = 6 families from suburban West Coast communities; 14 children; 10 children ages 7 to 11 years old

This convenience sample of families was recruited from a variety of community and health care provider contacts over a two-year period. Fliers that briefly described the study were distributed to contacts, and interested and eligible families were asked to contact the researcher. A snowball recruitment strategy was incorporated as well—meaning that one study participant might nominate or suggest another possible study participant. Interested families contacted the researcher through a recruitment site or another participating family. At the initial telephone contact with the family, elements of informed consent were discussed. All families who agreed to participate were sent a Committee on Human Research consent form to review, as a family, before the first meeting. At the first in-person interview, questions or concerns were addressed and informed consent was obtained.

Each family participated in five to six in-depth family group interviews that took place over three to four months. Interviews were conducted in the family home. Semi-structured, open-ended interview questions engaged family members in narrative accounts of specific health-related family and family member episodes and events. The final interview in the study took place with only the parents present. This provided an opportunity to discuss issues with the parents that might not be discussed if the children were present. An unstructured format was utilized for the final interview. Debriefing and feedback from the parents occurred at this time.

A relaxed tone for the interviews allowed family members to interact naturally. Using the home setting and relaxed tone permitted family dynamics to be observed during the interviews. Detailed field notes of observations of these family activities were kept. Observations of family dynamics during the interviews provided insight into the family's engaged practical involvement that is unreflective and often unarticulated (Chesla, 1995). These observations, recorded as field notes, were used to enhance and supplement the families' stories in the interpretation of the narrative-text.

Transcribed interview audiotapes and field notes became narrative-text analogs. Family diaries of physical health promotion activities over three nonconsecutive days were also kept and became part of the narrative-text. Parents and children were encouraged to contribute to the diaries.

Analysis and interpretation of narrative-texts was accomplished through three interrelated strategies used for IP, including thematic analysis, interpretation of exemplars, and paradigm cases. These strategies are well-described by Benner (1994). Four criteria for evaluating qualitative research—applicability, credibility, integrity, and consistency—guided this research project (Leonard, 1989; Sandelowski, 1986).

DINNERTIME AS A FAMILY GATHERING PRACTICE

Gathering practices, particularly family dinnertime, constitute one common theme in which health concerns showed up for the families in this study. Exemplar 10-1 illustrates three family exemplars of the theme and various sub-themes that are further described and discussed in this section. All names used are pseudonyms to protect anonymity of the participants. Health concerns and health-related activities are often deeply embedded in long-established practices in these families as their stories show.

> **Exemplar 10-1 Family Dinnertime as Exemplars of Family Gathering Practices**

- The Brannons: Dinnertime as a consistent family ritual
- The Switzers: Preserving dinnertime as an occasional all family ritual
- The Browns: Dinnertime as a disengaged activity (a non-practice)

Gathering practices in the family might include a myriad of activities whereby the family comes together to share their common life. These may be daily, weekly, occasional, and/or rare events, depending on the family. Family rituals may constitute gathering practices. Only the nuclear family might participate; or, extended family and even significant friends of the family may be included. These practices may occur in the family home or elsewhere.

Family dinnertime is a traditional gathering practice of many families that is integral to health-related activities and habits. Dinnertime is probably the meal that families most frequently take together as a family group, so for simplicity's sake, I use the term generically. "Dinnertime" could be any or all meals that the family takes together as a group.

Dinnertime is a time when families gather at the end of the day to share a common meal together and to have conversations about life in and out of the family. Conflicts may arise during dinner that may be resolved or be ongoing in the family dialog. At dinnertime, parents and children learn from and about each other, listen, and are listened to (Bellah et al., 1991). During dinner, children experientially learn certain patterns of life in the family and skills, activities, and habits for social comportment that they may take up as ways of being in social situations both in and out of the family. They also learn skills, activities, and habits perhaps for lifelong health and well-being. Dinnertime is routine in the family as a repetitive activity that is fairly consistent over time. It is also ritual in the way that it is a meaningful pattern of activity in the life of the family (DeVault, 1987). Just as family dinnertime can be part of family daily routine, it may be a celebration of family and part of family celebrations (Borgmann, 1984).

For many American families, dinnertime is a marginalized practice. A number of interconnected aspects of modern society play into this phenomenon: the rise in popularity of processed and prepackaged foods; fast-food and restaurant convenience and availability; the increasing proportion of two-career families; and the rapid pace of life, with a focus on individual fulfillment of goals and competitive success (Bellah et al., 1991; Borgmann, 1984). Underpinning all of these is the "rule of technology," which Borgmann describes as a "social paradigm" in which modern day life is "deeply entrenched":

> . . . it not only informs most human practices but . . . all of reality is patterned after the paradigm, and in this sense we can say that the paradigm has acquired an ontological dimension. . . . When the pattern is so firmly established it also tends to become invisible. There are fewer and fewer contrasts against which it is set off. . . . This relation to technology is neither one of domination by technology nor one of conscious direction of technology. . . . Living in an advanced industrial country, one is always and already implicated in technology . . . technology is the rule today in constituting the inconspicuous pattern by which we normally orient ourselves. (pp.104-105)

The engaged practice of the family meal—in terms of careful attention to the activities of preparation and partaking of it—is thus losing ground to the impoverished and disengaged activities of the commodification of food and eating, according to both Bellah et al. (1991) and Borgmann (1984). DeVault (1987) argued that in spite of technology, a certain amount of invisible work goes into feeding a family—including mealtime planning and organization—that cannot be replaced by technology. A major portion of this invisible work in the family is traditionally the mother's job, regardless of whether she works outside the home.

For all the families in this study, family dinnertime was a significant practice: It was a constitutive part of family life related to physical health of family members and the health of the family as a group. Its significance lies in the ways that families hold on to dinnertime as an important tradition; and in the conflict between dinnertime being an attentive, engaged family time, or a time of distracted and disengaged activity. In the balance of this chapter, I describe dinnertime practices in three families that exemplify the range between engaged practice and disengaged activity, the families' struggles to hold onto dinnertime as an increasingly marginalized practice, and what dinnertime means to the health of each family. In the following narratives, M stands for mother, F stands for father, D stands for daughter, S stands for son, and I stands for interviewer.

The Brannons: Dinnertime as a Consistent Family Ritual

For the Brannon family, dinnertime was preserved as a regular family ritualized routine when the whole family sat down for the dinner meal together.

> **MOTHER (M):** *Well, one thing I try to be consistent about is that we always sit down and all of us eat together, and I try to be very consistent about that.*

In a time when many people and families in our society are struggling with difficulties that arise for children in adolescent years, the Brannons (Charlie and Betsy) were already concerned about what kind of teenagers their two daughters, Eve (age 7) and Nikki (age 2) would become. They staunchly adhered to their family dinnertime practice, which was understood as constitutive for what makes a good teenager.

> *FATHER (F): That's also because of the philosophy that that's good for family values, too. . . . It's a good time to--you had read something somewhere where one of the traits of a teenager being stable was that they always had dinner with their parents and that was a family time together. Right?*
>
> *M: Yeah.*
>
> *F: It was one of the consistent things that in the past of teenagers growing up right, you know. So, that's part of it, too.*
>
> *M: Yeah.*

Both Charlie and Betsy grew up in families where dinner was eaten together as a family, but the legacy of Betsy growing up in a father-only family after her mother died when Betsy was 7 years old more strongly shaped the practice in their family.

> *M: And I always did it with my dad and that was probably not easy for him being . . . a bachelor. . . . Yeah, us being bachelors together. He always made a point of us having dinner together and having a real . . . nice meal. Not that it was tasty, but it, you know, nutritious meal together, talking to each other. I consider that. . . . I'm pretty rigid about that.*

It was not the nutritional content of the food that Betsy was so adamant about (although she *was* concerned about nutrition) but rather the quality of the time that the family spent together at the dinner meal. For her, a healthy dinnertime for the family meant a nurturing time and a time to pay attention to each other after a long day spent going their separate ways. For instance, watching television during dinner was absolutely forbidden. She recalled how early on in her relationship with Charlie this became an unspoken rule in the family that needed no further discussion.

> *F: Right. Yeah. My mother cooked every meal.*
>
> *M: I thought you were allowed to watch TV. . . .*

> **F:** *At some point, and it was later on when we were teenagers, we got these TV trays and then dinner became, you know… Remember those TV trays? Uh, it became more of a…you watched TV while you ate type thing and nobody talked. Uh, but earlier on, I recall that …I guess there wasn't that much TV around… .*
>
> **M:** *I remember when we were dating and I cooked a nice dinner after working a 12-hour day like he had, and, I mean, I'd come home and fix something nice and gone to the trouble of shopping and he wanted to eat it in front of the TV, and I was like, what do you mean you're going to eat this meal in front of the TV. [laughing] And uh, we don't do that.*
>
> **F:** *No, TV doesn't go on at all.*
>
> **M:** *And I'm rigid about that. . . . There's no TV. That's the time to talk. . . . And to me as a cook that's like the ultimate insult, too. Is to have somebody gobble down their food while watching TV. Not even taking the time to taste it or spend time with the cook. I feel like the maid then.*
>
> **I:** *Uh-huh, that your hard efforts aren't really appreciated.*
>
> **M:** *Yeah.*

Betsy's family legacy of dinnertime has evolved since she was a small girl, and she has extended it into her family of progeny. She staunchly defended preservation of dinnertime as time for family sharing and resisted any attempts to undermine the practice. Dinnertime is also a way of recognizing the effort put into the meal-planning and preparation as well as acknowledging the one who prepared the meal by attending with appreciation to the meal put on the table and avoiding distractions, such as television.

In addition, dinnertime is a time to recognize each member of the family and share their accomplishments, concerns, trials, and tribulations. "That little one" was a frequent topic of discussion because 2-year-old Nikki was recognized in the family as very strong-willed and assertive: a handful for Betsy to manage. Part of the dinner ritual was managing Nikki so that the rest of the family could enjoy the dinnertime sharing.

During the time the Brannon family participated in the study, I would arrive at their home about 6:45 in the evening for our scheduled interview. Usually the family would be just finishing dinner because Charlie, who commuted to the neighboring urban area, generally arrived home only shortly before that time. The family was always seated in the same pattern at the round dinner table in the bay window of the family room that adjoins the kitchen. Nikki was not present at the table. She sat in her highchair, about three feet away from, and parallel to, the rest of the family. Usually she was in her pajamas. When she finished dinner, she was taken back to her bedroom before we began our interview.

The fact that Nikki was not included as a member of the family at the dinner table was a matter of concern to me, but not one that I felt comfortable broaching with the family. However, from my perspective, she was not recognized as a full member of the family's dinner ritual. At our final interview, Charlie engaged in unsolicited discussion about how the family recognized Nikki at their dinner ritual.

> **F:** *You know, one of the things that's been bothering me about dinner recently is that Nikki is stuck in her chair and she's an outsider at dinnertime. Have you ever had that feeling? She's 2 years old and she's never been at our dinner table.*
>
> **M:** *Because the first time we let her sit at the dinner table we will never get her back in there [highchair].*
>
> **F:** *I know that, but shouldn't we at least bring her over to the table? In her chair?*
>
> **M:** *Okay, so we'll get Eve to move. . . .*
>
> **F:** *I'm sorry [to interviewer], this just made me think of . . . this.*
>
> **M:** *We'll get Eve to move to the back.* [F: *Yeah.*] *Okay, and we'll put Nikki. . . .*
>
> **F:** *We'll set the chair over. . . .*
>
> **M:** *. . .chair in the center.*
>
> **F:** *Yeah, cause don't you think that maybe . . . she's wondering why. . . . [M: Psychologically.] . . . you know, she's not part of the gang?*
>
> **M:** *Okay. Okay. It's interesting. I guess we have to include her.*

Charlie acknowledged a concern that their dinnertime had excluded Nikki as a full participating member of the family. Methodologically, this is an instance of how the interview can be an unintended intervention. In this situation, Charlie—through participation in the study—may have become more sensitized to the excluded member of the family and is now able to problem-solve with Betsy in how Nikki is recognized in the family. How a family member is recognized can be understood as a continually evolving process in the life of the family and family members.

Although Betsy was resistant to the suggestion, she agreed to entertain a way they could include Nikki while still keeping her in a space where she could be managed until she learned the skills to fully join the family at the table. Charlie spoke as an advocate for Nikki (who may herself recognize that she has to fend for herself to achieve full inclusion in the family) as he explained:

> **F:** *'Cause you don't—when I take her out to dinner, even though it's like McDonald's or something like that, she runs and gets herself the booster chair, herself, and goes and puts it in the thing so she can be part of sitting at the table. . . . So I just noticed that recently. [M: Okay.]*

In the family home, Nikki understands her place in the dinner ritual, but outside the home, the mores of the table are not as strictly observed, and Nikki asserts herself to be recognized as a full member of the family dinner ritual.

I had asked them earlier, as part of this final interview, how what they think or do might have changed as a result of participating in the study. Now I acknowledged with them that "something else has come about in the process of the interviews."

> **M:** *We're going to let Nikki sit with us at the table [laughing].*
>
> **F:** *Yeah, dinner table. Well, she is sort of out there by herself.*
>
> **M:** *Yeah, she is.*
>
> **F:** *And we sort of just like throw her food like she's a dog or something. You know, I'd started worrying about that. [laughing]*
>
> **I:** *When did you start worrying about that?*
>
> **F:** *Uh, in the last month or two, 'cause I found myself turning around and like throwing the food to her, and I was like, boy she's like a little dog over here. And you know she really should be part of the family.*
>
> **M:** *Yeah, we don't even make eye contact with her during dinnertime.*

> F: *No, and I don't think that's healthy. For her. Or us. That just bugged me in the last couple months.* [M: *Huh, okay.*] *Yeah, when she was a littler baby, it didn't bug me, but now that she's talking. . . .*

Dinnertime as a gathering practice and ritual in the Brannon family was a way they understood what it meant to be healthy as a family and as individuals. It meant being healthy in their whole person (physically, emotionally, and spiritually)—as well as whole family—through what happened at dinner in the past and in the present; and how it shapes their future possibilities as a family, especially as they anticipate their daughters' teen years. For the Brannons, dinner was an engaging and sustaining family-gathering practice.

The Switzers: Preserving Dinnertime as an Occasional All-Family Ritual

For the Switzer family, the engaged practice of dinnertime was more effortful. Although being together as a whole family for dinner was a practice that the Switzers were trying to preserve, it easily got sideswiped by individual interests and demands in the family. Tom, the father, who was a computer engineer, admitted that he had taken up the work ethic of his parents and tended "to get home a *little bit* later than the kids would like to eat. . . ." He got so engrossed in work—not because of what work demanded of him, but because of what he demanded of himself—that he might sacrifice dinner with the family, and sleep, for his work.

> F: *. . .And work happens not just at work hours, but there's a lot of late nights when I'm here in our study typing away, you know, on my own and stuff like that.*

Tom grew up in a family that was not at all focused on engaged family practices: a legacy that he was trying to flee from and reshape in his own family. He related a long, poignant story of his memories of a disengaged family life. Much was at stake for him in the way he took up being a father and a member of his family of progeny, yet he understood that part of his family legacy was deeply embedded and embodied in the way he took up his work outside of the family. This created conflicts for him and his family, which he and they struggled with in shaping their family life and certain family practices.

In contrast to the Brannons, where family dinnertime was taken for granted, dinnertime with the whole Switzer family present was often a source of conflict and took a concerted effort to schedule.

> **F:** *But yeah, it seems like with so many things going on, it's hard for us to just do things together and we actually . . . have sort of arguments about us not being able to do that. So one of the big issues in my life is trying to make sure I don't get too wrapped up in work so that I can actually come home at a reasonable time. So one of the reasons that Friday is a good night for you to come over and see us is like this is family night which means one of the nights I'm supposed to be home by 6:00 and we have to make a big production of it.*
>
> **I:** *So a Friday evening is a designated Friday, uh. . . .*
>
> **M:** *Family night.*
>
> **I:** *Sort of like a rule.*
>
> **M:** *Right, and the big part of that rule is that Tom will be home for dinner. . . . Because usually he's not unless something special's happening. Well, he's home on Wednesday nights too but that's because I go to school. So he's home for me to be gone for us not to pay a baby sitter.*

The ritual gathering and sharing time that included all family members was understood as important to their family life, but it was not a practice that the family was resolved to do on a nightly basis. Rather, it was reserved as an occasional practice. The regular nightly routine was that Mary and the two children, Eric (age 9) and Amy (age 7), ate dinner together.

For the Switzers, sometimes staying at home for dinner was considered a distraction to the family's gathering to share a meal, or to finding time when the whole family could be together because everyone was involved in individual pursuits, such as work, house chores, play, and other activities.

> **M:** *Well, the other thing that—I think that it's a valid one, that we go out to eat. That's recreational. It's eating, but it's a leisurely thing because nobody here is having to work for it and prepare it and cook it and all that. And that probably going out, being in the car to go to a restaurant, sitting together at a restaurant and talking or joking around, is something we're more likely to all four get together to do than go for a walk because somebody's somewhere else, like Amy was at the last one. And somebody else doesn't want to go, or Tom or I can't both go, so one of us takes the—I'll be more likely to take the kids with me on a walk than have all four of us go. Tom's less likely to want to go. And uh, so it's much more likely that we would go out to a restaurant to have a meal.*

Going out for a meal focused the family as a whole group—a time when they could be more attentive to each other for several hours. In this sense, the family's shared life benefited from the commodification of food in the form of dining out.

> **I:** *So can you think of ways that you feel that this involves family health and/or family member health?*
>
> **M:** *Well, they don't have to eat my cooking [laughter]. That's probably good for them once in a while. They're more likely to have a variety of things to choose from that maybe I don't cook. Like we're going to go out for seafood for Eric's birthday. I'm not a seafood cook at all. I don't think I'm skilled at it. So they can try different things that they wouldn't normally get at home. And it's good for our family health to be out together, you know, just, not physical as much as just our emotional well-being.*
>
> **I:** *Being together as a family.*
>
> **F:** *Yeah, to be together and do something different. Uh, to get out of the house and move away from a regular environment where there aren't all the distractions and all that.*

Going out to a restaurant provided everybody with a respite from chores and other distractions. It even provided a learning experience for the children. For instance, on one Sunday dinner outing, the family ate at a crêpe restaurant, and the children got to watch their crêpes being made. On these occasions when the children could choose from a menu, Mary got a break from dealing with their picky eating habits and the hassles that frequently accompanied her encouraging healthy food choices.

> **M:** *I wish the kids would eat a more balanced diet. That, I mean, when I talk about eating well, it's very easy, it's much easier for me to regulate my own intake than the kids because they're so picky, and they don't . . .like to eat, no, neither of them like the same thing and neither of them are very big on vegetables. And . . . they both love junk food and snacks, and it's hard to uh, do the food wars. We get into food wars more than I'd like.*

Mary, who has had weight concerns since adolescence, was on a weight loss–maintenance program and therefore, particularly sensitive to her own nutritional needs and aware of what her family needs. It was more difficult, then, for her to deal with her children's food likes and dislikes. Family dinnertime often presented other conflicts in the family. As was true in the Brannon family, the mother works to put a nutritious meal on the table, but she is not always able to satisfy all the family members' preferences and still prepare what she understands to be a well-balanced meal. The Switzers found that going out to dinner on occasion helped provide relief from the "food wars" and broadened the children's repertoire of foods they would taste and enjoy.

Although the Switzer family preserved dinnertime as an important family ritual, it only occurred as an all-family event through special occasions, or through special efforts to work around individual family members' pursuits, especially the father's work. Dinnertime for the Switzers was not embraced as a powerful and necessary ritual for what it means to be a healthy family and as positive for individual family members (i.e., what it means to be a "good" teenager) as it was in the Brannon family. Nonetheless, it was important for them that the father made the effort to participate in family dinner. If not, he ran the risk of extending a pattern for his children that was propagated by his own parents—that work is a more important commitment of his time than are his wife and children.

The Browns: Dinnertime as a Disengaged Activity

In the final exemplar, I describe how dinnertime for the Brown family (Rob, the father; Susan, the mother; and sons, 10-year-old John, and 4-year-old Bobby) was a threatened family practice: That is, it had become a disengaged activity for the family. Family dinnertime and other meals were not rituals of gathering and sharing for the Brown family to be relished and enjoyed. Rather, meals were obligatory activities steeped in dissatisfaction for the family, especially the parents. Breakfast, according to Susan, was a real "hodge podge, hit and miss, whatever's available—whatever you have time to fix, that's what you get." Dinner was no more satisfying for the family although Rob fantasized about how it might be a different and richer practice for the family.

> **F:** *I saw on TV some people get up in the morning and fix breakfast and sit down at a dining room table and eat breakfast together. I've never actually seen anyone do that, but I've heard that people do that. [laughs] We've been thinking maybe we should make a greater effort to sit down to dinner together because we don't do that as often as we like. Sometimes we think about it.*

Instead, the dinner ritual was described as a bad habit; rather than being comforting to the family sense of well-being, it was dis-comforting:

> **F:** *One of the things that I identified that need . . . could use changing in our lifestyle, which I've been unwilling to do, is like most Americans we're dominated by television. And uh it's easy to fix dinner, serve it, and we all go watch a television show. You know, whatever one we like at that particular time. And um, certainly that's what the kids want to do. And Susan and I haven't objected to that. . . . So I don't think that's the best family atmosphere, but it is like an addiction. And it's. . . . We're always together. But uh, watching TV.*
>
> **I:** *So your family dinnertime is really eating dinner and watching TV together. . . . So it's not like you're not together for your family dinnertime.*
>
> **F:** *Right. But it's not like we're interacting because we're watching TV.*

References to "an addiction" frequently came up in conversation with this couple, especially in relationship to eating habits. According to Rob, the family was addicted to watching television while they ate dinner. His rationale for an activity that he saw as deleterious to their family life was it was "easy," suggesting that the practice was a way of avoiding conflict even as it sometimes created it. Perhaps their dinnertime ritual of watching television is a way for family members to avoid engaging in conversation that may raise uncomfortable issues for them, allowing them to distance themselves from each other. Watching television together constitutes an impoverished form of gathering in which they remain individual viewers absorbed in their own worlds, rather than participants actively shaping a social space that acknowledges them as a family gathering, sharing and giving recognition to one another. However, this family does not seem to be able to muster the commitment and resoluteness to change.

The Brown family struggles with a dilemma that many American families confront. Both parents work, and often different hours of the day. Family members are often off in four different directions.

> **F:** *So and that will be for the whole semester [laughs] so it'll be that way. I won't be working every night. Sometimes I'll be out working. Typically Susan picks up the kids because she gets off work at 4:00, and I get off at 5:00 and work farther away. So there are sometimes two nights in a week where I'll pick them up because she's got something that she's doing, either work or internship or whatever. So . . . but most of the time she picks them up and then I get home about 6:00 or so, and we either go for some kind of fast food dinner or Susan fixes dinner. But uh one of our problems is getting home kind of late. . . . If I get home at 6:00 early, that's good. Any more. So uh. . . . But there are a couple of days when I leave work on time or early and*

> *get here and I pick up the kids because Susan is doing something in the evening. So sometimes the opposite of our morning schedule.*
>
> **M:** *It often seems like a relay race.*
>
> **F:** *Yeah.*

In the evening, after the family was gathered together at home—provided that either Susan or Rob was not working—Susan was often exhausted from a day of work, and fast food or something quick was all she was up to for the dinner meal.

> **M:** *And I'm not real domestic. I mean I try to keep the house as clean as I can. But I don't like to cook that much because I don't. . . . I don't like the idea of spending an hour or two hours in the kitchen after working all day. I'd rather uh (pause) have something really quick so that we can spend time—Rob and John are into* Star Trek, *so we watch that, or, you know, helping John with his homework.*

Susan was the main preparer of the dinner meal in the family. Despite the fact that she worked, she still came home to the second shift. She wished that she could be more organized and prepare some meals ahead of time on the weekends, but the thought of spending the weekends that way was almost as abhorrent as spending the time in the evenings to fix meals. Better yet, she "would like Rob to share the cooking more . . . and John, too." On occasion, Rob would cook, especially if Susan went out on strike.

> **M:** *Rob cooks when he wants to or if I absolutely refuse to. Sometimes I'll just come home and say I'm not cooking anything. Um. . . . One weekend—when I work on the weekends—usually the weekends aren't that difficult where I work—but this one particular weekend it was so . . . we had a bad day . . . I'm not sure when it was. Remember that day I came home and you'd made your chicken broccoli, and I came home and I got to lay on the sofa [Rob chuckles softly], and he fixed chicken and broccoli, and he made . . .what'd you, and you made uh, I don't know, you really did it up good [chuckles along with Rob].*

Susan indicates that Rob preparing a nice dinner for the family is a real gift, but in reality, she would find her tasks more satisfactory if there were a routinely shared effort by the whole family. Rob rationalizes why the family seems so stuck in a frustrating pattern in their life and evening routine:

> F: *Organization and planning everything out in advance has never been my strongest suit. I have struggled with disorganization. I'm the idea person. I'm not the detail person. [interviewer laughed] And um, you know, complete organization would help with all these things. Say O.K., what do we need for the weekend—go to the grocery store and buy it all. You know, that's not what we do. That's not the way we live our lives. But um, there was one other point about what gets in the way of our time. Like many people that commute here, it hurts us a lot. . . . So that uh eats up a lot of time for us even though it's not nearly what a lot of people have. [laughs] . . . But the organization is uh something that would improve planning all these things out, but uh it's like a deficit. So we have a time deficit so taking the time to plan everything out is something we haven't invested in because we feel we never have the time to even do that. So that would be a solution.*

The pervasiveness of technology is subtly at work in this family. On the one hand, it enables them to live far from work, but commuting takes time they might otherwise have to spend together as a family. Technology at many levels (automobiles, television, computers) shapes their understanding of what it means to be a family gathering and sharing—an understanding that is impoverished and shallow in the way that it distracts the family from sharing their life together at a more meaningful level.

Susan complained that "having free time to just sit down and talk, that's sort of a rarity in this house." Family time seemed scattered.

> M: *There's no consistency. There's no rhyme or reason to anything. It's just hit and miss. . . . Half hour here, an hour there. And so no, I don't like that. I wish that— and I think that we need to . . . somehow have more time.*

Time is a commodity for this family, and it is in short supply. The family was not very creative in arranging satisfying family shared time in their daily routines, rituals, and practices. Rather, they are stuck in a pattern of being conflicted and unfulfilled about the way their lives are going for them. They understand satisfying family time as something that needs to occur separate from daily routine of family and home maintenance and sustenance, rather than being integral to those daily activities and routines.

The Brown family, like all of us in contemporary Western life, is embedded in technological self-understandings that are played out in our everyday life in different ways. For the Browns, food is understood as something to be produced in an efficient manner or as a product for consumption (or conspicuous consumption, in the case of overeating). The family meal shared around the table as an engaged and attentive practice is being replaced by disengaged and distracted activity as they resort to fast foods or quick meals of processed and prepackaged food consumed in front of the television. Still, the parents talk wistfully about recapturing the engaged practice of dinner around the dining room table as a family sharing in their life together. The possibilities of recapturing this nearly lost practice will require the Browns to make choices between commitment and attention to family life or continuing in their often disengaged and distracted life. It is possible that, like the Switzers, they could start out by setting aside one or two evenings per week where they commit to a family night. In this way, they could actually experience the difference it might make to their family, rather than just "sometimes [thinking] about it." This may require some risk taking for the family to overcome what distances them from each other and prevents them from engaging in richer family gathering practices.

SUMMARY

Dinnertime, as a family gathering practice, differed in the three families in this study. Each family had a distinct way of taking up dinnertime as routine and ritual. Each family stands as an exemplar of ways to balance the traditional gathering practice of the evening meal with competing individualism and technological self-understandings that are intermingled with shared family life:

- The Brannons, who cling to dinnertime as paradigmatic of the healthy family past, present, and for future possibilities

- The Switzers, for whom dinner is important to family health as an occasional all family ritual that is preserved through a concerted effort

- The Browns, for whom dinner has become an impoverished and distracted activity consuming food in front of the television, but for whom the tradition of a shared and attentive family meal is held out as a possibility to enrich their family life

For each family, there is the shared background meaning of the good in the gathering practice of family mealtime, and this practice is understood as constitutive to a healthy shared family life. Although the practice may be increasingly marginalized in our society, these families illustrate the possibility for preserving or reviving this family practice. In fact, there are positive ways that technology helps the families to preserve dinnertime as a time when they can sit down at the end of the day and share their life together, even though it may mean a commodified version of what might have taken hours to prepare from scratch. The world of these families is often rapid paced, with parents commuting to high-intensity jobs. Consequently, it often takes a special commitment to preserve this and other family gathering practices. Sometimes, it may mean modifying the ritual by going out as a family for a meal at a restaurant, or picking up something ready-made at the store. It is possible for the family to preserve the sacred aspect of this ritual through this type of a modification. For other families, it may mean creating a special week-end breakfast ritual where the family gathers and shares in a celebratory fashion. However they are preserved, dinnertime and other mealtimes as gathering practices remain meaningful for families, nourishing their bodies as well as their shared family life.

References

Bellah, R. N., Madsen, R., Sullivan, W. M., Swidler, A., & Tipton, S.M. (1991). *The good society.* New York: Vintage Books.

Benjamin, J. (1988). *The bonds of love.* New York: Pantheon Books.

Benner, P. (1985). Quality of life: Phenomenological perspective on explanation, prediction and understanding in nursing science. *Advances in Nursing Science, 8*(1), 1-14.

Benner, P. (1994). The tradition and skill of interpretive phenomenology in studying health, illness and caring practices. In P. Benner (Ed.), *Interpretive phenomenology: Embodiment, caring, and ethics in health and illness* (pp. 99-127). Thousand Oaks, CA: Sage.

Borgmann, A. (1984). *Technology and the character of contemporary life.* Chicago: University of Chicago Press.

Bossard, J. H. S., & Boll, E. S. (1950). *Rituals in family living.* Philadelphia: University of Pennsylvania Press.

Boyce, W. T., Jensen, E. W., James, S. A., & Peacock, J. L. (1983). The family routines inventory: Theoretical origins. *Social Science and Medicine, 17*(4), 193-200.

Chesla, C. A. (1988). *Parent's caring practices and coping with schizophrenic offspring, an interpretive study.* Unpublished doctoral dissertation, University of California, San Francisco.

Chesla, C. A. (1995). Hermeneutic phenomenology in approach to understanding families. *Journal of Family Nursing, 1*(1), 68-78.

DeVault, M. L. (1987). Doing housework: Feeding and family life. In N. Gerstel & H. E. Gross (Eds.), *Families and work* (pp. 178-191). Philadelphia: Temple University Press.

Heidegger, M. (1962). *Being and time.* (J. Macquerrie & E. Robinson, Trans.). New York: Harper & Row. (Original work published 1927).

Kantor, D., & Lehr, W. (1975). *Inside the family.* San Francisco: Jossey-Bass.

Leonard, V. W. (1989). Heideggerean phenomenological perspective on the concept of the person. *Advances in Nursing Science, 11*(4), 40-55.

MacIntyre, A. (1984). *After virtue* (2nd ed.). Notre Dame: University of Notre Dame Press.

Plager, K. A. (1995). *Practical well-being in families with school-age children: An interpretive study.* Unpublished doctoral dissertation, University of California, San Francisco.

Plager, K. A. (1999). Understanding family legacy in family health concerns. *Journal of Family Nursing, 5*(1), 51-71.

Reiss, D. (1981). *The family's construction of reality.* Cambridge, MA: Harvard University Press.

Sandelowski, M. (1986). The problem of rigor in qualitative research. *Advances in Nursing Science, 8*(3), 27-37.

Taylor, C. (1991). *The ethics of authenticity.* Cambridge, MA: Harvard University Press.

Taylor, C. (1994). The politics of recognition. In A. Gutman (Ed.), *Multiculturalism, examining the politics of recognition* (pp. 25-73). Princeton, NJ: Princeton University Press.

Wolin, S. J., & Bennett, L. A. (1984). Family rituals. *Family Process, 23,* 401-420.

CHAPTER 11

Listening with Care to Teen Mothers and Their Families

LEE SMITHBATTLE

INTRODUCTION

In the late 1970s, I began visiting pregnant and parenting teens as a pubic health nurse in the Midwestern United States. Over the next 10 years, I learned first-hand of the wide gulf between the perspectives of teen mothers on being a parent and the clinical and scientific literature on early childbearing. This gulf has inspired a research program focused on understanding the meanings, concerns, caregiving practices, challenges, and possibilities experienced by teen mothers in family and community contexts. In this chapter, I review the findings from a longitudinal panel study that has followed a sample of teen mothers and their families every 4 years for 16 years. Each wave of the study was based on interpretive phenomenology. The findings challenge the scientific-clinical gaze and call for clinical practices and U.S. social policies that support teen mothers' growth in agency and purpose while also addressing the long-term adversities and stereotypes that place limits on becoming a coherent self and responsive parent. Pseudonyms are used throughout this chapter.

> *People would look at us as though we were scum of the earth. . . . Little did they know, my husband's working one or two jobs, we have our own home, our kids are not out breaking any laws. But they didn't care about that. They just had a lot of negative and mean things to say. (Cary, 35-year-old mother of four, who gave birth to her first child at age 17)*

THE RISE OF THE SCIENTIFIC GAZE ON TEENAGE CHILDBEARING

Beginning in the 1970s, teenage childbearing became the focus of intense scientific scrutiny, extensive social policy debates, and negative media coverage. The social ostracism that young mothers like Cary experienced reflected the growing power of the scientific paradigm to define teen mothering as a social-technical problem (Arney & Bergen, 1984). Early studies contributed to the scientific gaze by dissecting teen mothers' lives and parenting practices and imposing analytic frameworks and methodological screens that eliminate meaning and context (SmithBattle, 1994, 1995). Klein (1978) exemplified the results of this approach when he described teen mothering as a "syndrome," which includes ". . . failure to fulfill the functions of adolescence, failure to remain in school, failure to limit family size, failure to establish a vocation and be self-supporting, failure to have healthy infants, and failure to have children who reach their potential in life" (p. 1151-1152).

Many early studies on teen mothering supported this claim (Hayes, 1987). Although researchers were often careful to point out the methodological limitations of their work, an influential report by the National Research Council of the National Academy of Sciences determined that teen mothers "risked" their own futures and the health and development of their children (Hayes, 1987). The discovery of teen mothers' risks, deficits, and failures was no surprise because theories presumed teen mothers' deviance and overshadowed data that suggested otherwise (Furstenberg, 2002).

In the late 1970s, just as the scientific gaze was establishing an objective "truth" of teen mothering, I began visiting pregnant and postpartum women in their homes as part of a nurse-managed perinatal program for low-income families without health insurance. Employed as a public health nurse by a semi-rural health department in the Midwest, I made home visits before and after the women gave birth to promote maternal-child health and well-being. Many of the women I visited were teenagers. These families introduced me to a social landscape that was invisible to many Americans. This was *The Other America* described by Harrington in his 1962 book of the same title. Driving into neighborhoods and sitting around kitchen tables with families, I learned about lifeworlds quite different from my family's working-class background. The pregnant teens on my caseload had not planned to become pregnant, but unlike their counterparts of the 1950s and 1960s, they were now more likely to remain single and less likely to enter "shotgun" marriages or surrender their children for adoption (Fessler, 2006; Rains, 1971).

With or without marriage, mothering remained an important rite of passage to adulthood for girls with few educational or vocational options. As the rates of single motherhood increased among teens, the lives of their parents (hereafter referred to as "grandparents") were also altered as they faced the initial disappointment over a teenage daughter's pregnancy and the demands and challenges of caring for a teen mother and her child. But as I learned, neither grandparents nor teens on my caseload were aware of or even concerned about the risks of teen mothering that were enumerated by social scientists, and the losses that teens and families did describe were seen as short-term rather than long-term (Henderson, 1980). Their experiential understanding of teen mothering seemed far removed from the public and scientific discourse on teen mothers' failures and deficits.

My interest in teen mothers and their families was inspired by sitting around those kitchen tables more than 25 years ago. The home visits taught me invaluable lessons, none more important than the public health nursing (PHN) imperative "to begin with people as they are and the situation as it is." Sensitized to the wide gaps and contradictions between teen mothers' views and the professional-scientific discourse on teen mothering, I returned to graduate school to learn approaches that would not sacrifice teen mothers' meanings of pregnancy and parenting for theoretical, detached reasoning (SmithBattle, 2005).

Fully expecting to do a grounded theory study, I enrolled in the doctoral program at the University of California at San Francisco (UCSF) where Anselm Strauss and Leonard Schatzman had established a mecca for grounded theory. I could hardly believe my good fortune when I learned that the UCSF School of Nursing was the home of two qualitative traditions. This was qualitative nirvana! Although grateful for the courses taught by Strauss and Schatzman, I was quickly drawn to the interpretive phenomenological tradition. Philosophers in this tradition (Dreyfus, 1991; Heidegger, 1927/1962; Merleau-Ponty, 1945/1962; Gadamer, 1965/1975; Taylor, 1989, 1995) offered a persuasive account of how scientific practices separate the mind from the body and the person from the world. Their critique of realist ontology, which posits a reality separate from our practical understanding, helped me appreciate the web of scientific assumptions and procedures that silence and de-world teen mothers (SmithBattle, 2009a). Heidegger's view of the person as "thrown" into the world, as always situated and involved in activities and relationships, dissolved the Cartesian division between thinking minds and material objects and provided the ontological background for exploring how teen mothers' possibilities and constraints were a holistic expression of personal, family, and cultural worlds. Equally important for a novice researcher like myself, Patricia Benner, Hubert Dreyfus, Jane Rubin, and Judith Wrubel exemplified the openness to dialog and careful listening that allow others (be it persons or texts) to be seen in their own terms. Their example and expertise would be crucial for understanding teen mothers' lives and parenting practices as a meaningful response to local worlds of shared meaning.

How little did I realize that Benner's mentorship would create a clearing for a multigenerational study that has now spanned 16 years. In this chapter, I review the study's key findings and integrate the results from another study on teen mothers' first postpartum year (SmithBattle, 2007a, 2007b). To set the stage, I briefly describe the sample and research procedures of the longitudinal study; readers are referred to other publications for more thorough descriptions (SmithBattle, 1995, 1996, 1997, 2000a, 2005, 2006; SmithBattle & Leonard, 1998, 2006).

LISTENING TO FAMILIES OVER TIME

When I entered the doctoral program at UCSF, family studies of teen mothers were rare. Because pregnant teens were remaining single and often residing with their parents after giving birth, I designed the dissertation study (Time 1) to examine how family meanings, concerns, relationships, and caregiving practices reciprocally shaped the teen mother's care of her infant. I also want to discover the possibilities, constraints, conflicts, and resources for becoming a teen mother (SmithBattle, 1992).

These were quickly supplemented by another line of inquiry that surfaced in analyzing the teens' interviews:

- How did mothering alter the teen's sense of self and future?

- Did teen mothers understand their lives as restricted and foreclosed by mothering, as the clinical and research literature suggested?

- Or did their narratives reveal possibilities as well as constraints for becoming a parent and leading a meaningful life?

These questions were framed by my interest in problematizing the assumptions about early childbearing and improving our clinical understanding of what fosters or undermines the teen's transition to mothering.

Families were recruited from programs serving teen mothers in the San Francisco Bay Area. Mothers were eligible if they were non-Latina Black or Caucasian, younger than 19 years of age at delivery, and residing with a parent or surrogate parent at the time of giving birth to a first-born, healthy infant. To capture family meanings, relationships, and practices, a grandparent of the teen mother's child also had to agree to participate. After the teen mother and a grandparent agreed, the teen mother's partner was invited to participate with her permission.

The sample at Time 1 included 16 families and 39 participants (16 teen mothers, 19 grandparents, 3 partners of the mothers, and 1 sibling of the teen mother). Nine families were Caucasian, and seven families were Black. One family included a biracial teen mother, who had been adopted at birth. Families were diverse with respect to grandparents' educational levels, socioeconomic status (SES), and family structure. Household income ranged from a low of $10,800 for a family of five to a high of $70,000 for a family of four. Some families were very poor and lived in households that included three to four generations, and other families were middle class and nuclear in structure.

Families were enrolled in the first wave of the study after the teen's infant reached 8 to 10 months of age. I conducted a series of monthly family and individual semi-structured interviews over a three-to-five month period to identify coping practices and caregiving patterns. I also elicited the family's history from the grandparents. Monthly interviews were supplemented with four to six hours of monthly participant observations with each family in order to observe practices that would be difficult to report in an interview. Spending time with families in this way made it possible to notice emotional responses to events large and small, the comings and goings of family members, their involvement in the care of the baby, and the infant's reactions to family members. These sessions brought attention to how infant caregiving practices by the teens and family members played out in response to family routines and individual schedules such as working, going to school, or caring for other children. Data from Time 1 therefore included in-depth individual and family interviews and detailed field notes.

I returned to reinterview families every four years: 1993 (Time 2), 1997 (Time 3), 2001 (Time 4), and 2005 (Time 5). In follow-up studies, I interviewed mothers (and partners) twice, about one month apart, and grandparents once. Parents and grandparents were asked to describe meaningful and difficult episodes in being a parent or grandparent (Coping Interview). They were also asked to recall significant events that had occurred since the previous study (Life History Review).

I also asked mothers (and partners) to describe the oldest child, his or her interests, activities, schooling, peers, and any concerns they had about the child. At the second session with parents, I conducted another Coping Interview and then asked them (with their children whenever possible) to describe their family routines (Family Routines Interview). All studies were approved by a human subjects committee that reviews research protocols for the protection of human subjects.

At Time 4, I included the teen mothers' first-born children for the first time. They were infants when I began the study, but by Time 4, they were 12 to 13 years of age and attending 5th or 6th grade. Adding the children to the fourth wave of the study, I reasoned, would provide an opportunity to more fully examine family caregiving practices and relationships as they unfolded over time with accounts from grandparents, parents, and children. I was also keen on including children in future studies to see whether their lives supported the conventional wisdom that teen mothers' offspring are at high risk for educational failure, substance abuse, and early pregnancies. Of the 11 families who participated at Time 4, 6 children agreed to be interviewed. Four years later, the Time 5 study included 8 children (4 girls and 4 boys) who were 15 to 17 years of age, the approximate age at which I had first interviewed their mothers.

I began the children's private interview at Time 4 by asking them to tell me about the photos they had taken with disposable cameras that I provided one month earlier. At Time 5, I brought matted pictures of diverse subjects (e.g., nature scenes, people involved in activities, art objects) and asked children to select and talk about those pictures that "represented something about themselves." Beginning the children's interviews with photos at Time 4 and self-selected pictures at Time 5 provided an opening for probing about their activities, interests, and connections to family, peers, and school.

All interviews were tape-recorded, professionally transcribed, and corrected for accuracy. In analyzing the data from each time period, I listened carefully for meanings of the self, future, and parenting; commonalities and differences in teens' and grandparents' accounts of what was going well and poorly in caring for the teen's child; and turning points and continuities in identities, relationships, and caregiving practices. These data, along with my interpretive commentary, were archived in Interpretive Profiles that I created for each family at each time period.

Thankfully, I did not have to face the limits of my own understanding alone (SmithBattle, 1992). For the Time 1 study, Benner encouraged me to notice aspects of the text that I would have otherwise missed. Leonard (1993, 1994), who was interviewing older first-time mothers with career commitments at the same time that I was interviewing teen mothers, also provided valuable feedback as we immersed ourselves in our respective data sets. Because both groups of mothers differed by age and social location, our data offered sharp contrasts in how mothers were "thrown" into the world and were working out the constraints and possibilities of mothering.

As the teen mothering study took on a life of its own, Leonard continued to read selected interviews at each wave of the study. Her insights proved invaluable in confirming and refining interpretations as I compared cases and wrote research reports. On a few occasions, I also relied upon her knowledge of community resources for information to give to the families.

In spite of my efforts to maintain contact with participants, I have been unable to locate several families. In addition, two couples declined to participate at different times, and two grandparents have died. Because of the longitudinal design and the deep engagement required of interpretive research, losing participants for whatever reason is difficult and leaves me wondering about their fate. In comparing the baseline characteristics of the families at Times 1 and 4, the sample did not appear to have changed appreciably regarding the relative economic advantage or disadvantage of families (SmithBattle, 2005). In spite of attrition, 10 families and 28 family members participated at Time 5, including 10 mothers, 1 partner, 9 grandparents, and 8 first-born children. Mothers ranged in age from 31 to 35 years, and their first-born children were 15 to 17 years old.

RISKING THE FUTURE? TEEN MOTHERS' UNFOLDING SENSE OF SELF AND FUTURE

Findings from Time 1 revealed what the scientific gaze routinely overlooks: Teen mothering is an intelligible response to a lived world, and mothering provides a corrective experience for some teens. Here, I summarize the three patterns in how mothers understood the self and future at 1-year postpartum, and how these patterns configured their lives over time. One group of teen mothers was transformed by the world of mothering. In spite of childhood adversities and ongoing hardships, these teens made developmental gains and gained a sense of future and direction by reorganizing their lives around mothering. These teens exemplified the pattern of "inventing a future from an impoverished past." A second group of teens were not transformed by mothering. Their aspirations to improve their lives were continuously compromised by a capricious and oppressive social world. These teen mothers "inherited a diminished future." A third group of teens "pressed into an open future." These teens (and their families) held higher expectations for a promising future than the first two groups of teens. Their pre-pregnancy aspirations to finish high school and then to work or attend college were safeguarded by the emotional and financial support of their families and the availability of community resources such as good schools and subsidized day care. As I describe below, each of these patterns challenged the scientific gaze and the pervasive belief that mothering jeopardizes the futures of U.S. teens.

Inventing a Future from an Impoverished Past

Although the majority of the teens in the study had drifted into pregnancy from a background of childhood adversities, the group of teens who invented a future from an impoverished past described mothering as a fresh start—a catalyst for gaining responsibility and a sense of direction. Mothering provided a moral ground that anchored and reorganized their lives, and provided meaning, identity, and purpose (SmithBattle, 1994, 1995). LaKeisha, for example, had dropped out of high school prior to her pregnancy and described her interests in terms of "getting the newest clothes, going to parties, just hanging out or running the streets, trying to find boys." Her world changed with mothering:

> "I want to set a good example for my son so that he can grow up to be somebody."

L: *That's not important no more. . . . Now that I am a mother, I care about what I be in the future. Before I just wanted to live, day by day, and didn't worry about whatever happens in the future, it would just happen. Now I think ahead of time.*

LS: *Can you give me an example?*

L: *School. I really wasn't interested in school. I didn't like it. Now I'm willing to go and try to graduate. . . . School's more important now. Besides my son, school is next.*

LS: *Was it hard to hard to make this change?*

L: *I just changed slowly. Didn't realize I wasn't doing those things no more.*

"I wanna be a good mother" and "I wanna have a good future" were defining features of these mothers' stories. Their new aspirations revealed and contributed to a growing sense of self and future. They reported reinvesting in school; abstaining from cigarettes, drugs, or alcohol; becoming more patient; and avoiding risky situations such as fighting with peers or shoplifting. They also began to reevaluate their friends and their own behavior by new standards that were consistent with their vision of being good parents and examples for their children. As LaKeisha said, "I want to set a good example for my son so that he can grow up to be somebody." Completing high school was seen by these teens as the first step to additional schooling or job prospects to support their children (SmithBattle, 2007a). They also rejected welfare as a long-term resource because of the poor example it would set for their children.

Rather than "risking the future," mothering propelled these teens into a more promising future. Tammy put it even more bluntly, "I believe being a mother saved my life." Others agreed that the responsibilities of mothering placed their lives on a more meaningful path. Loving a child provided a moral compass that righted their course and helped them to imagine and create a better life for themselves and their children. These mothers were no longer adrift.

Participating partners, who were a few years older than the mothers, reported similar life-changing experiences. Tim said that fathering changed his life "360 degrees around." After he became a father, he found stable work to support his family and avoided the fate of his high school friends who became involved in drugs and crime (SmithBattle, 1992, 2008).

How did women in this group fare over time? Follow-up studies have shown that the existential possibilities these women first found in mothering were sustained over time and contributed to developmental gains in emotional responsiveness and in family caregiving practices. They gained a moral voice, a sense of agency, and a long-term perspective from mothering; and these gains extended into the domains of paid or volunteer work and adult love (SmithBattle, 2005). In spite of challenges and occasional setbacks, mothering provided a "narrative backbone" that contributed to a coherent life story.

Inheriting a Diminished Future

A second group of teens had also drifted into pregnancy, but these teens inherited a diminished future that was unaltered by mothering. Their backgrounds revealed more chaos, despair, and emotional voids than the first group of teens. They recalled few, if any, positive memories from childhood, and their current situations provided little emotional validation or support that might correct for grim childhoods. Compared with the first group of teens, these teens were more likely to have desired children from very young ages to compensate for emotional absences. Mothering did not transform their sense of self or future but contributed to the despair that prefigured the pregnancy (SmithBattle, 1993, 1995). These mothers continued to drift through the first-year postpartum.

Tamika was a paradigm of this second pattern. She began her first interview at Time 1 with a stark description of being:

> . . . *a wild person, always hanging out, running here, running there. Drinkin'.* (SmithBattle, 1993, p. 242)

Tamika's mother stated bluntly that her two oldest children, including Tamika, were "lost, that they won't survive" (SmithBattle, 1993, p. 239). In surveying her community where crime and drugs were rampant, and graduation rates from high school were dismally low, this grandmother noted that "the future stops dead at adolescence" (SmithBattle, 1995, p. 26). Tamika's interviews and actions validated her mother's bleak assessment. She remained wild and rudderless, often placing herself or her baby in dangerous situations. Her hopelessness reflected the lack of possibilities and social exclusion (SmithBattle, 1995, p. 26):

> **LS:** *What do you hope for tomorrow?*
>
> **T:** *I guess just for my baby to live. . . . I guess just for her to wake up in the morning.*
>
> **LS:** *What about for yourself? Is there anything you hope for yourself?*
>
> **T:** *Not really.*

Tamika's story revealed a highly predetermined situation and a legacy of hopelessness that silenced the self and eroded the moral agency to act on her own behalf or on behalf of her child. This theme persisted 4 years later when her efforts to extricate herself from a dangerous social world were consistently undermined, for example, when her brother "loaned" her car to drug dealers to maintain his drug habit (SmithBattle & Leonard, 1998). When the police called Tamika to inform her that they found her stolen car and that a gang member had been killed in it during a gang shootout, she abandoned the vehicle rather than risk being the target of a revenge killing. Tamika's seeming passivity and resignation was a tailored fit to a capricious social world.

The thin capacity for relationship and emotional responsiveness to the baby that I observed among this group of teens reflected an embodied response to a leveled world. Mothering did not provide a fresh start or a new direction but entailed overwhelming constraints that reinforced prior feelings of rejection and despair. Because these mothers often relied heavily upon their families for survival and childcare, their attempts to flee or isolate themselves proved difficult or unworkable. Their stories revealed how oppressive situations and relationships eclipsed a sense of future, dampened the mother's moral voice, and thwarted their efforts to improve their situations (SmithBattle, 1995).

> **"I thought teen moms were stupid before I became one."**

One might suppose that this group of teens confirms the "risking the future" discourse on teen mothers, but this conclusion fails to appreciate how the futures of these teens were foreclosed *before* becoming pregnant. In follow-up studies, these women continued to drift through their 20s and early 30s. They moved passively through life experiences with little forethought, reflection, or imagination (SmithBattle, 2005). Their stories depicted a sense of hopelessness and the self-understanding that they could do little to influence events and project themselves into the future. Mothering continued to show up as a source of relentless conflicts and vexing frustrations. At Time 5, the two women in this group had experienced partner abuse and additional unplanned pregnancies, and relied heavily on their mothers for parenting their children. Compared with the first group, they lacked the narrative structure that gives life meaning and direction. They continued to experience the future as closed (SmithBattle, 2006).

Pressing into an Open Future

A third group of teen mothers pressed into an open future at Time 1. Unlike the first two groups, these teens imagined a promising future *before* becoming pregnant. They had no intentions of becoming pregnant as a teen and expected to graduate from high school and then attend college or work. One teen said, "I thought teen moms were stupid before I became one." Their coping stories did not focus on overcoming difficult pasts. Mothering nevertheless strengthened their focus on the future as they aspired to support themselves and their child. These teens would seem to have the most to lose from an unintended pregnancy, but their futures remained open by their family's emotional and financial support and by the greater availability of community resources, such as good schools, college advising, and subsidized day care (SmithBattle, 1995).

To summarize, all three groups of teens challenged the scientific gaze that early mothering "risks the future." For the first group, mothering was a corrective experience that contributed to the development of a coherent sense of self and future. These mothers and their partners described more gains than losses as young parents. Loving a baby became a *reason* for planning the future and provided a "narrative spine" for their unfolding lives, sometimes against great odds. The lives of the second group were not risked by mothering but by existential despair, oppression, and danger. These mothers did not describe gaining ground as a self or mother. Their thin sense of agency reflected longstanding disconnections and a capricious or dangerous social world. The goals of mothers in the third group were never in doubt or challenged by the pregnancy. They achieved personal goals by weaving complex schedules together with the help of family and community resources. These patterns highlighted how mothering requires a coherent social world and relationships that foster a sense of self and future.

FAMILY RELATIONSHIPS AND CAREGIVING PRACTICES AT TIME 1

A second aim of the Time 1 study was to examine how family relationships and caregiving practices reciprocally shaped the young mother's coping and care of her baby. In the first study, two patterns of family caregiving were identified by closely examining the coping narratives of teen mothers and grandparents (SmithBattle, 1996). In *adversarial caregiving*, grandparents leaped in and took over the care of the teen's infant. Their over-involvement in the care of the baby thwarted the development of maternal skill and the maternal-child relationship. In the most extreme cases, grandparents appraised themselves as the parents of the teen's baby, perpetuating long-standing family problems and mistrust. Frozen in past relationships, these families experienced intense competition over "Whose baby is this?" Power struggles were common and could easily escalate, as one grandparent said, into "World War III."

These grandparents reported histories of having been emotionally abandoned or abused as children. Married grandparents described longstanding marital problems. In Ann's case, her baby provided the glue that held her parent's tenuous marriage together. Even when Ann's brothers warned their parents that they were taking over and excluding Ann from the care of her baby, Ann's parents lacked the practical and relational skills to reset their course (Smith-Battle, 1996). Mothers like Ann were invalidated and excluded, and made statements like: "I can't do anything right," or "There are too many parents here." As grandparents took over infant care, mothers became more resentful and rebellious, giving more reason for grandparents to take over. Some teens withdrew from the care of the baby altogether, reinforcing the grandparents' convictions that their daughters were irresponsible mothers. Ann left home and conceived another pregnancy quickly to have a child of her own. Other mothers, like LaKeisha and Tammy, left home with their babies to escape conflict and to develop caregiving practices without family interference.

The second pattern of *responsive caregiving* involved grandparents who did not take over the infant's care but "leaped ahead" to support the teen's development as a mother (SmithBattle, 1996). In this family situation, grandparents provided an indispensable experiential cushion for the teen mother to learn her baby. Because they respected the teen's relationship to her baby and her ability to learn from experience, grandparents did not expect the teen to be completely independent or dependent upon them. Family practices of sharing infant care in a flexible manner and approaching conflicts through dialog supported a relatively smooth transition to mothering. Mothers said things like, "The help I get from my parents is neither too much or too little. It's just right." And grandparents appraised their daughters as devoted mothers.

Adversarial and responsive caregiving patterns revealed circular family interactions and relationships that organized teen mothers' possibilities and constraints for mothering (SmithBattle, 1996, 1997). As I learned in follow-up studies, these early patterns reflected family caregiving legacies, which mothers extended, revised, or rejected.

THE DEVELOPMENT OF FAMILY CAREGIVING LEGACIES

Family caregiving legacies emerged as a strong theme in shaping teen mothers' concerns and struggles in caring for their children in follow-up studies. Drawing on Heidegger's (1927/1962) understanding of temporality, and Plager's (1999) description of family legacies, family caregiving legacies showed up as the lived understandings of family care that are carried in memories, stories, emotional predispositions, relational skills, and family habits (SmithBattle, 2000a, 2006). According to interpretive scholars, our understanding of the past involves embodied meanings that shape our experience of the present and future (Benner & Wrubel, 1989; Leonard, 1994; Richardson, Fowers, & Guignon, 1999). Vogel (1994) elaborates:

> *History is not something over against a subject but is the lived context from out of which one's limited possibilities emerge. That history is personal does not mean that it is the product of an individual's meaning-constituting will. The individual is always already social and historical, yet free to thoughtfully respond to her heritage or to lose herself in it. (p. 50)*

We are always responding to our "thrownness" and to the multiple meanings available in our pasts. With respect to parenting, our understanding of how we were parented provides the resources and possibilities for the parents we can become. The longitudinal data revealed three patterns in how mothers responded to their pasts and, in particular, to their family caregiving legacies.

Elaborating a Positive Legacy

Mothers who appraised their parents as good parents took up parenting from a stable ground. They emulated their parents and relied on an experiential cushion of positive memories and experiences to respond to the particularity of their own child (SmithBattle, 2006, 2007b). Their coping stories did not focus on inventing parenting practices in opposition to their pasts.

Jenna was a paradigm of a teen mother who drew on positive memories from childhood and supportive relationships with both parents for extending and revising family caregiving legacies. When I asked Jenna, "Do you think you'll be like or unlike your mom as a parent?", her reply revealed an openness and resourceful response to the possibilities available in her legacy:

> *I think I'll be like her, but then not like her. . . . How should I say this? There's certain things that I'll be like her, but . . . I'll put a whole new spin on it, I think. [laughter] You know. It's like I can't really follow in her footsteps and be the mother exactly how she was, but I can only do my best to try and then, you know.* (SmithBattle, 2003a, p. 373-374)

Mothers who lacked positive caregiving legacies were more likely to reject the past and responded by either submitting to their family caregiving legacy or by doing things "different from the way I was raised." These patterns are described more fully in the following sections.

Losing Themselves in the Past

At Time 5, the two mothers with a thin sense of self and future submitted to the past. What set these women apart from the full sample was their stark assessment that parenting had *not* changed them as persons. One mother reported, somewhat wistfully, "I would like to say it has [changed me] but I don't think it has." Neither mother offered stories of reinventing themselves or of putting much effort into parenting, especially because grandparents early on in the child's life had leaped in and assumed many parenting responsibilities. From the outset, mothering did not sharpen their priorities or propel them into a new direction. Their limited engagement in mothering dampened their ability to act. Both women appropriated the past by losing themselves in it.

From her first set of interviews, Maya stood in the shadow of her mother, Vera. She consistently deferred to Vera, making comments like ". . . [my mother] reminds me of the things that I need to know" and "lets me know if I'm doing something wrong" (SmithBattle & Leonard, 2006, p. 355). Maya never expressed anger, regret, or disagreements with Vera until Time 5, when she offhandedly remarked that she wanted to avoid her mother's harsh parenting practices. Because she had rarely disclosed emotions or much about her childhood over the full study, I was even more surprised when she reported, in a tentative voice, that the interviews were the only arena for discussing her feelings.

While Maya had been voiceless over the full study, Meg became more cynical and angry with each follow up. Although she admitted having little recollection of her childhood, she described being hit by her mother up until she was 12 years of age. At Time 2, she related that she had hit her 4-year-old son hard enough to create a welt but resolved at that time to never hit her children again. She kept this pledge, but she also admitted at Time 5 that

> *I have an extremely short temper and an extremely verbally abusive mouth. And it's hard for me because I don't whip my kids. I know I don't have that shut off [valve]. If I whip them, it's not a spank, so I don't do it. But verbally it's no better. So I know that I need to find a happy medium. . . . I mean I'm not comfortable . . . a lot of my children's issues are my issues. There's no excuse but the environment that I'm in is a lot different. . . . I 100% believe . . . [that] you are products of your environment, without a doubt.*

Meg conveyed an inevitability about repeating the past. As her first-born son was about to become a teenager, she expected him to have a "bad attitude." She did not see herself as playing much of a role in the path he would take, conceding that "[because of the] things that I put my mom through, [his bad attitude] is just expected." Parenting increasingly receded as she emotionally withdrew from her older children and invested in work and other projects to escape conflicts at home. Because Meg's mother had also emotionally withdrawn from Meg's children by Time 5, there was very little center to hold the family together. Meg astutely commented, "There's a black cloud over this house constantly."

Responding Resourcefully to a Negative Caregiving Legacy

LaKeisha admitted that "it's hard to break the habits you're in" (SmithBattle, 2000a, p. 90). In spite of their shabby past, she and other women showed that repeating the past was not inevitable. These women shared strong, mostly negative memories of childhood that established clear landmarks and guidelines for how *not* to raise their own children:

> *When I was growing up, my mom was smoking, my sister, my brother, everybody. So when peer pressure came, I figured it's supposed to be like that, you know? I had to smoke or drink, it's a part of life. And I wanted my kids to feel that it's not a part of life. You don't have to. . . . That's what I end up telling them all the time.*

> *I'm kind of glad that I have a little insight [about my past] and . . . try to help [my kids] with difficulties because that was one of the things with my childhood. A lot of the things I notice of my childhood I try to or I have been doing the opposite. I didn't have hugs and kisses and sweet and nice words, so I try to give them everything that I was so desperately wanting as a child.*

Although grandparents' flawed practices established clear guidelines for what to avoid as parents, LaKeisha and other women also relied on trial and error; conscious deliberation;

positive memories from childhood; or corrective experiences with a therapist, partner, or others to alter their family legacies. LaKeisha drew on early positive memories with female kin to create loving relationships and family practices that were otherwise missing in her past. At Time 3, she recalled a pivotal experience with a beloved aunt (at age 3) for fueling the development of responsive practices with her young children:

> *What happened was my auntie showed me how [to bake cookies], and I tried before by myself a couple of times and they didn't taste right. But this time I had [my oldest son] read the directions. I explained to him what a teaspoon and what one cup was, and so he read the directions and [followed them] and then he gave it to [next child] to pour in the bowl. . . . So it was kind of a family thing. And then the cookies came out and they tasted good. And I really enjoyed that. I think [they] did too. . . . And they asked me the other day when I was going to make some more. So that made me feel good that I could do something that somebody liked. (SmithBattle, 2000a, p. 90)*

LaKeisha's attempts to repair the world were a fragile but notable accomplishment given the constraints in her past and current situation at Time 3 (SmithBattle, 2000a). By Time 5, her delicate attempts had developed into well-established practices and responsive relationships that supported her goals of creating "good" children and a family "team" (SmithBattle & Leonard, 2006). When she referred to her early childhood memories with her aunts again 8 years later at Time 5, I was curious to know how she evaluated their impact on her life. So I asked, "Do you think you draw on those experiences [with your aunts]?" She responded by recalling a recent experience with her own niece:

> *. . . [My niece] is the oldest of 6 girls and she has it kind of rough. I remember this one time she had spent the night and we had so much fun. We did our toenails and did our hair, and we took walks around the park and school and we talked about everything. And before she left, she was like, "I don't want to go." And I was like, "Yeah but we can do this again." "Yeah, but I don't want to go, I wish you were my mom." And right there I recall myself saying that to my auntie. So it kind of blew me back and I was like wow, it was a good feeling. It was a sad feeling when I thought about being in her shoes, but it was a good experience for me that I was able to make someone else feel like that. Because I think without that good, I could have been totally dark. I mean there is some dark sides in me but I think without that, I could've been totally dark.*

LaKeisha drew primarily on positive but sparse memories from childhood, and Tammy created a new caregiving tradition in opposition to her past by learning new relational skills from a longstanding relationship with a therapist. She described how embodied responses to harmful childhood experiences became available during moments in therapy for insight and correction (SmithBattle, 2006). That she has largely succeeded in coming to terms with her past and has created new family practices testifies to her gritty resolve to avoid what had been done to her:

> **T:** *I want to raise [my daughter] the way that I wish I had been raised [to have] the chance that I should have been given.*
>
> **LS:** *And how hard has it been to do that?*
>
> **T:** *Really, really hard. I don't believe I could have done it without counseling and confirming with someone else the things that I believed and how I felt, knowing why I feel the way that I feel about certain things. . . . I've been the only one that's been able to do it in my family. And it's been f****** scary. Really scary. But just by seeing [my daughter's] actions, her attitude, everything, it's reconfirming that I'm doing the right thing.*

Tammy drew on a corrective relationship with a therapist, and LaKeisha relied on life-saving memories from childhood to develop new skills and a more coherent caregiving legacy. Cary relied primarily on her husband's family legacy for recovering caregiving practices from her own past that were worth preserving, and discarding what had been hurtful (SmithBattle, 2008). All three mothers demonstrated grit and grace in creating more positive legacies with their own children.

MOTHERS' AND CHILDRENS' LINKED TRAJECTORIES AT TIME 5

Because the oldest children of the teen mother participants were 15 to 17 years of age at Time 5, I was interested in how they were negotiating the challenges of adolescence. As I describe here, the mothers' sense of self and future, as well as their responses to the past, had powerful ramifications for the development of their oldest children.

Creating a Future

At Time 5, mothers who had developed a coherent sense of self and future shared strong behavioral expectations for their children and coherent family practices that promoted their children's long-term development (SmithBattle & Leonard, 2006). These women cultivated the child's connections to family and school and affirmed the child's personhood through dialog, even when these practices had been lacking in their childhoods. Separate interviews with the teens affirmed that they felt recognized by their mothers. Only one of these teens was doing poorly in school, but his learning disabilities, which had never been addressed, posed a significant academic challenge. None of these teens were truant from school or had been involved in the juvenile system. The two teens in this group who were known by their mothers to be sexually active were in long-term romantic relationships and using birth control effectively. These teens were negotiating adolescence from a family cushion of safety and recognition. They were not adrift in an empty world.

Repeating the Past

The two women (Maya and Meg) who continued to drift through their 20s and 30s lacked the sense of self or agency to help their children connect to school or respond to the demands of the world. They also lacked a long-term perspective to ground their children's lives. Because both women had resided with their mothers over most of the 16 years, ongoing family conflicts and arbitrary rules made it difficult for mothers and grandmothers to develop a more coherent caregiving tradition. Although grandmothers had described positive relationships with the oldest grandchild in earlier studies, by Time 5, these relationships had frayed, and grandmothers had largely withdrawn from a parenting role.

With family relationships tenuous and conflicted, Maya's daughter, Trina, and Meg's son, Mike, had drifted into risky situations. They were truant from school and had had several pregnancy events between them. Trina, a 16-year-old girl, was also on probation for shoplifting. Her alienation was vividly portrayed in her response to a picture that she selected to represent her life. The picture was of a masked person with the caption "The invisible."

> *I'm drawn to [this picture] because . . . that's how I feel with my life, like nobody sees me, nobody appreciate my feelings. I feel like I'm just not even there. . . . People just pass by me and just don't care about how I feel or how my life is, and they don't help me out in my situations that I need to be helped to make my life better. (SmithBattle & Leonard, 2006, p. 356)*

Both Trina and Mike had little sense of where they were headed. They were absorbed into the perils of an adolescence without responsive relationships and a cushion of safety and landmarks to guide them. Like their mothers, they were cast adrift in a world with little meaning or direction.

RESTORING MEANING AND DIALOG

Since beginning the longitudinal study in 1988, a growing number of empirical studies have challenged the conventional wisdom that teen mothering "risks the future" (Furstenberg, 2007; SmithBattle, 2009b). As researchers have adjusted for previously unmeasured background factors (e.g., growing up in poor neighborhoods, attending inferior schools, doing poorly in school, having parents with limited education and income) by using powerful statistical techniques and innovative comparison groups, teen mothers' childhood disadvantage has been shown to have a more powerful effect on long-term outcomes for teen mothers and their children than young maternal age (see Fessler, 2003; Furstenberg, 2007; Geronimus, 2003, 2004; Luster & Haddow, 2005; Quinlivan, 2004; SmithBattle, 2000b). Although small differences in some maternal-child outcomes exist when different ethnic groups are compared, the evidence suggests that young maternal age contributes very little to negative outcomes (Geronimus, 2004; Turley, 2003).

As crucial as these findings have been in challenging the stereotypes of teen mothers, there is less recognition for how the search for an objective truth excludes meaning and the discovery of situated possibilities and constraints (Benner & Wrubel, 1989). In this study, the recovery of meaning led to the discovery of patterns and variations in the lifeworld and caregiving practices that help to explain the outcomes that have been of continuing interest to social scientists, clinicians, and policy makers. The narrative findings also highlight the clinical imperative to affirm meaning and validate the possibilities that teen mothers discover in mothering (SmithBattle, 2009a).

CULTIVATING MEANING AND DIALOG IN CLINICAL PRACTICE

The discovery that mothering can be a critical turning point and a catalyst for developing existential dwelling skills (see Weiss, 1996) legitimizes the clinical skills that cultivate meanings available in the situation. In two studies of public health nursing practice, my colleagues and I (SmithBattle, Drake, & Diekemper, 1997; SmithBattle & Diekemper, 2001) found that

PHNs who relied on dialog and narrative understanding moved beyond the objective norms of the scientific gaze to validate young mothers' joys, strengths, difficulties, learning, and their growing agency. The seasoned PHNs we interviewed offered clinical narratives that highlighted the relational skills and contingent responsiveness to the other that cultivate a sense of hope and worth and deepen possibilities. A nurse who exemplified these skillful practices referred to the teen mothers on her caseload ". . . as diamonds in the rough. I see more potential in them maybe than they see for themselves" (SmithBattle, 2003a, p.374). Here is how she described her visits with a 13-year-old mother:

> *I give her all the education that I can and we sit down and we have talks about life. What would you like to see happen to you in the next five years? What would you like to become? And I've told her, just because you have a child does not mean that your goals and your dreams have to be put to the wayside. . . . And I always encourage her because she's a fabulous mother. Wonderful mother. But we talk about how her life has changed because of it. She tells me how she can't go out with her girlfriends. She can't hang out at the "Y" anymore. She gets lonely. We talk about her relationship with this young man and we talk about everything. And she knows that I'm an up-front, straight-from-the-hip kind of person. And we're working on this plan for her life. Her next step. Now that she's finished summer school, she starts high school. That's a whole different chapter in her life. (SmithBattle, 2003a, p. 374)*

In this and other clinical narratives, PHNs demonstrated the ethical sensitivity and the clinical wisdom (Benner, Tanner, & Chesla, 1996; Benner, Hooper-Kyriakidis, & Stannard, 1999) that help the mother voice concerns and aspirations that may be inchoate and undeveloped. Affirming the teen's identity as a mother and sharing her moral vision of the good contributed to an enlarged horizon that is especially crucial for teens with a dim sense of future. As we learned, nurses coached and mentored these vulnerable teens to support their budding priorities, such as returning to school, leaving an abusive partner, developing new habits of care for the self and baby, and avoiding risky situations. Developing attentive relationships with teens who had few prior experiences of trust and care required a refined sense of timing and the advocacy skills that help teens overcome personal and bureaucratic barriers to community resources (SmithBattle, 2000a, 2003a, 2005). Although we did not interview the teen mothers who were followed by nurse informants in these studies, I suspect that in many cases, these highly skilled PHNs provided the corrective experiences that promote the develop-

> *". . . as diamonds in the rough. I see more potential in them maybe than they see for themselves."*

ment of a coherent narrative, especially for teens bereft of partner and family support, who struggle to repair the past and to develop new caregiving legacies on their own.

The steadfast responsiveness of expert PHNs and their development of attuned relationships far exceed the clinical application of prescriptive protocols, standardized languages, or the formal reasoning characteristic of scientific-professional discourse. Their careful attention to process, particularity, and relationship (Benner, 2000a, 2000b, 2004; SmithBattle, 2003a, SmithBattle & Diekemper, 2001) offers a strong endorsement of the clinical maxim that I first discovered in visiting families many years ago: "Begin with people as they are and the situation as it is." Excellent nursing practice also confirms the thought of Levinas: "The other (autrui) is not an object of comprehension first and an interlocutor second. The two relations are intertwined" (cited in Nortvedt, 2001, p. 39). Levinas' fundamental concern with our ethical responsibility to the other reminds us of the limits of the scientific gaze; so long as teen mothers are viewed as "object[s] of comprehension first," we easily overlook the meaning (or the lack of meaning) that structures teen mothers' unfolding lives *and* the clinical practices and ethical sensitivity that cultivate meaning, care, and possibility.

CONCLUSION

It's difficult at any age to become a parent. Just because you become a parent at a young age, it doesn't mean life is over. Cary

In spite of growing evidence that teen mothers' lives are disadvantaged slightly, if at all, by an early birth, public ostracism and professional stereotypes of teen mothers remain common. The depiction of teen mothering as the start of a downward trajectory—that "life is over"—conveys more about our scientific biases and cultural blind spots (about human beings in general, and race, poverty, and sexuality in particular) than about teen mothers themselves (Geronimus, 2003, 2004; SmithBattle, 2000b, 2003b). Teen mothers and their families carry a heavy burden for our "dubious conceptions" (Luker, 1996). In scrutinizing teen mothers for the ways that they fail to measure up to parenting and life-course norms, we overlook their possibilities and resilience and the social sources of many of their difficulties.

The lens that we adopt to understand and explain teen mothering inevitably shapes our clinical and policy responses. Do we see teen mothers as "children raising children?" This frame argues for removing their children at birth (personal communication, Westman, December, 16, 2006). Are they economic pariahs feeding at the welfare trough? This view blames and punishes teen mothers for the structural conditions of poverty (Geronimus, 1997, 2003; SmithBattle, 2003b). If we reject these two frames, and adopt the position that teen mothers are "diamonds in the rough," then we might listen carefully, respond with humility, and capitalize on the meanings and corrective experiences available in mothering, even when these possibilities are fragile and long-term outcomes are unknown. When we listen carefully, teen mothers can help us to appreciate more fully that we are "thrown" into the world, living out the constraints and possibilities available to us in our family and cultural legacies. Our lives may be held in place by sturdy cables from the past or by tattered threads (SmithBattle, 2000a). But even in the context of fragile beginnings and threadbare traditions, we may rise to the occasion to discover new meanings, or we may continue to drift in a capricious world. Our lives may reveal grace and grit, possibility or despair.

ACKNOWLEDGMENTS

I owe each of the study participants a huge debt of gratitude for sharing their lives with me. Victoria Leonard, RN, PhD, has remained a steadfast friend from the time we began our doctoral studies, and her consultation on each wave of the longitudinal study has been invaluable. I could not have done this work without her. Edna Dell Weinel, RN, MPH, and Patricia Benner, RN, PhD, FAAN, have been the best mentors. Rebecca Lorenz, Janet Palmer, and Judy Smith, doctoral students in the School of Nursing at Saint Louis University, provided helpful comments on a draft of this manuscript. I am also grateful to funding organizations, including the National Institute of Nursing Research (NR1F31NR06266 and NR04700R29); the American Nurses Foundation; Sigma Theta Tau International (STTI); the Graduate School and School of Nursing, Saint Louis University; Delta Lambda and Alpha Etta chapters of STTI; the Fahs-Beck Fund for Research and Experimentation; the Century Club of the School of Nursing, University of California at San Francisco (UCSF); and the Graduate Division, UCSF. Pseudonyms are used throughout this paper.

References

Arney, W. R., & Bergen, B. J. (1984). Power and visibility: The invention of teenage pregnancy. *Social Science & Medicine, 18*, 11-19.

Benner, P. (2000a). The quest for control and the possibilities of care. In M. A. Wrathall & J. Malpas (Eds.), *Heidegger, coping and cognitive science: Essays in honor of Hubert L. Dreyfus* (Vol. 2., pp. 293-309). Cambridge, MA: The MIT Press.

Benner, P. (2000b). The roles of embodiment, emotion and lifeworld for rationality and agency in nursing practice. *Nursing Philosophy, 1*, 1-14.

Benner, P. (2004). Seeing the person beyond the disease. *American Journal of Critical Care, 13*, 75-78.

Benner, P., Hooper-Kyriakidis, P., & Stannard, D. (1999). *Clinical wisdom and interventions in critical care*. Philadelphia: Saunders.

Benner, P., Tanner, C. A., & Chesla, C. A. (1996). *Expertise in nursing practice: Caring, clinical judgment, and ethics*. New York: Springer.

Benner, P., & Wrubel, J. (1989). *The primacy of caring: Stress and coping in health and illness*. Redwood City, CA: Addison-Wesley.

Dreyfus, H. L. (1991). *Being-in-the-world: A commentary on Heidegger's Being and Time* (Division I). Cambridge, MA: The MIT Press.

Fessler, K. B. (2003). Social outcomes of early childbearing: Important considerations for the provision of clinical care. *Journal of Midwifery & Women's Health, 48*, 178-185.

Fessler, A. (2006). *The girls who went away*. New York: Penguin.

Furstenberg, F. (2002). How it takes thirty years to do a study. In E. Phelps, F. Furstenberg, & A. Colby (Eds.), *Looking at lives: American longitudinal studies of the twentieth century* (pp. 37-60). New York: Russell Sage Foundation.

Furstenberg, F. (2007). *Destinies of the disadvantaged: The politics of teenage childbearing*. New York: Russell Sage Foundation.

Gadamer, H. (1975). *Truth and method* (Wahrheit und Methode, 2nd ed., 1965) Translation edited by G. Barden & J. Cumming. London: Sheed and Ward.

Geronimus, A. T. (1997). Teenage childbearing and personal responsibility: An alternative view. *Political Science Quarterly, 112*, 405-430.

Geronimus, A. T. (2003). Damned if you do: Culture, identity, privilege, and teenage childbearing in the United States. *Social Science and Medicine, 57*, 881-893.

Geronimus, A. T. (2004). Teenage childbearing as cultural prism. *British Medical Bulletin, 69*, 155-166.

Harrington, M. (1962). *The other America*. New York: Macmillan.

Hayes, C. D. (1987). *Risking the future: Adolescent sexuality, pregnancy, and childbearing* (Vol. 1). Washington, DC: National Academies Press.

Heidegger, M. (1962). *Being and time*. (J. Macquarrie & R. E., Trans.). New York: Harper & Row. (Original work published 1927).

Henderson, G. H. (1980). Consequences of school-age pregnancy and motherhood. *Family Relations, 29*, 185-190.

Klein, L. (1978). Antecedents of teenage pregnancy. *Clinical Obstetrics and Gynecology, 21*, 1151-1159.

Leonard, V. W. (1994). A Heideggerian phenomenologic perspective on the concept of the person. In P. Benner (Ed.), *Interpretive phenomenology: Embodiment, caring, and ethics in health and illness* (pp. 43-64). Thousand Oaks, CA: Sage.

Leonard, V. W. (1993). *Stress and coping in the transition to parenthood of first-time mothers with career commitments: An interpretive study*. Unpublished doctoral dissertation, University of California, San Francisco.

Luker, K. (1996). *Dubious conceptions: The politics of teenage pregnancy*. Cambridge, MA: Harvard University Press.

Luster, T., & Haddow, J. L. (2005). Adolescent mothers and their children: An ecological perspective. In T. Luster & L. Okagaki (Eds.), *Parenting: An ecological perspective* (pp. 73-101). Mahwah, NJ: Lawrence Erlbaum.

Merleau-Ponty, M. (1962). *Phenomenology of perception*. (C. Smith, Trans.). London: Routledge & Kegan Paul. (Original work published 1945).

Nortvedt, P. (2001). Clinical sensitivity: The inseparability of ethical perceptiveness and clinical knowledge. *Scholarly Inquiry for Nursing Practice: An International Journal, 15*, 25-48.

Plager, K. A. (1999). Understanding family legacy in family health concerns. *Journal of Child and Family Nursing, 5*,

51-71.

Quinlivan, J. A. (2004). Teenagers who plan parenthood. *Sexual Health, 1,* 201-208.

Rains, P. (1971). *Becoming an unwed mother.* Chicago: Aldine.

Richardson, F. C., Fowers, B. J., & Guignon, C. B. (1999). *Re-envisioning psychology: Moral dimensions of theory and practice.* San Francisco: Jossey-Bass.

SmithBattle, L. (1992). *Caring for teenage mothers and their children: Narratives of self and ethics of intergrational caregiving.* Unpublished doctoral dissertation, University of California, San Francisco.

SmithBattle, L. (1993). Mothering in the midst of danger. In S. L. Feethan, S. B. Meister, J. M. Bell, & C. L. Gilliss (Eds.), *The nursing of families: Theory/research/education/practice* (pp. 235-246). Newbury Park, CA: Sage.

SmithBattle, L. (1994). Beyond normalizing: The role of narrative in understanding teenage mothers' transition to mothering. In P. Benner (Ed.), *Interpretive phenomenology* (pp. 141-166). Thousand Oaks, CA: Sage.

SmithBattle, L. (1995). Teenage mothers' narratives of self: An examination of risking the future. *Advances in Nursing Science, 17*(4), 22-36.

SmithBattle, L. (1996). Intergenerational ethics of caring for adolescent mothers and their children. *Family Relations, 45,* 56-64.

SmithBattle, L. (1997). Change and continuity in family caregiving practices with young mothers and their children. *Image, 29,* 145-149.

SmithBattle, L. (2000a). Developing a caregiving tradition in opposition to one's past: Lessons from a longitudinal study of teenage mothers. *Public Health Nursing, 17,* 85-93.

SmithBattle, L. (2000b). The vulnerabilities of teenage mothers: Challenging prevailing assumptions. *Advances in Nursing Science, 23*(1), 29-40.

SmithBattle, L. (2003a). Displacing the "rulebook" in caring for teen mothers. *Public Health Nursing, 20,* 369-376.

SmithBattle, L. (2003b). Understanding teenage mothering: Conventional and unconventional wisdom. *Prevention Researcher, 10*(3), 1-4.

SmithBattle, L. (2005). Teenage mothers at age 30. *Western Journal of Nursing Research, 27,* 831-850.

SmithBattle, L. (2006). Family legacies in shaping teen mothers' caregiving practices over 12 years. *Qualitative Health Research, 16,* 1129-1144.

SmithBattle, L. (2007a). "I wanna have a good future": Teen mothers' aspirations, competing demands, and limited school support. *Youth and Society, 38,* 348-371.

SmithBattle, L. (2007b). Learning the baby: Findings from an interpretive study of teen mothers. *Journal of Pediatric Nursing, 22,* 261-271.

SmithBattle, L. (2008). Gaining ground from a cultural tradition: A teen mother's story of repairing the world. *Family Process, 47,* 521-535.

SmithBattle, L. (2009a). Pregnant with possibilities: Drawing on philosophical thought to recast home visiting interventions with young mothers. *Nursing Inquiry, 16,* 191-200.

SmithBattle, L. (2009b). Reframing the risks and losses of teen mothering. *MCN American Journal of Maternal Child Nursing, 34,* 122-128.

SmithBattle, L., & Diekemper, M. (2001). Promoting clinical practice knowledge in an age of taxonomies and protocols. *Public Health Nursing, 18,* 401-408.

SmithBattle, L., Drake, M. A., & Diekemper, M. (1997). The responsive use of self in community health nursing practice. *Advances in Nursing Science, 20*(2), 75-89.

SmithBattle, L., & Leonard, V. W. (1998). Adolescent mothers four years later: Narratives of the self and visions of the future. *Advances in Nursing Science, 20*(3), 36-49.

SmithBattle, L., & Leonard, V. W. (2006). Teen mothers and their teenaged children: The reciprocity of developmental trajectories. *Advances in Nursing Science, 29*, 351-365.

Taylor, C. (1989). *Sources of the self: The making of the modern identity*. Cambridge, MA: Harvard University Press.

Taylor, C. (1995). *Philosophical arguments*. Cambridge, MA: Harvard University Press.

Turley, R. N. (2003). Are children of young mothers disadvantaged because of their mother's age or family background? *Child Development, 74*, 465-474.

Vogel, L. (1994). *The fragile "we": Ethical implications of Heidegger's "Being and Time."* Evanston, IL: Northwestern University Press.

Weiss, S. M. (1996). *Possibility or despair: Biographies of aging*. Unpublished doctoral dissertation, University of California, San Francisco.

CHAPTER 12

Life-Course Considerations for Adolescents Born with Spina Bifida: Toward Authentic Care and Transparency of the Other

CHRISTINE KINAVEY

INTRODUCTION

Benner's (2000) account of the phenomenon of care lays claim to our "being connected regardless of the quality or content of that connection" and underscores nursing's imperative to engage in authentic care (p. 293). "Authentic care" is a form of solicitude or societal caring that allows the Other to be revealed, grasped, and readily understood (Benner, 2000; Heidegger, 1926/1962):

> *This kind of solicitude pertains essentially to authentic care–that is, to the existence of the Other, not to a "what" with which he is concerned; it helps the Other to become transparent to himself in his care and to become free for it. (Heidegger, 1926 /1962, p. 159)*

In Heideggerian phenomenology, authentic care of the Other denotes not the objectification or "othering" associated with viewing individuals as radically independent from one another, but an existential being-with Others in a manner that keeps our shared humanity central to our existence. These notions of authentic care are relevant to our experience and understanding of disability and chronic illness, which situate others in particular ways across the life course.

Benner's (1994; 2001b) rendering of the phenomenon of care—specifically, how ontological structures of care and particular care-giving practices foster and/or thwart health over the life course—serves as the ground for my research on adolescents born with the physical disability of spina bifida. Ontological structures of care can be understood as existential scaffolding or "webs of interlocutors" that sustain and facilitate connection and concern in our lifeworld inclusive of relationships, language, commitments, identity, recognition, and possibility (Benner, 2001a; Taylor, 1985b).

THE LIFE COURSE OF SPINA BIFIDA

Spina bifida describes a group of multiple complex congenital anomalies and abnormalities involving imperfect development of the neural tube and related structures (Kaufman, 2004). Although the primary lesions involve the spinal portion of the central nervous system (CNS), there are an array of manifestations and sequelae affecting seemingly disparate structures and functions, including the brain, bony spine, extremities, bowel, and bladder (Kaufman, 2004). In addition to the physical and cognitive (biological) effects, there are a host of psychosocial challenges, including body image concerns, low self-esteem, social isolation, depression, and stigma (Blum, Resnick, Nelson, & St. Germaine; 1991; Kinavey, 2006; Simeonsson, McMillen, & Huntington, 2002). Long-term biological, psychological, and/or social (biopsychosocial) effects are still relatively unknown because longevity is a more recent phenomenon (Bowman et al., 2001; Liptak, 2003). As a result of advances in medical technology, approximately, 90% of babies born with spina bifida are now expected to live to be adults (Spina Bifida Association, 2008).

Biopsychosocial Possibility and Spina Bifida

In interpreting the experience and meaning of living with the physical disability of spina bifida, it is important to consider biological and psychosocial effects as well as biological-environmental interactions (Engle, 1977, 1983; Rolland, 1994; Rolland & Williams, 2005). Psychosocial factors have a direct bearing on physiologic and pathological states and vice versa. Adopting a biopsychosocial developmental orientation toward biological disorders provides a more meaningful framework by which to understand the disability or illness experience over the life course and at particular stages of development (Engle, 1977, 1983; Rolland & Williams, 2005).

From a phenomenological standpoint, we are "thrown" (born) into a world already in progress: a world with shared values and practices, language and history that give it meaning and structure as well as shape self-understanding (situatedness). Being situated means that we are always experiencing our future in temporal relationship to our present and past. Because we are always already situated, there are limits to our ability as individuals to constitute our particular lifeworld (Benner, 1994; Taylor, 1985a). "Situatedness" both opens up and closes down possibilities with regard to self, world, and other. This is not to say however, that we can never discover new possibilities nor dwell in new lifeworlds; we can, in the midst of transformations.

The self is closely intertwined with embodiment, comportment, affectivity, and perception (Merleau-Ponty, 1962/1946). Our bodily self can be understood at once as an individual and a social being, as an object and a social agent, reconciling biological and social phenomena (Lyon & Barbalet, 1994). Because we live both in and as our bodies, we are always perceiving and experiencing ourselves and one another as bodily selves (Lyon & Barbalet, 1994; Todes, 2001). Opening to a particular lifeworld, the lived body faces a myriad of possibilities and circumstances, including its own finitude. Bodily intentionality directed toward self, other, and things provides the opportunity to "traverse the boundary between finitude and transcendence" so that we might situate our possibilities in our bodily limitations as well as our embodied possibilities (Barnard, 1995, p.39): in other words, challenging bodily limitations with the hope of expanding possibilities while heeding corporeal limitations and thereby closing down possibilities, with the hope of preventing more incontrovertible limitations in the future.

Discourse on Disability and Self

Despite advances in the quest for civil rights for persons with disabilities over the past 30 years, including recognition as a social minority, physical disability continues to be highly stigmatized within our culture (Kinavey, 2006, 2007; Nussbaum, 2004; Wendell, 1996). Signs of oppression toward persons with disabilities can still be located in inaccessible built (that is, architectural) structures, higher rates of poverty and unemployment, continued biomedical categorization of difference as deviance, and marginalization within society.

Negative images of people with disabilities linger within the cultural consciousness as a consequence of ignorance, fear, and past exclusion from greater society. Integration as individuals and as a minority group continues to be hampered by sociopolitical structures that are at best unwelcoming and at worst hostile (Gill, 1997; Olkin, 1999; Toombs, 1993). Sociopolitical structures include culturally, ethnically, and religiously influenced values and beliefs as well as social, political, and economic structures and processes that are constitutive of our understanding and experience of disability.

An Interpretive Approach to Studying Spina Bifida

This study sought to investigate the experience of disability and its meanings in relation to self, world, and other for adolescents born with spina bifida by using a phenomenological (interpretive) ethnographic approach as informed by Benner (1994), Dreyfus (1997), Geertz (1973; 1988), Heidegger (1926/1962), Jackson (1996), Kleinman (1988), Merleau-Ponty (1946/1962), and Taylor (1988). Phenomenological ethnography is representative of a particular type of ethnography that focuses on meanings, habits, skills, and practices in the world of study participants. Within a phenomenological framework, individuals can never entirely escape the influence of background, including cultural and personal practices, meanings, and belief systems. Everyday concerns and practices shape—and, in turn, are shaped by—understandings of self and other. Individual possibilities and opportunities are strongly tied to what is socially and culturally available (*situated possibility*).

Study Sample

A purposive sample of 11 late-stage adolescents living with spina bifida was recruited from two large medical centers in northern California with spina bifida–specialty clinics. Individuals were included if they

- Were between 18 and 24 years of age (mean age, 21 years)

- Had a neural tube defect in the form of spina bifida

- Did not have a history of mental retardation

This age group was targeted because most late-stage adolescents have the cognitive ability to be self-reflective. Late-stage adolescence (18 years to mid-20s) occurs for those individuals thought to be delayed in their acquisition of adult roles as a consequence of educational goals or other social factors, including chronic illness and physical disability (Elliott & Feldman, 1990; Hallum, 1995; White, 1997). The sample included 7 female and 4 male participants. Five study participants were Caucasian, 5 were Hispanic/Latino, and 1 was of White-Latino mixed ethnicity. Seven study participants lived at home with their parents, 3 participants lived off-campus with other college students, and 1 lived with her boyfriend. Two were seniors in high school, 7 were in college, 1 was enrolled in a vocational training program, and 1 was employed full-time.

With respect to medical history, 8 study participants had a neural tube defect in the form of myelomeningocele, 2 with lipomyelomeningocele, and 1 with lipoma with a sacral agenesis. Seven of 11 participants required cerebrospinal fluid diversion (ventricular shunting) during infancy for hydrocephalus. Ten of 11 study participants catheterized their bladder a minimum of four times per day with only 1 participant being able to void independently; 5 of 11 wore disposable underwear (diapers). Six of 11 study participants had ambulatory capability (2 using a combination of crutches and leg braces, and 3 using leg braces only); 5 of the study participants were full-time manual wheelchair users. Additionally, two other participants used a manual wheelchair for traversing longer distances. Study participants were recruited over a period of 7 months. Approval for human subject research was obtained from both institutions.

Study Data Collection

Forty-three, 1-hour interviews were conducted with 11 study participants over a 7-month period (mean number of interviews per participant = 4; mean time to complete interview series per participant = 8 weeks). The interview guide was developed, in part, on the basis of pilot interviews with adults living with spina bifida as well as issues raised in the literature and in clinical practice. Interview questions were open-ended and designed to elicit narratives about the experiential worlds of adolescents born with physical disability in the form of spina bifida. The interview guide was divided into 11 main categories with several questions under each. See Table 12-1 for a listing of the interview categories and sample questions.

Naturalistic field observations were undertaken in the community to ascertain how the structural (built) environment affects accessibility, mobility, and sociability for individuals living with physical disability. Field observations with study participants included traversing college campuses and attending classes, riding county transit buses and university shuttle buses, visiting faculty offices and bookstores, and being a passenger in cars with hand controls, furthering understanding of day-to-day world.

Study Analysis

Narrative accounts and field notes of the experiential worlds of late-stage adolescents born with spina bifida were interpreted and reported here. Analysis of narratives from each adolescent and analysis of narratives between adolescents were conducted over the course of the study. Themes and exemplars of narrative, illustrating the every day world, were identified and are put forth as the findings that substantiate interpretive conclusions (Benner, 1994).

Table 12-1 Interview Categories and Sampling of Questions

Life Narrative	Tell me a little bit about yourself: When and where you were born, what growing up was like, how things were with your parents, whether you have brothers or sisters.
Recent and Current Experience	Describe those people closest to you. How, if at all, does living with spina bifida impact on those relationships?
Belief Systems	How, if at all, has the experience of having spina bifida affected you? Have your viewpoints changed over time?
Friendships/Intimate Relationships	Please describe your closest friend(s). How did you meet this individual? What kind of relationship do you have with this person? What kind of things do you do with this person now?
Disability/Illness Experience	When you were very young, did you have any spina bifida–related challenges, such as controlling your bowels and bladder? Walking? Participation in group activities/games/sports? Tell me about that and how you think those experiences affected you later in life.
Life History	What are some of the things you liked best about your adolescence? Can you tell me more about that? What were some of the hardest things about your adolescence? Can you tell me more about that?
Family History	How does your father/mother respond to your having a physical disability? Has that changed over the years? How does your sibling(s) respond to your having a physical disability?
School and Peer Relations	I am interested in hearing about your experiences as a teenager living with spina bifida. Are there particular memories or stories that stand out in your mind that you can share? As an individual living with spina bifida, what do you think is one of the biggest assumptions/misconceptions that your peers have about you? Tell me about that.
Body and Sexual Experience	What were your earliest sexual experiences, if any? How did you feel about your body and your sexuality at the time? Has that changed?
Self-Help and Empowerment	Have you participated in any disability-related support groups/recreational activities/camps? When? For how long? How (if at all) did this group or activity assist you?
Career/Vocation/Future Planning	Can you describe your dreams and goals for your life? Have there been particular things along the way that helped to get you where you are today?

Study Findings

Study participants described commonalities with respect to the experience of disability and its meanings for adolescents born with spina bifida. The theme of social marginalization with visible disability is discussed here. These study findings are part of a larger research project. For example, differences in how study participants claim disability in relation to self-understanding as well as biopsychosocial developmental challenges for adolescents born with spina bifida are published elsewhere (Kinavey, 2006, 2007).

Exemplars of narrative center on how sociopolitical structures, including an unwelcoming physical (architectural) and social environment, promote isolation and marginalization in youth born with the physical disability of spina bifida. The term *marginalization* implies peripheralization, or degraded social status of an individual or group by a dominant, central majority (Hall, 1999).

Over the past three decades, there has been a trend to move the education of children with disabilities from special education classrooms into regular mainstream education. This "mainstreaming" of youth with disabilities via passage of the Individuals with Disabilities Education Act (IDEA) was intended to break down barriers and facilitate inclusion. Although advantageous on many fronts, it has yet to fulfill the promise of true integration, particularly as it relates to socialization and developmental opportunities for these children (Simeonsson et al., 2001). As demonstrated in the following abbreviated narrative, mainstreaming youth with physical disabilities from special education into regular mainstream education may have paradoxically stigmatizing effects in the absence of retooled sociopolitical structures expressly designed to ensure a "horizon of shared significance" (Taylor, 1991) within the public education system.

Kevin, in his mid-20s as of this writing, recalled being mainstreamed into regular education classrooms at the beginning of 4th grade. This transition was experienced as heralding in a sense of difference.

> *Special Ed. to mainstreamed. . . . I don't really remember much, except to say that, I had friends, a lot, a lot of friends, people that actually, I guess since they were all in the same boat, really cared and understood. . . . And, I went from a situation where everyone was basically in the same boat [special education], to the situation where I was kind of different [regular education].* (Kinavey, 2007)

The metaphor Kevin used to describe the experience of special education ("all in the same boat") paints a picture of lost community. There is an awareness of feeling at home in the world among a group of similar others that vanishes with placement into regular education. Separated from his core group of friends, and thrown into a situation where everyone else is "able-bodied," Kevin began to feel disenfranchised. A sense of being "other-than-normal" took hold. Although technically "mainstreamed," Kevin was not truly integrated into the classroom or the school.

> *Because I was mainstreamed at such an early age, I kind of lost that, lost it a little bit, lost that, we're, in this together, kind of thing. I became, as we say in the anthro class, "the other." . . . I was part of this group but I wasn't part of that group. Part of group A saw me as part of group B, and group B saw me as part of group A, and so, I was in kind of no-man's land. (Kinavey, 2007)*

Kevin used the word "other" in a postmodern context, signifying a form of stigmatized difference or marginalization that distanced him from his classmates. Kevin has lost his sense of shared humanity because he is so actively seen as completely "other" in the mainstream class. Losing his sense of "place," and relocated far from the cultural center, Kevin subsisted along the margins.

> *Recess was kind of interesting, because they had the big kids' yard down on the bottom level. And, because my legs aren't that strong, I could only make it to the little kids' yard. . . . I was on crutches back then. And so, the few times that I was able to make it down to the big kids' yard, I was kind of outcast anyway. . . . 'Cause I couldn't participate in the basketball or much of anything, really.*

The spatial arrangements of the play yards reinforced for Kevin his difference from others of his age group. Even when through great effort he was able to access the "big kids' yard," he found himself excluded from participation. Recess is an important avenue of social learning in which children learn to negotiate situations of competition, conflict, and ambiguity through games and unstructured play. Unable to participate, Kevin found himself sidelined.

> *I was very unpopular, back then, and, when lunchtime would come, I would walk out to the lunch tables outside and they'd say, "Oh, here comes 'It.'" So I was the boy called "It." (Kinavey, 2007)*

Having a name by which we are known is fundamental to our sense of self. Nicknames can serve as bonds indicating closeness, or as ways of distancing. Being called "it" suggests an objectification that rendered Kevin even more "other": a thing.

Sixth grade and entry into middle school was especially traumatic, exacerbating his sense of otherness. Kevin recalled being betrayed by his only friend, someone with whom he had confided in about his bladder incontinence and the need to wear diapers.

For a while there, I did have a friend [rueful chuckle], if you can call him that. Uh, but then, as time went on, you know, I took him into my confidence and I told him, and I don't know if it was shortly after that . . . um, [that he] joined the dark side, if you will, and he joined in the teasing. . . . I don't remember this, but my dad told me . . . that this kid pulled my pants down, in class.

Neither the school administration nor his teacher offered a safe harbor. Kevin recounted one humiliating incident after another. On one occasion, he was forced to crawl across the length of the classroom in order to retrieve his crutches after they were tossed aside by his peers as a practical "joke." Kevin was unable to stand or walk without his crutches.

School had just let out, and um, stayed around in the room, and a couple of other kids stayed, and he suddenly grabbed my crutches, and tossed them over, to the other side of the room. So I had to, crawl. 'Cause what else could I do? Crawl to get the crutches, and, um, it was [voice breaks] humiliating.

Symbolically, Kevin was infantilized in front of his peers, forced to crawl to achieve mobility. At this point, his parents decided to take him out of school to protect him from further harassment and humiliation. He never returned to that 6th grade classroom, or the school for that matter. He was home-schooled the rest of the school year. Twelve years later, he is still haunted by these events.

Adolescents born with the physical disability of spina bifida come to know and experience stigmatized difference over time and in relationship with others, especially their peers. Study participants' narratives uncovered repeated instances of encountered hostility that fostered isolation and marginalization while maneuvering through the physical and social environment.

Study participants were all well versed in the extant assumptions and misconceptions associated with having a physical disability in the culture:

That we're helpless. Just because we're slightly encumbered by this wheelchair or crutches . . . that we're invalids, we're weak! That we're whiny people. That we complain a lot . . . that we're always demanding special treatment. That we're not really sexual creatures. . . . That we don't have the same wants and desires.

They described being ignored and/or rejected by their classmates as a consequence of stigmatized physical difference.

> *Kids weren't always comfortable being around me or making friends with me, or even talking. (Kinavey, 2006)*

Adolescence, particularly early adolescence with its emphasis on peer group affiliation and conformity, is especially challenging for youth experienced as "different" by their classmates (Eder, 1995; Spencer & Dornbusch, 1990).

> *Adolescence was really, really hard. . . . It was the first time for me, personally, that it dawned on me, that I was different. And, how that affected like, my relationships with people and stuff like that. It's the first time I realized that there were going to be certain people who didn't want to really deal with me, because I had a disability.*

Flirtations and dating rituals, so common at this developmental age and stage, were frequently unavailable to study participants.

> *It started in 7th grade. Everyone started pairing off. And I mean, everyone. Like, the entire cool crowd had a significant other. . . . Everyone was with someone, and I wasn't. Everyone was interested, or had someone interested in them, and I didn't.*

Adolescents requiring a wheelchair for mobility are at even greater risk of being isolated and marginalized as a consequence of an unwelcoming architectural environment. For example, most single-family homes in the United States are not wheelchair accessible, discouraging invitations to and participation in age-appropriate, developmentally significant socialization opportunities, such as after school get-togethers, birthday parties, and sleepovers.

> *Sleepovers. . . . Just something I would never do . . . they never had an accessible bathroom in those houses. Never had widened doors and wheelchair-accessible anything.*

Additionally, stigma attached to the wheelchair intensified differences with peers, further reducing socialization opportunities. Originally intended to facilitate mobility and access, wheelchairs often have a paradoxical, more chilling effect (Murphy, 1990).

> *We started playing with each other. And then, a few months later they decided that all of a sudden they didn't want to be friends anymore. And one of the girls said,*

"Well, we can't play with you 'cause you're in a wheelchair . . . and you can't do the things that we do and we want to do, and you know, we want to play just with us."

DISCUSSION OF ADOLESCENT NARRATIVES

Study participants' narratives enlarge upon and deepen our understanding of the experiential world of adolescents born with spina bifida: a world complicated by biologic difference and impeded by sociopolitical structures undermining opportunities for socialization and belongingness. Exemplars of narrative reveal deeply rooted negative cultural connotations about disability that contribute to an understanding of disability as "difference" and persons with disabilities as stigmatized "other."

Stigma in association with bodily difference is a melding of attribute and stereotype (Goffman, 1963). Mostly, it serves a discrediting function in that the stigmatized attribute reinforces the appropriateness of the normalized trait. Thus, the stigmatized feature assumes a less-than-human quality, neutralizing other positive characteristics that the individual might possess, opening the door to a variety of discriminatory practices. Feelings of inferiority within stigmatized groups are often created and maintained via social isolation.

Social isolation and marginalization are ongoing concerns for youth with spina bifida. With the advent of early adolescence and entry into middle school, visible physical disability poses even greater social liability as differences become more highly charged and less well-tolerated, placing youth with stigmatized physical difference at risk for alienation from their peers (Eder, 1995; Yeo & Sawyer, 2003). The more that an individual differs from his/her peers, the more difficulty he or she can have in forming relationships and making friends (Rubin, Bukowski, & Parker, 1998). In addition, primary and secondary effects associated with spina bifida may further restrict socialization opportunities in this population, exacerbating their sense of otherness.

Youth with spina bifida often require physical aids for locomotion such as wheelchairs, crutches, and/or leg braces; may walk with an exaggerated, propulsive gait (if they are ambulators); frequently have a neurogenic bowel and bladder requiring diapers; are at risk for obesity as a consequence of decreased mobility; and can experience learning disabilities from brain formation abnormalities (Arnold Chiari II malformation). Mobility restrictions, inaccessible architecture, fear of bowel and bladder accidents, body image concerns including sexual desirability, and stigma all contribute to reduced social interactions: hence, limited opportunities for friendship development. Friendships and peer relationships are thought to be protective, offering youth a mechanism for emotional support; the potential for practicing sex-role behaviors and attitudes; a medium for the development of a moral and social consciousness, and modeling for building and improving self-esteem (Harter, 1999).

Youth with stigmatized physical differences are frequent targets of hostility manifested by bullying and victimization at school (Kinavey, 2006; Witt, Riley, & Coiro, 2003). Peer ridicule and rejection as a consequence of stigmatized bodily difference amplifies feelings of inferiority and increases isolation. In one of the first U.S. population–based studies examining psychosocial adjustment in youth with disabilities ages 6 to 17, psychosocial difficulties most frequently cited involved peer relations and encountered hostility (Witt et al., 2003). Bullying victimization contributes to increased behavior and school adjustment problems in young children and increased internalizing problems with age, including adolescent and adult-onset depression (Arseneault et al., 2006).

The scarcity of similar others both at home and at school for youth with disabilities, combined with children/adolescents' proclivity for forming friendships with others like themselves, deserves greater consideration from health professionals, educational specialists, and children's policy advocates, particularly as it relates to curriculum development. At present, one of the major tenets of the disability movement—the concept of community belonging—is under-appreciated and under-represented within primary and secondary education. And yet, community belonging has been a very effective tool in the adult disability movement in terms of breaking down barriers, challenging current discourse, reversing stigma, and providing a forum for constructing a positive identity as individuals and as a minority group (Gill, 1997; Hahn, 1997; Ville, Crost, Ravaud, & Tetrafigap Group, 2003). Instituting a form of community belonging early, prior to the start of middle school, would provide youth with disabilities a peer group of similar others and promote sociopolitical resilience by offering more social resources, coping, and adaptation skills.

IMPLICATIONS FOR NURSING PRACTICE

Individuals are constituted through repeated exposure to the political, economic, and social systems with which they interact, including everyday beliefs and practices surrounding health, illness, and disability (McCubbin et al., 1993). Understanding how ontological structures of care and specific care-giving practices impact opportunity, ability, and participation for youth born with physical disability can assist health care professionals, educators, and children's policy advocates in devising strategies aimed at maximizing biological, psychological, and sociological health while preventing disability's secondary effects. Although we have long advocated for a biopsychosocial approach in providing care to individuals living with disability and chronic illness, we continue to prioritize biomedical outcomes over psychosocial effects (Scherger, 2005; Yeo & Sawyer, 2003).

Ontological care relates to the extent of connection and concern that human beings experience in their lifeworld (Benner, 2001a). Benner (2001a) emphasized that, "Understanding ontological care as world and person-disclosing enables us to reflect on specific caring practices that may support or undermine the person's self and world-defining concerns (ontological care)" (p. 358).

> *"Understanding ontological care as world and person-disclosing enables us to reflect on specific caring practices that may support or undermine the person's self and world-defining concerns."*

Caring sets up a world and creates the possibility for disclosure. Authentic care or solicitude can facilitate transparency of the "Other" so that individuals can be clearly seen and readily understood in their uniqueness and alterity (Levinas, 1985). Benner (2000) argues "the best of nursing practice is infused with an understanding of caring as actions that nurture, foster growth, recovery, health, and protection for the vulnerable" (p. 300). Greater emphasis needs to be directed toward humanizing and emancipating the physical and social environment for youth with disabilities to promote transparency, self-understanding, and belongingness while maximizing developmental opportunity, ability, and participation over the life course. This means shaping ontological structures of care and ontic care-giving practices in ways that recognize, acknowledge, and champion the equal value of different modes of being in the world.

References

Arseneault, L., Walsh, E., Trzesniewski, K., Newcombe, R., Caspi, A., & Moffitt, T. E. (2006). Bullying victimization uniquely contributes to adjustment problems in young children: A nationally representative cohort study. *Pediatrics, 118*(1), 130-138.

Barnard, D. (Ed.). (1995). *Chronic illness from experience to policy*. Bloomington, IN: Indiana University Press.

Benner, P. (1994). *Interpretive phenomenology: Embodiment, caring, and ethics in health and illness*. Thousand Oaks, CA: Sage.

Benner, P. (2000). The quest for control and the possibilities of care. In M. Wrathall & J. Malpas (Eds.), *Heidegger, coping, and cognitive science: Essays in honor of Hubert L. Dreyfus* (Vol. 2, pp. 351-369). Cambridge, MA: The MIT Press.

Benner, P. (2001a). The phenomenon of care. In S. K. Toombs (Ed.), *Handbook of phenomenology and medicine* (pp. 351-369). Dordrecht, Netherlands: Kluwer.

Benner, P. (2001b). The roles of embodiment, emotion and lifeworld for rationality and agency in nursing practice. *Nursing Philosophy, 1*(1), 5-19.

Blum, R., Resnick, M., Nelson, R., & St Germaine, A. (1991). Family and peer issues among adolescents with spina bifida and cerebral palsy. *Pediatrics, 88*(2), 280-285.

Bowman, R. M., McLone, D. G., Grant, J. A., Tomita, T., & Ito, J. A. (2001). Spina bifida outcome: A 25-year prospective. *Pediatric Neurosurgery, 34*, 114-120.

Dreyfus, H. L. (1988). Husserl, Heidegger, and modern existentialism. In B. Magee (Ed.), *The great philosophers: An introduction to western philosophy* (pp. 254-277). New York: Oxford University Press.

Dreyfus, H. L. (1997). *Being-in-the-world: A commentary on Heidegger's Being and Time*. Cambridge, MA: The MIT Press.

Eder, D. (1995). *School talk: Gender and adolescent culture*. New Brunswick, NJ: Rutgers University Press.

Elliott, G. R., & Feldman, S. S. (1990). Capturing the adolescent experience. In S. Feldman and G. Elliott (Eds.), *At the threshold: The developing adolescent* (pp. 1-13). Cambridge, MA: Harvard University Press.

Engel, G. L. (1977). The need for a new medical model: A challenge for biomedicine. *Science, 196*, 129-136.

Engel, G. L. (1983). The biopsychosocial model and family medicine. *Journal of Family Practice, 16*, 409-413.

Geertz, C. (1973). *The interpretation of cultures*. New York: Basic Books.

Geertz, C. (1988). *Works and lives: The anthropologist as author*. Stanford, CA: Stanford University Press.

Gill, C. J. (1997). Four types of integration in disability identity development. *Journal of Vocational Rehabilitation, 9*, 39-46.

Goffman, E. (1963). *Stigma*. New York: Simon & Schuster.

Hahn, H. (1997). An agenda for citizens with disabilities: Pursuing identity and empowerment. *Journal of Vocational Rehabilitation, 9*, 31-37.

Hall, J. M. (1999). Marginalization revisited: Critical, postmodern, and liberation perspectives. *Advances in Nursing Science, 22*(2), 88-102.

Hallum, A. (1995). Disability and the transition to adulthood: Issues for the disabled child, the family and the pediatrician. *Current Problems in Pediatrics, 25*(1), 12-50.

Harter, S. (1999). *The construction of self: A developmental perspective*. New York: Guilford Press.

Heidegger, M. (1962). *Being and time*. (J. Macquarrie & R. E., Trans.). New York: Harper & Row. (Original work published 1927).

Jackson, M. (1996). *Things as they are: New directions in phenomenological anthropology*. Bloomington, IN: Indiana University Press.

Kaufman, B. (2004). Neural tube defects. *Pediatric Clinics of North America, 51*(2), 389-419.

Kinavey, C. (2006). Explanatory models of self-understanding in adolescents born with spina bifida. *Qualitative Health Research, 16*(8), 1091-1107.

Kinavey, C. (2007). Adolescents born with spina bifida: Experiential worlds and biopsychosocial developmental challenges. *Issues in Comprehensive Pediatric Nursing, 30*(4), 147-164.

Kleinman, A. (1988). *The illness narratives: Suffering, healing, and the human condition*. New York: Basic Books.

Levinas, E. (1985). *Ethics and infinity*. (Richard A. Cohen, Trans.). Pittsburgh: Duquesne University Press.

Liptak, G. S. (2003). *Evidence-based practice in spina bifida: Developing a research agenda*. Washington, DC: Spina Bifida Association of America.

Lyon, M. L., & Barbalet, J. M. (1994). Society's body: Emotion and the "somatization" of social theory. In T. J. Csordas (Ed.), *Embodiment and experience*. Cambridge, UK: Cambridge University Press.

McCubbin, H. I., Thompson, E. A., Thompson, A. I., McCubbin, M. A., & Kaston, A. J. (1993). Culture, ethnicity, and the family: Critical factors in childhood chronic illnesses and disabilities. *Pediatrics, 91*(5 Pt 2), 1063-1070.

Merleau-Ponty, M. (1946). *The phenomenology of perception*. (C. Smith, Trans.). London: Routledge & Kegan Paul. (Original work published 1962).

Murphy, R. F. (1990). *The body silent*. New York: W.W. Norton.

Nussbaum, M. C. (2004). *Hiding from humanity*. Princeton, NJ: Princeton University Press.

Olkin, R. (1999). *What psychotherapists should know about disability*. New York: Guilford Press.

Rolland, J. S. (1994). *Families, illness, and disability: An integrative treatment model*. New York: Basic Books.

Rolland, J. S., & Williams, J. K. (2005). Toward a biopsychosocial model for 21st century genetics. *Family Process, 44*(1), 3-24.

Rubin, K. H., Bukowski, W., & Parker, J. G. (1998). Peer interactions, relationships, and groups. In N. Eisenberg (Ed.), *Handbook of child psychology* (Vol. 3, pp. 619-700). New York: John Wiley & Sons, Inc.

Scherger, J. E. (2005). The end of the beginning: The redesign imperative in family medicine. *Family Medicine, 37*(7), 513-516.

Simeonsson, R. J., Carlson, D., Huntington, G. S., McMillen, J. S., & Brent, J. L. (2001). Students with disabilities: A national survey of participation in school activities. *Disability and Rehabilitation, 23*(2), 49-63.

Simeonsson, R. J., McMillen, J. S., & Huntington, G. S. (2002). Secondary conditions in children with disabilities: Spina bifida as a case example. *Mental Retardation and Developmental Disabilities, 8*, 198-205.

Spencer, M. B., & Dornbusch, S. M. (1990). Challenges in studying minority youth. In S.S. Feldman & G.R. Elliott (Eds.), *At the threshold* (pp. 123-146). Cambridge, MA: Harvard University Press.

Spina Bifida Association (2008). *Can children with spina bifida grow up and live a full life?* Retrieved November 7, 2009, http://www.spinabifidaassociation.org/atf/cf/%7BEED435C8-F1A0-4A16-B4D8-A713BBCD9CE4%7D/Spina%20Bifida%20low%20litJune%202008.doc

Taylor, C. (1985a). *Human agency and language. Philosophical papers* (Vol. 1). Cambridge, UK: Cambridge University Press.

Taylor, C. (1985b). The person. In M. Carrithers, S. Collins, & S. Lukes (Eds.), *The category of the person: Anthropology, philosophy, history* (pp. 257-281). New York: Cambridge University Press.

Taylor, C. (1988). *Human agency and language: Philosophical papers*. Cambridge, UK: Cambridge University Press.

Taylor, C. (1991). *The ethics of authenticity*. Cambridge, MA: Harvard University Press.

Todes, S. (2001). *Body and world*. Cambridge, MA: The MIT Press.

Toombs, S. K. (1993). *The meaning of illness: A phenomenological account of the different perspectives of physician and patient* (Vol. 42). Dordrecht, Netherlands: Kluwer Academic Publishers.

Ville, I., Crost, M., Ravaud, J.F., & Tetrafigap Group. (2003). Disability and a sense of community belonging: A study among tetraplegic spinal-cord-injured persons in France. *Social Science & Medicine, 56*(2), 321-332.

Wendell, S. (1996). *The rejected body*. New York: Routledge.

White, P. H. (1997). Success on the road to adulthood. Issues and hurdles for adolescents with disabilities. *Rheumatic Disease Clinics of North America, 23*(3), 697-706.

Witt, W. P., Riley, A. W., & Coiro, M. J. (2003). Childhood functional status, family stressors, and psychological adjustment among school-aged children with disabilities in the United States. *Archives of Pediatrics & Adolescent Medicine, 157*(7), 687-695.

Yeo, M., & Sawyer, S. M. (2003). Strategies to promote better outcomes in young people with chronic illness. *Annals, Academy of Medicine, Singapore, 32*(1), 36-42.

CHAPTER 13

Our Patients: Heretics, Believers, Agnostics, and Ecumenists

RICHARD MACINTYRE

INTRODUCTION

In 1985, I was a 33-year-old gay man living in San Francisco and a registered nurse who just tested positive for human immunodeficiency virus (HIV). This chapter is a demonstration of how interpretive phenomenology helped me develop a much richer understanding of my own community. Maybe it was because I was a nurse, but gay men who were positive for HIV but without symptoms of acquired immune deficiency syndrome (AIDS) stopped me everywhere to talk with me about the new disease—on the sidewalks in San Francisco's Castro district, at the gym, in bars, and cafés.

People were taking very different stances. Some advocated regular medical monitoring; others warned against assuming a "sick identity." Some adapted holistic health practices; others focused intensely on the meaning of their own lives. For my doctoral research, I interviewed 17 people whose stories were representative of the hundreds that I had been hearing. This chapter tells how understandings of HIV shaped identities, social relationships, and health practices in my community. Four different orientations to HIV and its treatment emerged in this study, but these four positions are not inflexible or airtight categories; each is constituted and sustained by a dialogue between the stances, and are therefore presented here as a conversation between participants who take different stances. (Benner, 2009)

SITUATING METHOD

The research in this chapter avoided predetermined methods, following Rorty (1982) and Taylor (1989), the ethnography of the illness experience of Benner and Wrubel (1989), and the interpretive ethnography of Geertz (1972/1987). Too often, the literature on qualitative methods seemed paradigmatically confused—both fleeing from and clinging to logical positivism and a drive toward making truth claims. Interpretive research is neither idiosyncratic nor subjective but rather offers alternative accounts and understandings that open up our worlds and tell those at the margins that they are not alone, and to those in the mainstream that the marginalized are not completely different and "other."

My own research sought a deeper understanding of how a community of urban, HIV-positive gay men was interpreting its antibody status and its T-cell counts in the late 1980s and early 1990s just prior to the availability of protease inhibitors. Patricia Benner encouraged me to "follow the story," which included eliciting stories and experiences from people in the community and writing the best-possible interpretation. During this interpretive work, a religious metaphor emerged that helped me sort the participants into four major orientations or relationships to the health care system. However, I did not make this metaphor a central organizing framework for my dissertation (Sex, Drugs and T-cells, 1993) or for the book that that came afterward (Mortal Men, 1999). Mostly, I was afraid that the metaphor might upstage the stories themselves rather than serving as a means to understand those stories. Today, I'm more confident that the metaphor has the potential to help health care professionals better understand how people cope with a number of chronic illnesses, and not just HIV/AIDS.

The four major orientations to the health care system offer metaphors for how people orient themselves in relation to the dominant religion in a culture:

- Heretics hold values or adhere to practices that conflict with the dominant understandings of the health care system and the medical model of disease.

- Believers share the values and participate in the practices of the dominant health care system in a culture, just as they might share the values and rituals of a dominant religion.

- Agnostics maintain a distance from both the dominant and alternative medicines.

- Ecumenists seek to integrate values and practices from a variety of traditions in service of health and healing.

A note must be made on the use of quotation marks. When I began the process of writing and rewriting that is central to interpretive work, I took the liberty of rearranging and editing the participant's statements. Part of the interpretive work involved with turning a conversation into a text involves reorganizing the conversation into a story that will be coherent to the reader. Listeners are more forgiving than readers because they can always interrupt to ask questions. I often corrected grammatical errors, eliminated repetitive statements that did not enhance or emphasize something significant in the story, supplied antecedents when only a pronoun was given, and so forth. Therefore, the use of quotation marks was used in the manner of a fiction writer to offset dialog. As the process continued, I found myself removing much of my own voice in the conversation when it was not contributing to the story, letting the participant speak for himself. My own voice appears in the interpretation and is mostly directed at the reader. Thus, quotations are not verbatim but are always based upon actual statements of the participants.

BEFORE COCKTAILS: WAR AND RELIGION

The 1970s were innocent years of liberation and indulgence: years when Eros taught gay men to celebrate their sexuality and establish relationships. An old photo captured me, two ex-lovers, a recent fling, and my new lover all giggling hysterically at a mechanical bear. Confetti and birthday hats date the event as my 25th birthday in 1977. I had an old T-shirt that lamented, *So many men; so little time*. Five years later, the god of death arrived and taught us compassion, and how to love through grief.

As a nurse, I spent most of the 1980s and 1990s caring for friends and loved ones with AIDS. Ordinarily, doctors and nurses don't know their patients as well as I knew many of mine. The long-term loving relationships I had with them made it possible to blend the personal and the professional, and I learned a lot about caring in the process (see MacIntyre, 1996; 1999). But the newly liberated and often still-angry young men in my community were not always easy to understand. Some went to the doctor and did what they were told. Others articulated understandable reasons for not seeking medical attention. Some seemed to stake out ideological positions in response to what I thought were basically biomedical or clinical questions. A few seemed to conflate theories of government conspiracy and corporate greed into explanations for why AIDS existed in the first place, and why there was still no cure. Because this was my community, I wondered whether anyone would be able to comprehend the complexity and variety of our issues and concerns when I was in trouble.

I began my doctoral studies with Patricia Benner (see Benner, 1989) because her work promised to help me develop a richer and more sensitive understanding of my community of HIV-positive gay men. Because I was a nurse, gay men with HIV frequently asked for my opinions on monitoring and treatment decisions, and I felt obligated to offer the most intellectually defensible and individually relevant advice possible. To do this, I had to discover how population-based science intersected with the artful expression of life that varied so much from person to person. I had to take the sidewalk discussions in our community more seriously. I had to pay closer attention to what HIV meant in individual lives. My research included field notes on casual conversations as well as 17 taped interviews of gay men with relatively asymptomatic HIV.

Metaphors of war and religion were central to the interpretations that I drew from my data and have continued to shape my understanding—not only of people with HIV or AIDS, but of how most people coping with chronic disease relate to the health care system and the professionals charged with ministering to their needs.

Biomedicine has unabashedly taken up the metaphor of war, but the ways in which it takes up the metaphor of religion are less obvious. For decades, scholars from a variety of disciplines have discussed the parallels between Western biomedicine and state religions. The idea that science is the religion of the 20th century is reflected throughout our culture. These parallels are no where more apparent than in the medical sciences. Goethe feared that the world was turning into one giant medical institution (cited in Zola, 1984), and Reiff (1979) believed that "the hospital is succeeding the church and the parliament as the archetypal institution of Western culture" (Rieff, 1979, p. 355). That our health care system has taken over many responsibilities that once adhered to the church is clear. Today, the modern hospital supervises our births, our suffering, and our deaths. More importantly, the biomedical industry supervises the production of truth through officially sanctioned research. Like the Catholic Church of the Middle Ages, the biomedical industry has become a monolithic power that structures not only what we understand as "knowledge" but also the way we feel about and understand ourselves in relation to sickness, suffering, and death (Foucault, 1963/1975).

I found that the participants in my study, like most people, orient themselves to the powerful structures in society that define and organize their experiences with pain, suffering, and death in four major ways. Some adhere to the central understandings of medical research centers, hospitals, and the health care industry. These people are the "believers" and are akin to members of a European State Church. The metaphor does not work as well in the United States where there is no single, official church. However, for some European countries (such as Italy, Great Britain, and Norway), the metaphor plays well. For example, the relationship of the Catholic Church to the Italian State is outlined in Article 7 of its Constitution and governed by the Lateran Pacts (1929). In Great Britain, the Church of England is the official church, and the monarch is the head of the Church. And the Evangelical Lutheran Church of Norway is the Norwegian State Church, of which 83% of Norwegians are members (The Church of Norway, 2009). Members of the state church generally share similar notions of truth, values, and understandings about birth, death, pain, and suffering.

Like members of a European State Church, those with strong beliefs in Western medicine share conscious and unconscious ideas about the body, medical science, and illness care that are consistent with dominant cultural understandings. They seek care from licensed professionals and have hope in the products of Cartesian medical science—a science that emphasizes the search for those single causative agents of both health and illness.

The other three religious and medical positions are defined by their relationship to the dominant State Church or health care system.

Those who hold views that are largely antithetical to the dominant medical paradigm can be understood as *heretics*, some because of their holistic thinking and others who cite economic factors rather than objective science as the driving force behind modern medical treatment (see Moss, 2007). In the stories that follow, the heretics are presented first, followed by the believers. *Agnostics* are skeptical of both allopathic and alternative approaches to health and illness. They are not "unsure" like religious agnostics, but generally certain that the longstanding human desire to beat death resulted in both allopathic and alternative medical practices being overvalued. They were often my favorites with a strong sense of their own identities and what seemed to me like immense courage. Finally, there are those like me who take a cross-cultural approach to health care, attempting to integrate ideas and practices from complementary and alternative traditions with Western medicine. They are the *ecumenists*, people who appreciate multiple approaches to healing and who might be inclined to visit a variety of care givers both inside and outside the official health care system.

The Heretics

War is the most overt metaphor in modern medicine, and it is employed in response to most diseases. Modern medicine is not alone in this regard. The metaphor of war has signified and guided our response to a number of medical and social problems. Lyndon Johnson started a war on poverty. Richard Nixon declared war on cancer. Retired generals wage a war on drugs. Emmanuel Dreuilhe (1988) wrote a moving book about a war against AIDS fought on the battleground of his own body. Social liberals admonished us to "fight AIDS, not people with AIDS."

In a culture of war, pacifists are the chief heretics. My friend, Jason, was forever on guard against mucus-producing dairy, cancer-inducing additives, and any chemical that did not make people high. He often spoke of making peace with the virus:

> *Remember how we always used to say that perhaps the thing to do was to get into harmony with the virus? Maybe we should say, "Okay, Virus, as soon as I die, you're dead, so we just have to live here together." I try to be at peace with it. But battling against the thought that I'll eventually die from AIDS is like swimming upstream. We're still living in the belief that we're all going to die from it. The hundredth monkey has not yet thought that HIV is a manageable condition. It's a mental concept. I wonder how long people would live if they weren't tested at all. Now I watch my T cells go down, and I think, uh-oh, they might never go back up again. With that attitude, our chances are cut in half. I really believe that getting tested is not for everybody because you have to be willing and able to overcome your fears.**

**All exemplars in this chapter are excerpted from MacIntyre, R. (1999).* Mortal Men. *New Brunswick, NJ: Rutgers University Press. Reprinted with permission.*

I wondered how Jason's battle was going and whether there was anything that might be done to help him. A number of his friends shared the belief that not everyone with HIV would die from AIDS—perhaps not as fervently as Jason did, but with less apparent anxiety. Even so, people were dropping dead all around us, and I was convinced it wasn't all because of their minds. When I asked Jason how we might create a consciousness of hope without denying the fact that we were living with a deadly virus, Jason jumped into a discussion of support groups that revealed a serious belief in mental powers.

> *I don't think that any of those support groups really work. It's a bunch of people getting together who feel that they've got to somehow struggle to survive. I don't even want to think about having to survive. Once you get down to the level of finding out you've got something, once you start fighting to survive, then you've put into existence that there's something that's trying to kill you.*

I thought Jason was taking the positive-thinking, mind-over-matter philosophy too far. I told him I figured that chances were greater than 50/50 that I would die from AIDS, and I wasn't putting anything "into existence" by saying so. He exploded, and we argued for a while.

> **J:** *Well, that's just what I've been trying to not figure. I can't understand why you'd want to think that! Because deep down you know that whatever you believe is what you're creating in your life. So don't believe that. A million people are HIV positive, and so far only a tenth of those are sick. If we all believe we'll eventually die from AIDS, then we certainly will.*

RM: *I don't believe I'll die from AIDS. I'm just saying my chances of dying from it are rather high. What else am I going to die from?*

J: *You could die of old age, for heaven's sake. You could never die of AIDS. You could never even contract it. As soon as we find out we're HIV positive, we just wait until the day that something starts happening to us. More than any other disease, I think you have to have a positive attitude with HIV. You can't sit around thinking that you're going to get sick. I think the ones who focus on sickness and dying the least are the healthiest ones to face death. Take Bart. To me, he's the ultimate example of how to deal with HIV. He's known he's been positive for four years, and it doesn't affect him the least bit.*

JM: *Why should it? He's got 900 T cells and is totally healthy.*

J: *So am I! I'm healthy, too! My doctor says "T cells, T schmells. You're not a T cell." What about healthy people who don't have HIV? How do you know that their T cells don't go down to 100 when they get something and then go back up to 1,000? They don't monitor T cells in all those people, so that could be a common occurrence. This is the problem with an unknown situation like this, but we start living in fear and thinking it's something bad. Like right now, I'm sitting here thinking I have to make some effort in the next two weeks to get my T cells up. I have to start getting my rest. I have to not be stressed. Let me see, maybe I shouldn't go to work today and rest instead. But if I don't, then I'll go in tomorrow and things will be really tense. Then I think maybe I'll quit my job, but maybe I can't because it might affect my T cells, and that would mean I'd have to get on AZT [azidothymidine] and I don't know how I'll react to AZT. So everything is based around my damn T cells, including building the house in Hawaii! And that's ridiculous! My doctor says not to worry about my T cells, but I'm getting a lot of outside pressure here. I get barraged with information—from my doctors, from you, and from all of my other friends who love me.*

Jason had tried to avoid the numbers game altogether, but after he and his lover succumbed to our admonitions to take the test, retreat was impossible. T cells came to have a number of meanings for him, not all of which were consistent with each other. On one hand, T cells were meaningless and artificial definitions of health. Even though Jason had only 300 T cells and suffered from lymphadenopathy, night sweats, and chronic upper respiratory infections, he didn't see himself as being any less healthy than Bart, who had no symptoms at all and 900 T cells. On the other hand, Jason thought that T cells were a "good measure of viral progression," and he also felt challenged to raise them. He wasn't the only one who felt this pressure.

Although health professionals did not expect people to raise their own T cells, many felt responsible for doing just that. The sense of personal responsibility for raising one's T cells was not just confined to people with "holistic" attitudes like Jason's. In 1995, an old friend came up to me at the gym and asked whether I thought his workout would affect his T-cell count. At first, I thought he was asking whether workouts were good for people with HIV, and I was ready to encourage him to keep it up, but then it became clear he was having blood drawn later in the day. He wanted today's workout to raise today's T-cell count. It wasn't at all uncommon for men in my community to attempt to raise their T cells a few days prior to having them drawn.

Others wanted to know the worst news as soon as possible in order to make treatment decisions at the most efficacious time—whenever that was. This is the rational model. The medical purpose for monitoring T cells is either to facilitate treatment decisions or to document an individual history that might facilitate treatment decisions in the future. However, people don't always interpret their blood tests within the medical model. Like other lab values, T cells also indicate prognostic probabilities and therefore function as a measure of one's health, and even of one's life, taking on a meaning–laden message.

One of the only ways to get out from under the enormous pressure and sense of responsibility for low T-cell counts was to periodically assert that they were meaningless. For men like Jason, T-cell counts tended to function as report cards. The ambivalence these men felt about T cells was similar to that of students who cram or hope for good grades while at the same time maintaining that grades are meaningless. Jason had asserted that testing was not for everyone, and I was already wondering whether the group of us that pushed Jason and his partner into taking the test had done the right thing.

Another group accepted the war metaphor but questioned the strategy, particularly our overinvestment and consequent reliance upon the offensive weapons of medical intervention. To these more holistically minded folk, our preoccupation with advanced weaponry diverted attention from defensive concerns—the health, well-being, and combat readiness of our immune systems; the availability of fresh food and water; and related psychological and environmental conditions. My friend, Damian, related that an experimental medication he was on never produced a change in his T cells:

> At that point, I began to think that this had more to do with taking care of myself and less to do with taking that stuff. I cleaned up my act, wasn't drinking or smoking or doing anything. I was working out and running and taking care of myself—more stringently and more disciplined than I had ever done in my life, and after two months, my T cells went up to over 500.

Another friend, Eric, insisted that instead of waiting for pharmaceutical intervention, we should focus on constructing a balanced life that he defined as

> . . . eating well, being happy, getting touched, having sex, feeling good about yourself, feeling good about others. In our society, that's very hard to do. Instead of putting so much energy into the techno-medical aspect of everything, we need to make this a functional, livable society. We need to stop putting all of our life energy, expertise, intelligence, and care into medicine and work on creating a healthier society, and that means reducing alienation, anger, violence, drug addiction—all those things which cause ill health.

Some argue that medical science is developing a more objective and ultimately more humanistic approach to human problems. Critics like Eric counter that medical authorities have been no less dogmatic in their pronouncements on the causes and treatments of human problems than religious authorities have been, and that the result has been an even greater objectified and dehumanized understanding of life. The power of the medical profession in the lives of everyday people is often experienced without being consciously understood. As a sociologist, Eric understood power dynamics. His analysis of the modern doctor's office reflected his deep distrust of physicians and is a good example of how many people might experience an office visit.

> Think about what happens when you go into a doctor's office. You are dealing with crucial issues, with life and death. Enter a person who *has been given all the magical powers that our society bestows on anybody. They're almost religious.* He is wearing—usually he, male authority—is wearing a white robe, you know. Wash your hands and stuff like that. The power dynamics are that you're coming in and asking for divination. You are being told what your status is, what your condition is. You're nervous because your very integrity as a person is threatened. Then you're told that you're near death, and it's given the full weight that our society can give it.

Eric's real heresy reflects a distrust of the power and status of professionals that has surfaced throughout history, from the Protestant reformation's assault on the authority of the Roman church to the Puritan assault on the authority of the English church, to our modern self-help movements that range from 12-step programs to selling homes without real estate agents, writing wills without attorneys, and staging memorial services without funeral directors. Eric distrusts the professional authority, worries about the unequal power dynamic between physician and patient, and advocates for a more-level playing field between patients and their professional caregivers.

> *What I personally feel is that the status and the role of doctors and the medical profession need to be reduced to that of a plumber. The general public needs to know more about medical information so that everybody knows enough about common sense medical and health issues to figure things out and make their own decisions. Then go to a mere plumber-type of person, a doctor, to like prescribe the stuff or to set the bone or to do the T cells or whatever. Until the roles become that equal, I think getting involved with the medical world is dangerous.*

Eric's position may seem extreme, but it shares medicine's instrumentalist and techno-understanding of the body. In Eric's world, the priestly and caring activities required by patients should be provided through social services and safety nets with physicians providing simple technical expertise. Illich (1982) did not worry so much about social systems and professional power dynamics but rather that our reliance on professional strangers to manage our pain, suffering, and death was abrogating too much of our essential humanity. That diseases, pain, suffering, and death are not simply enemies to be conquered but rather a central feature of our common humanity is highly unorthodox and overly philosophical in an empirically focused science.

The adequacy of alternative systems of beliefs and practices to sustain medical heretics through health crises varies. Eric's distrust of medicine's authority presents a significant challenge for his health care providers. In the absence of nurturing social services and the presence of symptoms, patients like Eric will feel alienated by physicians who assume the detached nature of a plumber.

Eric and Illich (1982) distrust the doctor-priest, but patients like Jason will embrace any doctor-priest who shares their holistic ideology that can range from thoughts and feelings affecting health to positive thinking raising T cells. For some, these ideas were empowering. For others, these ideas formed imperatives and obligations for self-healing that were often not achieved, deepening a sense of disease as personal failure. They exacted an unachievable demand for self-control over the body. For Jason, I was concerned about the extent to which his holism might be functioning as a means to cope with abject fear—fear that was not permitted within his mind-body ideology.

Unorthodox views or heresies are neither inherently empowering nor delusional. They are not necessarily instances of enlightened thinking or of denial. The same general idea can function in widely different ways, and it is incumbent upon healers to understand the function of their patients' ideologies if they intend to provide more than instrumental care. As Taylor (1993) notes, conflicting theories often function simultaneously and with different possibilities.

The Believers and the State Church

The best way to understand a dominant paradigm is often through investigating the ideas and practices that develop in opposition to it. The primary alternative to the dominant Western construction of health and illness is loosely identified as holism and provides a framework for practices now referred to as complementary and alternative therapies. This alternative paradigm is not just about ideas, but economic and social power struggles as well. According to Lowenberg (1989), holism functions in opposition to the tradition of Cartesian dualism, which is the philosophical foundation of Western medical practice. Although the holistic movement can sometimes romanticize nature, Western medical science tends to see nature—and especially death—as the enemy. Holism struggles to make death acceptable while fully embracing life, and constructs a metaphor of harmony. Western medicine pits life against death and constructs a metaphor of war. The metaphors are oppositional and dualistic rather than interrelated or continuous.

Several men in my study would find the constructs of holism as articulated by Lowenberg (1989) to be closer to their notions of self and world than they would biomedical materialism. Conversely, others clearly embraced the construction of HIV and AIDS that came from the medical establishment. Their ideas seemed less dramatic than Eric's anti-medical stance or Jason's mind-over-matter holism, in part because they are largely consistent with dominant medical understandings and practices.

In fact, the orientations to Western medicine articulated in this study do not seem like ideologies at all. These men are believers but not in the fundamentalist Protestant sense. The "pro-medical" position is more akin to membership in a European State Church that comes with birth or citizenship. Membership has not been renounced to avoid paying church taxes, but beliefs are not world-defining as they are for the truly devout. However, like anyone with a life-threatening illness, these men would resist any limits placed upon receiving medicine's sacraments. Matthew's and Ron's stories are emblematic of those who looked for Western doctors with an aggressive approach to treatment.

RM: *Have you done anything in terms of lifestyle changes or anything as a result of being HIV positive?*

M: *I started taking acyclovir four years ago because I thought AIDS was eventually going to be associated with herpes. I'd never had it, so I figured, why bother getting herpes? My doctor said acyclovir wasn't harmful, so I've been taking it since 1986. I've tried various things. I took that muck you put in the blender, AL-721 (a mixture of lipids extracted from egg yolks thought to inhibit HIV; see ClinicalTrials, 2005). I did that for about a year. I've tried various things. I still do acyclovir, and I started AZT two months ago.*

RM: *Your T cells are about 700. How did you decide to start taking AZT?*

M: *. . . from the research coming out. My doctor seemed to think that when you get below 500, you should start AZT. They have an attitude of "when, not if." It's like they're waiting. It's sort of creeping up on you. I figure as long as it's going to be eventual—and they keep telling me that eventually my T cells will drop—I might as well just start it now.*

RM: *Your physician recommended you start AZT with 700 T cells?*

M: *No. He said there's no research, no statistics to show that it does anything, especially for people with more than 500 T cells. The only studies were in the 200 to 500 level. Granted, it was significant, but the sample was so small that he didn't consider it relevant. But I disagree. I know a number of people who are taking AZT and have had dramatic increases in their T cells, which I find strange.*

RM: *Did you just feel like you should be doing something?*

M: *Well, it's not just feeling that I should be doing something. I have this horrible feeling that at some point, we'll find out that we all should have been taking AZT all along, and now it's too late. You should have been doing this two years ago or whatever. I guess I figure I should do something. AZT is all that's out there at the moment that's approved, and it seems to be relatively nontoxic or relatively safe. I had a friend who was just killed by ddI [didanosine]—from pancreatic failure. I don't have those worries about AZT. I had my blood work done again this week, and my red and white cells are fine.*

Matthew was a man who thought things through for himself. He generally accepted the medical establishment's appraisal of the situation: "They have an attitude of when, not if." However, his decision to begin using pharmaceuticals earlier than his physician recommended was not uncommon. His physician's research training included concepts of significance and T-cell parameters, but Matthew wasn't a researcher and was not overly concerned with what seemed like fine points of his physician's reasoning. Matthew wasn't interested in AZT because it symbolized hope. Instead, he had a rather pragmatic fear that while waiting for confirmation of a medication's effectiveness, he might miss the boat. A number of men in my community were anxious to begin taking medicines sooner rather than later. Health professionals often try to weigh potential benefits against potential side effects, but withholding medications from patients who want them can be difficult.

Ron's story depicts a reversal in the usual state of affairs. Ron describes himself as a "real medical person," and his response to recommended support groups and meditation was perhaps predictable.

RM: *We had the test around '85, and you had it done around '87. Why did you wait?*

R: *There was no known treatment. They'd just tell you to clean up your act. I always knew that drinking and drugs and late nights were bad for you. I'd already started to clean up my act. But the minute I found out that AZT was available and was effective for treatment, my partner [James] and I decided to go down and take the test. We didn't want to take AZT unless we were actually positive. But the minute we knew there was some kind of positive action we could take, besides just living a good clean life, then it made sense to take the test. I figured that finding out I was positive wouldn't be such a disaster since there was something I could do about it. I never had much doubt in my mind. I figured I maybe had a 10 or 20 percent chance of being negative. I wasn't surprised I was positive. I wasn't happy about it, but I wasn't surprised.*

RM: *What was it like for you?*

R: *I think I would've been okay, but two things scared me to death. First, they sat me down at the clinic and were so heavy about giving me the results that it scared me. Then they suggested that I go to a support group at Project Inform. That turned out to be the most horrible experience of my life. It was about twenty or thirty people who all sat around and talked about how great life was before AIDS—and that* *they would all be dead in a year. So instead of being supported, I ended up cheering everybody up. I felt good about that, but it was a bunch of defeatist people wondering how they were going to tell their parents and worrying that their parents would wind up taking care of them. The whole feeling was death. There wasn't one person in the group who was thinking that they might live a normal life span. Except for me. My doctor said he wished I hadn't gone, but the people at the clinic practically forced me to go. They made it sound like it was standard procedure and that it would be really helpful. They made me feel like if I didn't do it, I wouldn't be doing everything possible to help myself. The whole testing procedure up to that point was fine.*

RM: *It sounds like the counselor was too caught up in his own feelings about HIV to appreciate where you were coming from.*

R: *They could've handled it differently. They sat me down like it was the biggest thing in my life and made me feel like everyone they tested in the last several weeks came up negative. I really got the impression that they were singling me out. I sort of went in knowing I was going to be positive. I went out totally broken. A few days later I went back, and they made you do meditation and all that kind of stuff. Then I felt guilty because I'm not into meditation and self-healing and all that stuff. I'm a kind of a real medical person. I would've preferred their saying that they're doing this research and they have this drug and that drug. Even if it wasn't true, that would have made me feel better. You're supposed to go like once a week, but I just went one day. It scared the hell out of me, and I never went back. And from that moment on I felt better and better and better.*

Some have argued that medical information is never neutral and that the metaphors surrounding AIDS have been as deadly as the virus. This is an interesting position in light of Ron's reaction to the HIV test. Ron had approached the HIV test within a context of hope. As a medically sanctioned intervention, AZT provided the impetus and the courage for him to take the test, but that was not the context in which Ron was received by the more "holistically" oriented health care system in his city. Neither the counselor nor the people at the support group shared Ron's faith and hope in Western medicine. The psychosocial-spiritual interventions they offered in its place were as comforting to Ron as a bottle of AZT would have been to those who believed it was poison. Nonetheless, those who generally trust Western medicine have access to a culturally sanctioned system of care that is mostly alienating for heretics.

The Agnostics

Some of the HIV-positive gay men I interviewed seemed to find heavy anchors in their own self understandings and to resist most forms of intervention, especially early in the disease process. These men clearly understood the limits of Western medicine but were not seeking alternative treatments or philosophies. As with other diseases, those who stay relatively healthy have much more freedom to choose or refuse treatment. Serious symptoms tend to force people into existing structures for care and treatment where dominant cultural understandings prevail. When they got sick, they did what they were culturally prepared to do—visit the doctor.

The freedom from symptoms and the freedom to refuse culturally sanctioned therapies for asymptomatic HIV infection create a degree of ambiguity, ambivalence, and even hostility among some with asymptomatic HIV infection. This is especially true in such cities as San Francisco and New York where health and illness are understood from a variety of different perspectives. Family, friends, and physicians often push different treatments and approaches and sometimes undercut the patient's choices.

Dick did not begin his story with taking the HIV test, but rather his experience with loss.

> *The thing that affected me most at the time, probably more than anything that's ever happened in my life, was the death of Peter. He was from New Zealand, and I met him here in the US through a mutual friend. We became the very, very best of friends. He was the human being with whom I had the closest relationship in my life. It was way more than lovers. It was just this incredible connection in so many ways. I think we sort of had sex once, but it was just kind of peripheral to something else that was going on. We were extremely close. We saw each other every day. We knew everything about each other's lives. He had boyfriends, and I had boyfriends, and we knew all about and talked to each other about our boyfriends—so we were more intimate with each other than we were with our respective lovers. It would take me more tape than is available and more time than I have to try to describe the wonderfulness of that relationship. Experiencing how pure a love between two men can be stands as the high-water mark in my life. I am very fortunate to have had that experience in life with a man. I think if you get one of those, you're very lucky. If it happens more than once, you're exceptional.*
>
> *I am basically a fairly positive person who likes himself and likes his life and is fairly self-confident and enjoys having a good time. Yet the first year after Peter died was*

the longest year of my whole life. I was miserable all the time, and life was just black. Then over the period of the second year it got grayer, progressively lighter, and in the last half year or so, I think that I got a hell of a lot happier. Not like I was before, because before Peter died I had a sort of childish innocence based on ignorance. I no longer feel that sort of youthful notion that everything's going to get better as I go along: that I'm in the prime of my life, that I'm going to conquer the world. Now I realize that death happens and things end, but I think that one can know that and be happy anyway.

To draw on an old Catholic metaphor, it's sort of like the fall from grace. Before they got knowledge, Adam and Eve had this sort of blissful ignorance where everything was always perfect and they didn't know anything other. But then they got knowledge, which changed everything and got them thrown out of the good situation they were in. That's sort of what happened to me. Now I know what death is. I have the knowledge of death, so I feel older and wiser. I'm certain that I will never have the innocent quality of happiness I had before I knew of death, but I think it is still possible for me to be happy anyway.

Dick's concise account of regaining a kind of happiness after losing the love of his life suggests Kierkegaard's idea of world-defining commitments, which Kierkegaard (1843/1971) thought were vitally necessary to any rich and full life. Dick's story included a long section where he explained why he could not even imagine a new relationship. For Dick, love was not an abstract concept or a force that somehow attached itself to a beloved object. Love was a particular embodied experience, so when Peter died, love and his way of being in the world died as well.

To avoid commitments like Dick's love of Peter is to avoid life itself, but world-defining commitments come with a price: They must eventually be mourned. Trying to distinguish between the happiness he felt before and after coming to know death was not simply an abstract philosophical issue for Dick. It was about distinguishing who he was as a man who had lived, loved, and mourned. Dick was not alone in this struggle. Freud (1917/1955), Kierkegaard (1849/1983), Becker (1973), and Wilbur (1986) all worked on making sense of mourning and mortality without recourse to overly simple religious or New Age explanations. Dick's sophistication in dealing with his own grief did not mean that he was ready to start contemplating his own mortality on a day-to-day basis, though.

D: *If I've been gradually dropping T cells over the last few years, I don't really want to be reminded of that fact or have it verified. I knew I was antibody-positive when I got the test, and after taking it, I was bummed out for a long time. I suspect that my T cells may be declining. Maybe they are; maybe they aren't. What I ask myself is, what practical good will it do me to know? What benefit is to be gained? What unpleasantness is to occur? Profit/loss. Let's look at this the way I look at everything else.*

RM: *Okay—tell me what the balance sheet shows.*

D: *And the balance sheet says there's not a great deal to be gained because if your T cells are going down there isn't a thing you can do about it. It's not like it would confirm or deny that I have some disease that can be effectively treated. I could take a highly toxic drug called AZT that will eat my bone marrow and build for me the "ill person" Zeitgeist by putting me on this permanent prescription that I'll never get off. And this would also identify me as an HIV-er to the insurance companies to whom I have to send the AZT bills, which would get me put on the list of people who should be executed or sent to concentration camps or whatever. So all of that is to be lost. And identifying myself as a sick person—both publicly and to myself—would seriously hurt my sense of well-being. I stand to lose that if I get into searching for confirmation that I have some preliminary manifestation of AIDS.*

D: *So part of me laughs at myself and says, "Honey, you are in heavy denial; you're trying to preserve this fragile illusion that you're really not sick or that you really don't have AIDS, an illusion that's getting progressively more fragile." And maybe I am, but that's what it takes for me to get up every day and keep living. If I start counting T cells, that will probably lead me to start taking medicine. If I start counting T cells and taking medicine, I'm going to become like some hypochondriac old lady who gets worried and obsessed and then wants to talk about it all the time. It's boring!*

D: *I want to spend my energy making sure that the quality of my life, however much longer it's going to be, is as high as I can possibly make it. I do work that I really enjoy. I love being a teacher because I feel like I can start people out doing something that will continue after I'm gone. I may have somebody for only one day, but I may be able to plant some kind of seed or light some kind of spark in them that will make their life better. I think that's kind of neat. I feel like I'm giving a little something back for all the good things I have taken from living. I've had a* *wonderful, marvelous, incredibly lucky life. I've met wonderful people and have had things happen to me that I had no reason to think I deserved. So I want to do those sorts of things instead of sitting around fussing over whether my T cells went up or down.*

RM: *Do you know anybody who is monitoring T cells, taking AZT, and not being a hypochondriac?*

D: *No. One of my friends has been watching his T cells decline for a long time. As a result, he started taking AZT. We were sitting around, and he was describing how much weirder and worse he feels now that he's started taking a strange and powerful new drug. So, yeah, watch your T cells decline, take AZT, feel weird, get the idea planted in your head that you're sick, pay too much attention to yourself. It just gets in your way. It gets in the way of doing whatever else you try to do in your day.*

RM: *Okay. Have you been presented with the evangelical medical appeal?*

D: *My friend the doctor tried to give me that. I just buried him last month in New York. So, heal thyself, physician. Yeah, I've had people do that and turn around and die themselves. Chinese herbalists—dead. Western medicine—dead. Clean living, bodybuilding, good diet, lots of exercise—dead. Every damn one of them. So anybody can get evangelical in my face about anything they want, and I'll listen to them and go, "Yeah, okay, fine. Show me a live one, and we'll talk."*

Dick seemed to reject both biomedicine and the narrative accounts of survival in our community, and his approach seemed needlessly myopic and even deadly. It flew in the face of my rationalism and my idealism. Although Dick had little hope in medicine or New Age holism, he could not wholly abandon hope because he knew that he needed hope to keep living. But his hope was tempered by his experience, which was that HIV invariably led to AIDS and that AIDS invariably led to death. I was concerned that his personal experience with HIV was nonetheless essentially hopeless, at least as far as either alternative interventions or Western medicine was concerned. However, Dick's hopes were neither about medicine nor prolonging biological life. Dick's hope was about preserving what was valuable to him in his own life. This is often a difficult position for nurses, physicians, and loved ones to understand—and when they don't, the patient suffers.

The Ecumenists

Asymptomatic, HIV-positive gay men have found themselves at the intersection of a number of competing approaches to health and illness, including Western biomedicine, traditional ethnomedicines, and a variety of complementary and alternative modalities. At the center of this competition are theories about the immune system: not only the mechanics of its defenses against microbes and cancers, but also its relationship to lifestyle and social issues. In addition to seeing their physicians, people in the HIV-positive community are also visiting acupuncturists, ingesting herbs, and joining gyms. Gay men, especially those with asymptomatic HIV infection, still seek out a variety of approaches to treat it. Even the most medically minded among us were experimenting with things like AL-721—"that 'muck you put in a blender'—along with their AZT. Nathan, a psychiatrist, embraced both Western and alternative approaches.

> I went to see an AIDS specialist who did skin testing. I'd already finished two years of medical school, so I knew what skin testing meant. She kept shaking her head, and the message I got from her was, "You are typical; you are doomed." I didn't have any reaction to the skin tests, and rather than realizing that that was a bad sign, I just totally blocked it out. I canceled my appointment, and the nurse told me I had to come in and have my skin test read. And I just said, "Don't worry. I'm fine. I'm fine." I've never had a case of denial that extreme in my life. I forgot I had ever done the test until a whole year later. It terrified me because it meant I had no immune system. Then one day after I was back in medical school, I was doing skin testing on somebody. All of a sudden I remembered my own skin test, and the result, and I was horrified.
>
> Then in the spring of '87, I went for a routine physical, and my white count came back at 3.9 [low]. My doctor said I had to get tested because this was an indication that something might be wrong, and there was really no excuse not to get tested at this point. So I agreed to go ahead and finally get tested. I felt I really had to face it and was fully prepared for a positive result. What I wasn't fully prepared to find out was that my T cells were only 226. So what happened actually was that I got the results of the T cells before I got the results of the HIV test.
>
> What freaked me out so much was that I wasn't familiar with the numbers, and I really didn't know what they meant. I had just learned about what the ranges were. I had heard that 200–400 was ARC [AIDS-related complex]. So immediately

> *in my mind, I had ARC. Anything under 200 meant you were vulnerable to opportunistic infections. I didn't know anything about how T cells could stay in the same place for a long time. Actually, I didn't know anything. Even being a doctor, I didn't know anything. So what I thought that meant was that any day I would come down with AIDS. It was like, "Sorry I have to tell you this, but you only have a year to live."*
>
> *None of the other doctors knew what they meant, either. I learned about these lab values through my own experience, through what I learned from other people, through watching my own numbers. It wasn't from having learned it from a textbook or from an article, because even now [1990], nobody really knows.*
>
> *Then I had my T cells rechecked, and they were 315 a week later. So I learned my first lesson about T cells from that. They could vary 100 points. It didn't really mean anything necessarily.*

Nathan's comment that "it didn't really mean anything necessarily" was repeated several times by the men in my study but rarely meant the same thing twice. For Nathan, it meant that he wasn't necessarily going to get sick and die within the year. His interpretation of the skin testing was not scientific but symbolic. The negative result indicated not a compromised immune system but no immune system at all.

Even physicians occasionally interpret laboratory tests within personal, rather than rational, frameworks. In fact, nobody understands laboratory tests in perfectly rational and abstract terms all of the time. Nor should we. Despite our culture's having come to idolize the rational over the past 300 years, much of life is lived outside neat rational abstractions in the rather messy world of personal and social meanings and concerns. This is not to say that all personal meanings should be accepted without argument, but rather that personal and social meanings often collide with the rational constructs of health professionals. Nathan seemed to seek some common ground between the personal and social meanings that HIV had in his community and his professional understandings, often by moving back and forth between his feelings and his science. Having no immune system whatsoever was way too dangerous to Nathan's sense of self, so he "forgot" for a whole year that he had taken the test, which was perhaps the most rational response possible.

When Nathan received his first T cell count, he did not rationally choose the meanings that he assigned to his results. Before giving him the result over the phone, his physician asked whether he was sitting down, and Nathan interpreted the result in the context in which it was given. The medical technology to measure CD4 counts (or the levels of T-helper cells, the primary target of HIV) was available in 1987, but the stories in this project showed that we did not have the experience necessary to make much sense of them. Neither his medical education nor his psychiatric residency did much to reduce Nathan's terror or the symbolic interpretations that grew out of it. So he turned to "alternative things."

N: *I decided to start researching everything I could possibly do for myself. AZT wasn't a possibility at that time. It was still just experimental. There were really no treatments at that point. I've always been somewhat holistically minded, so within a week after being in a major depression, I was out there doing a whole list of things. First, I started doing complete vitamin therapy,"* [laughing] *"like several hundred dollars on vitamins. I started doing acupuncture, Chinese herbs. I started jogging regularly, meditating, visualization.*

N: *Six months previously, I had started reading* A Course in Miracles, *which is the first spiritual work that ever touched me in any way. It had been collecting dust in a corner, so I pulled that out again. I started reading things like Louise Hay, Dr. Bernie Siegel, a lot of inspirational things about mind over body. I joined a support group at the Center for Attitudinal Healing, which I attended for fifteen months.* [laughing] *That was it. Then I took six months off from my residency while I was instituting all of these things. I came out to my supervisor and training director. I told them what was going on, and they were very supportive. So I was given the time off with pay, which was really nice.*

RM: *Jesus! You did it all. What was that like?*

N: *It was empowering. It gave me the feeling that I could have control over this, particularly when I read things from Louise Hay and Bernie Siegel. I also attended seminars and whatnot. I got it into my mind that I'm not going to be a victim of this. I can take charge. I can have control over this. And my theory at the time—it's changed significantly since then—was that if I don't want to die, I'm not going to die. I can will this thing into submission.* [laughing] *And I needed to feel that at the time. Everything I was doing for it—the meditation, the vitamins, the herbs—made me feel like this was my way of controlling it. As long as I was doing those things, this thing was not going to get me. I felt real positive about that.*

N: *Throughout the first year, I gradually started dropping all the things I had started. I didn't feel like going for acupuncture anymore. The herbs were a pain in the ass—boiling that shit every morning, and the smell was horrible. Not to mention* *the expense! All those trace minerals and enzymes; all this shit. Then I started doing AL-721. I did that for an entire year. The only thing it probably did was put weight on me. I finally boiled it down to a multivitamin, multimineral, E and C.*

N: *But again, all those alternative things were important because they gave me confidence psychologically. I wasn't just sitting there doing nothing. As time went on, I realized I'm still alive and not getting sick. But I needed to do all those things before to give me a sense of power. When I regained confidence that I wasn't ready to drop dead, I was able to stop doing a lot of those things.*

RM: *So what finally convinced you to take AZT?*

N: *I had a very rigid, pushy, by-the-book internist who said, "You just have to do this." But the same day I was told I needed to be on AZT, I was told I needed to go on Pentamidine and that I should fill out a durable power of attorney. So I really flipped out. When he gave me the forms for the durable power of attorney, I felt like I was getting a death warrant to sign, whereas a friend of mine immediately filled them out because he said it made him feel much better.*

RM: *It gives some people a sense of control.*

N: *Yeah, but that was the same day my ANC [absolute neutrophil count] was 800. My doctor believed in full-strength AZT, and then thought, because of the ANC, that I was in too terrible a state to be on full-strength AZT! I was tied to a schedule of getting my arm stuck every two weeks, an M.D. visit every two weeks, and a once-a-month Pentamidine appointment. I thought I'd never be able to stop thinking about AIDS.*

When Nathan started taking AZT, it wasn't because he found his doctor's arguments reasonable or convincing. It wasn't really because he was convinced that it would help. Unlike some of the men I interviewed, Nathan never said that AZT gave him hope. Nathan began AZT to comply with an older gay physician's insistence, and in the process, was able to let go of some of his denial. He also felt that he had given AZT some of his "power" and that if he stopped taking it, he'd feel very vulnerable and trapped. It made him feel "lousy," and in a few months, he told his doctor he would rather die than take the full dose of AZT. Nathan called me later that day to tell me how "pissed off" his doctor was.

He was so pissed off that he dictated his notes right in front of me. He turned on the Dictaphone and said, "Patient refuses to take 500 mg as recommended. Will only take 300 mg even though I told him there is no evidence that 300 mg"... blah, blah, blah—as if life waits for evidence. You know, I never thought the AZT did much at all. There never was a bump in my T cells.

A couple of years later, Nathan had two T-cell counts in a row that were below 200. "I got horribly depressed. I thought this is it. It's inevitable. There are two of them now." He started Prozac, and his T cells went back to above 200. On the advice of his new physician, Nathan stopped the AZT. He tried two new antivirals. DDC (dideoxycytidine) gave him canker sores, and ddI gave him diarrhea. Two months later, his T cells went up a bit more. For the next few years, Nathan stayed away from antivirals altogether. When protease inhibitors were available in 1996, he started taking what was known as "the cocktail"—generally three different antiretroviral medications. In 2005, he became impressed with Harold Foster's work and added selenium, NAC (N-acetyl cysteine), glutamine, and tryptophan.

CONCLUSION

While Nathan went back and forth between Western and alternative medicine, the playing field for the holistic and biomedical positions is hardly level. Western medicine isolated HIV and defined AIDS. Western biomedical understandings have dominated public discussions, shaped the structure of HIV and AIDS services and research, and became the credo of almost every major AIDS organization. A century ago, Robert Koch (1878/1880) and Claude Bernard (1865/1957) took different positions on the relative role microorganisms played in human diseases. Koch focused on microbes, whereas Bernard argued that microbes were everywhere and that health was dependent on the human terrain or milieu intérieur.

Some gay men with asymptomatic HIV heeded Bernard's warning against the "single minded fervor of the microbe hunters," especially because the early drugs used to fight HIV were often both ineffective and dangerous. Some of these men focused on stress reduction, drug and alcohol use, nutrition, exercise, and meditation. Others developed fantasies about being able to control their HIV and T-cell counts with right living and right thinking, becoming examples of the "blame-the-victim" critique that Western medicine has leveled against the holistic health movement. Some, like Nathan, took an ecumenical approach.

However, the vast majority of gay men embraced Western medicine. We grew up in a culture informed by the notion that diseases are caused by single, identifiable, and measurable agents. People who accepted the dominant, medical construction of AIDS understood that the illness was caused by a chance encounter with a virus. The religious and political right, however, construed the epidemic as the scourge of an angry God or the consequences of an immoral agent—"the wages of sin is death" approach.

A more holistic approach to AIDS would have included psychosocial and behavioral issues, such as the rampant promiscuity, alcoholism, and drug use in the gay community, but the battle lines had been drawn. The religious and political right proclaimed our guilt and picketed our funeral services, while the biomedical establishment insisted that the virus was morally neutral and would infect whomever it could. The cause of AIDS became a black-or-white issue: a blame-the-victim mentality parading as personal responsibility, or a blame-the-virus mentality parading as hard science. Given those choices, it is no surprise that most people with HIV felt more comfortable with the latter.

When the scientific establishment did address psychosocial and behavioral issues, it was almost always within a viral framework. Researchers seemed to conclude that studying behavioral issues that were not directly related to contracting HIV (and the social structures that sustained them) might be construed as being homophobic or blaming the victim. The viral framework had the distinct advantage of appearing objective, amoral, and nonjudgmental, and most humanists and academics opted for the "HIV is the cause of AIDS" equation.

Over time, however, as people accumulated more experience living with HIV, the assumption that the virus held all the cards seemed too simplistic, disempowering, and unduly pessimistic. In addition to pursuing traditional holistic approaches to sustaining health (e.g., nutrition, exercise, acupuncture, herbs, and micronutrients), many gay men started reappraising specific social structures and practices in their community. The gay liberation movement had forced gay men out of the closet and into a world where they were compelled to develop new identities and ways of understanding themselves. That all this gay liberation and gay identity construction took place within a largely hostile and homophobic culture immersed in its own narcissism and hedonism has not been fully appreciated. A sexuality and sensuality that had been repressed and restrained throughout adolescence (and for eons) suddenly exploded.

Not all practices that develop around liberation movements are valorous or healthy. Some take a serious toll. The idea that some of the behaviors associated with gay liberation contributed to the decimation of gay men's immune systems continues to be both psychologically untenable and economically unprofitable. It is far more comforting for patients and far more profitable for the medical industry to attribute the entire epidemic to a chance encounter with a virus.

Yet the notion that lifestyle might affect who remains asymptomatic and who progresses to AIDS has been part of the conversation among gay men with asymptomatic HIV for well over two decades. This hasn't been an easy conversation. The major "party boys" did seem to drop dead first, but lots of us knew men who had lived cleaner lives but were already dead. Thus, questions about the effect that drugs, alcohol, stress, depression, and promiscuity might have on disease progression persist in the gay community, both consciously and subliminally. These questions aren't simply attributable to unresolved feelings of guilt, self-loathing, or internalized homophobia. Although emotions often accompany such questions, rational minds will pose them independently. But the questions have been hard to answer.

Science does not know how people with asymptomatic HIV can prevent their conditions from turning into AIDS. Even the fine print on the pharmaceutical advertisements admits that we don't know whether antiviral medications will prolong the asymptomatic period. We also don't know whether reducing stress, abstinence from drugs and alcohol, eating right, exercising, or meditating will prolong the asymptomatic period. Some studies show that cigarette smoking hastens and some micronutrients slow progression to AIDS, but these conclusions are not uniform. After all this time, we don't even know whether condom use between HIV-positive partners will prolong life. And even though science has not answered these questions definitively, people with asymptomatic HIV answer them every day, within the contexts of their own lives, experiences, and beliefs.

Whereas most of the top AIDS researchers gave lip service to the existence of "co-factors," the role that these and other non-HIV-related factors might play in the progression of HIV to AIDS has not been systematically investigated, although some progress is being made. The war against AIDS has mostly involved a single strategy: Seek out the virus wherever it may be lurking and kill it. The single-minded focus on the virus is not confined to the medical establishment. When Rotello (1996) suggested that 2,000 or more sexual partners per decade may not be a biologically sustainable norm in any community, many accused him of being homophobic. Nonetheless, the views of dissident and often marginalized academics and community leaders who suggest that other factors besides the virus should be considered are seriously entertained by many gay men living with HIV. Foucault's work (1963/1975; 1975/1979; 1976/1979) on the relationship between scientific truths and the structures of power that develop and sustain them has inspired serious thinkers to reconsider the biomedical construction of HIV/AIDS. Those who have lived with asymptomatic HIV infection over the past two decades have had to chart their courses between these larger cultural arguments about health, microbes, and disease.

On the surface, comparisons between religion and medical science can seem strange, but the struggles between religious and medical authorities are over the same turf—the nature of reality or truth. One prescribes the methods required to investigate objective reality; the other prescribes the rituals required to understand revealed truth. However, big differences exist between modern medicine and the modern church. In the Western world, rejecting modern religion is increasingly possible (Taylor, 2007), but it is as hard to walk away from modern medicine as it was to walk away from the church of the Middle Ages. The sacraments of health care can be withheld, as they frequently are in the United States, but the importance of health care cannot be denied. Nonetheless, heathens and heretics have never been completely extinguished, and the AIDS dissident movement always intrigued me.

Over the past two decades, I came to appreciate that being a nurse is somewhat like being a nun. Nuns are told what to profess by a religious hierarchy, whereas nurses obtain their doctrine from an industrial or academic one; yet, the truths perpetuated by our religions and sciences are far more orderly than the real world in which people live—worlds of crisis, chaos, and ambiguity. Nuns and nurses tend to live closer to the people than do their more powerful priest and physician counterparts, and both nuns and nurses often wind up mediating relationships between their neighbors and the larger powers that govern modern life. Nuns now offer communion, and nurse practitioners dispense medications. Both minister to parishioners and patients in ways that used to be the singular province of priests and physicians.

Today, many nurses act as apologists or even evangelists for the medical status quo. Many nurses—especially those in academic positions—demonstrate a deep reverence toward the modern systems charged with developing scientific knowledge. They are contemptuous toward the "*n* of one": the anecdote, the individual patient. Other nurses, though, revere the sanctity of specific human lives in addition to statistical data based upon populations and aggregates. Our challenge is to remain simultaneously respectful and skeptical of both positions.

Healing care requires an understanding of particular patients and population-based science. If we approach everyone as if they were members of our own church—if we fail to distinguish between heretics, believers, agnostics, and ecumenicists—we miss the mark. If we cannot comprehend why our most compliant patients might also visit the alternative clinic down the street, we must struggle to enlarge our concept of the population we treat.

Aristotle's (350 B.C.E/1994) concept of the virtuous mean can be helpful here: Aristotle postulated that human virtues can be found between their two opposing vices (and it has always been easier to identify pathological states than healthy ones). Aristotle's most famous example is perhaps the virtue of courage falling between the vice of cowardice and the vice of recklessness, and a bit closer to recklessness than cowardice. In health care, the virtue of healing can be found between the vices of shamanism and scienticism. The most sensitive healers will move away from one vice or the other depending upon their own tendency to favor one over the other, their institution's tendency to favor one over the other, and the patient's beliefs and orientation to health and the health care system.

References

Aristotle (1994). *Nicomachean Ethics*. (W. D. Ross, Trans.). The Internet Classics Archive. (Original work published 350 B.C.E.). Retrieved November 25, 2009 from http://classics.mit.edu/Aristotle/nicomachaen.mb.txt

Becker, E. (1973). *The denial of death*. New York: Free Press.

Benner, P. (2009). Personal communication.

Benner, P., & Wrubel, J. (1989). *The primacy of caring: Stress and coping in health and illness*. Menlo Park, CA: Addison-Wesley.

Bernard, C. (1957). *An introduction to the study of experimental medicine*. (H. C. Greene, Trans.). New York: Dover Publications. (Original work published 1865).

ClinicalTrials (2005). A study of AL721 in HIV-infected patients with swollen lymph nodes. Retrieved November 25, 2009 from http://www.clinicaltrials.gov/ct2/show/NCT00001012

Dreuilhe, E. (1988). *Mortal embrace: Living with AIDS*. (L. Coverdale, Trans.). New York: Hill and Wang.

Foucault, M. (1975). *The birth of the clinic: An archaeology of medical perception.* (A. M. Sheridan Smith, Trans.). New York: Vintage Books. (Original work published 1963).

Foucault, M. (1979). *Discipline and punish: The birth of the prison*. (A. Sheridan, Trans.). New York: Vintage Books. (Original work published 1975).

Foucault, M. (1979). *The history of sexuality Volume 1: An introduction*. (R. Hurley, Trans.). London: Penguin Books. (Original work published 1976).

Freud, S. (1955). Mourning and melancholia. In James Strachey (Ed.), *Complete psychoanalytical works* (pp. 237-258). London: Hogarth Press and the Institute of Psycho-Analysis. (Original work published 1917).

Geertz, C. (1987). Deep play: Notes on the Balinese cockfight. In P. Rabinow & W. M. Sullivan (Eds.), *Interpretive social science: A second look* (pp. 195-240). Berkeley: University of California Press. (Original work published 1972.)

Illich, I. (1982). *Medical nemesis: The expropriation of health*. New York: Pantheon Books.

Kierkegaard, S. (1971). *Either/Or Volume I*. (D. Swenson & L. Swenson, Trans.). Princeton, NJ: Princeton University Press. (Original work published 1843).

Kierkegaard, S. (1983). *The sickness unto death*. (H. Hong & E. Hong, Trans.). Princeton, NJ: Princeton University Press. (Original work published 1849).

Koch, R. (1880). *Investigations into the etiology of traumatic infective diseases*. (W. W. Cheyne, Trans.). London: The New Sydenham Society. (Original work published 1878). Retrieved November 25, 2009 from http://books.google.com/books?id=mCEJAAAAIAAJ&dq=Robert+Koch+investigations+into+the+etiology+of+traumatic+infective+disease&printsec=frontcover&source=bl&ots=DPSg8Ms6g0&sig=l1kRq8RCR9M68HiQfT9Qn_Aus7o&hl=en&ei=QcURS4zHIIfIsQPQ5eiQDw&sa=X&oi=book_result&ct=result&resnum=1&ved=0CA8Q6AEwAA#v=onepage&q=&f=false

Lateran Pacts (1929). Retrieved November 25, 2009 from http://www.aloha.net/~mikesch/treaty.htm

Lowenberg, J. S. (1989). *Caring and responsibility: The crossroads between holistic practice and traditional medicine*. Philadelphia: University of Pennsylvania Press.

MacIntyre, R. (1994). *Sex, Drugs and T-Cells: Symbolic meanings among gay men with asymptomatic HIV infection*. University of California, San Francisco, 1993. Ann Arbor, MI: UMI. Order # 9406617.

MacIntyre, R. (1996). Nursing loved ones with AIDS: Knowledge development for ethical practice. In S. Gordon, P. Benner, & N. Noddings (Eds.), *Caregiving readings in knowledge, practice, ethics, and politics* (pp. 141-153). Philadelphia: University of Pennsylvania Press.

MacIntyre, R. (1999). *Mortal men: Living with asymptomatic HIV.* New Brunswick, NJ: Rutgers University Press.

Moss, R. W. (2007, April 1). Patents over patients. *The New York Times*, p. 12, Section 4.

Reiff, P. (1979). *Freud: The mind of the moralist*. Chicago: University of Chicago Press.

Rorty, R. (1982). *Consequences of pragmatism*. Minneapolis: University of Minnesota Press.

Rotello, G. (1996). *Sexual ecology: AIDS and the destiny of gay men*. New York: Dutton.

Taylor, C. (1989). *Sources of the self*. Cambridge, MA: Harvard University Press.

Taylor, C. (1993). *Explanation and practical reason*. M. Nussbaum & A. Sen (Eds.), *The quality of life* (pp. 208-231). Oxford: Clarendon.

Taylor, C. (2007). *A secular age*. Cambridge, MA: Harvard University Press.

The Church of Norway. (2007). Retrieved November 25, 2009, from http://www.kyrkja.no/english/engelsk.cfm?artid=5276

Wilber, K. (1986). *Up from Eden: A transpersonal view of human evolution*. Boston: Shambhala Publications.

Zola, I. (1984). Healthism and disabling medicalization. In P. R. Lee, C. L. Estes, & N. B. Ramsay (Eds.), *The nation's health* (2nd ed., pp. 160-169). San Francisco: Boyd & Fraser.

CHAPTER 14

Dwelling in the World: Realms of Meaningful Involvement in Late Life

SARA MANNY WEISS

INTRODUCTION

By midlife, most people have had some experience that throws off balance their taken-for-granted sense of what the world is about and their place in it. This may involve the birth of a child, the loss of a parent, a serious injury or illness affecting oneself or a loved one, the devastation of losing one's home to fire or natural disaster, or the tragedy of violence in one's community.

Less significant or extreme circumstances can also call into question a person's ordinary grasp in day-to-day life. A move to a new home in a different community can precipitate varying degrees of disruption in a person's practices and understandings of what is salient. A more transitory experience of this disequilibrium may occur when visiting a foreign country where the language isn't familiar, the currency has a substantially different value from that of one's own country, and the manners and customs of the people don't immediately make sense. Although these kinds of changes can occur at any time, they may increase toward the end of life when one's health, social matrix, and conditions of daily life are at increased risk of being disrupted in dramatic and significant ways.

As explicated in the works of Benner (1984a, 1994a), Benner & Wrubel (1989), Dreyfus (1991, 1992), Heidegger (1927/1962), Taylor (1985a, 1989, 1991a, 1991b), Wrubel (1985), and others, one's usual concerns, habits, traditions, practices, and familiar patterns of relating and getting the expected responses from one's environment are the very things that make a person understandable as who he or she is. This notion of the situated relation between the person and his or her world—that a person both constitutes and is constituted by one's existential involvement in the world—is the condition for the possibility of meaning to arise at all. In this sense, meaning is not located in or created by the individual, but rather is given by cultural and social parameters that define and delimit what it is to be a person in the particular situation.

To the extent that we participate in day-to-day life through familiar habits, routines, and practices that mean something to us, we are defined by this involvement. This is the notion of human beings as "self-interpreting" (Benner & Wrubel, 1989; Heidegger, 1927/1962; Taylor, 1985a). To be disconnected from these taken-for-granted ways of knowing oneself and navigating in the world leaves a person essentially "without a place to dwell." Heidegger (1927/1962) used the word "dwelling" to illustrate the fundamental mode of human being-in-the world and to emphasize that this relation is not of a subject to an object. Dreyfus (1991) also used a synonymous word—"inhabiting"—to illustrate how *Dasein* (human being) and the world are mutually constituted: "When we inhabit something, it is no longer an object for us but becomes a part of us and pervades our relation to other objects in the world" (p. 45).

> *"When we inhabit something, it is no longer an object for us but becomes a part of us and pervades our relation to other objects in the world"*

Polanyi (1962) made this idea clearer by pointing to how visionary discoveries in the sciences and creativity in the arts occur in the process of "dwelling" or "losing [one] self" in the wonder of astronomy, or in the music of a symphony, for example, as opposed to a detached relation characterized by observing and analyzing objective facts about such fields.

In this chapter, I make visible some of the existential skills of "dwelling in the world" that are challenged during the late stages of life. The discussion will address the relational fabric and context of people's lives that allows meanings to be sustained when familiar ways of comporting oneself—the embodied, skillful know-how that comes from "inhabiting" the world—break down because of illness, debility, losing loved ones, or relocating, for instance. Some things that can impair a person's capacity to dwell-in-the-world will also be discussed. The paradigm case approach to data explication and analysis (Benner 1994b; Leonard, 1994) will be used to make these points.

The two paradigm cases discussed in this chapter were drawn from an interpretive phenomenological (IP) study of older adults' lived experience of aging. Both people presented were community-dwelling octogenarians whom I interviewed at their homes on four occasions each over a period of two to three months. The interviews lasted approximately one-and-one-half hours per visit. The interview guide designed for the study elicited demographic and health data, information on how participants conducted their day-to-day lives and coped with health events, and their life stories. The life story part of the interviews drew from experiences the participants identified as salient to how they had come to be the people they were at the time of the interviews.

> *I would rather live, I would rather be strong, I would rather be young. But there are no choices here.*

PARADIGM CASE #1: ANN

Ann was meaningfully engaged in lifelong traditions and practices despite failing health. An 80-year-old former university professor, she lived in an urban house where she had lived for decades. Her disability of chronic arthritis and advanced congestive heart failure had progressed to the point where her pain, dyspnea, and weakness were ever-present in varying degrees. She had difficulty walking even the length of her house at times. Her deterioration in the year preceding these interviews was particularly dramatic following surgery for colon cancer and two episodes of pneumonia, one requiring hospitalization. However, she responded to the situation with equanimity and acceptance:

> *I accept it because that's the way life is. I also am perfectly aware that if I were to fight and struggle, I wouldn't accomplish anything and I'd feel worse. Actually I don't like being in pain. I don't like being stressed, so I try and do the best I can to sort of quiet it down. I would rather live, I would rather be strong, I would rather be young. But there are no choices here.*

Ann did not experience her debility as defeat nor an occasion to give up in spite of the recognition that many physical capacities she once took for granted are irretrievably gone. She adapted to her limits with day-to-day strategies that made the best use of her physical resources and preserved her enjoyment of everyday life:

> *I think, considering my limitations, I enjoy what I do when I can do it. This last year has been a great change in my life since my surgery and my pneumonias and things. And it isn't a question of being satisfied, I just do the best I can with what I've got. I mean, my disabilities are such that I have very few choices. And I just enjoy myself with what I have at hand. I have a rich mental life. That probably is what makes the difference. And I have a very rich social life, don't forget.*

Despite being essentially homebound, Ann was by no means a social isolate. She received frequent phone calls and had visitors almost daily from among her many friends, relatives, and acquaintances. For years, she invited international students at the nearby university to live with her in exchange for what she called "goods and favors." Besides benefiting from their companionship and practical assistance for household chores and meal preparation, Ann and the students provided *each other* intellectual stimulation, with Ann assuming the role of sage or mentor to many of them. Over the years, these relationships expanded her ever-enlarging network of caring and appreciative friends.

When Ann was alone—and she was much of the day—she found numerous possibilities for pleasurable activity. She continued to read scholarly works and wrote numerous memoirs and two children's books over several years before I interviewed her. Reading romance novels and listening to classical music were additional sources of enjoyment. In recent years, Ann's avocational interest in "armchair biology" was expressed primarily through her extensive collecting and reading of all the available writings by and about a famous scientist, particularly focusing on the sociological aspects of the man and the development of his theories. This could be understood as a vibrant extension of her former career as an academic. However, instead of pursuing this interest for scholarly reasons, she engaged in it for the pure pleasure it gave her:

> *I have many, many books about him and all of his writings. So I can amuse myself at my own level. I don't plan to do anything with any of this except enjoy myself.*

Ann often needed, by necessity, to acquiesce to the "will of the body" (Frank, 1991). Over the course of the interviews, she experienced increased weakness which she attributed, in part, to a viral illness, yet overall she interpreted this and her frequent heart palpitations and chronic ankle edema as evidence that she was on a downward trajectory. Her ongoing sense of where she was physically took into account both what her condition precluded as well as what possibilities for meaningful life her body still allowed:

> *I think I'm past the stage where I will be writing anymore because my powers are failing. Not because I couldn't write, but I haven't got the energy to put my mind to it. I still try to do as much as I can in the world, that is. I am really helpful when I can be without being pathologically helpful. I never interrupt anybody and say, "I think you should do so and so." Least of all, my own children. But they do come to me for advice, and I give them my most considered opinion as I do anyone else who will ask me. And I'm not at all offended if no one takes my advice.*

She knew and respected her body's willfulness, trusting in its wisdom (Frank, 1991) as it was part of the natural order of things:

> *I didn't really think I was going to make it to a very old age because I had used my body so badly. I'd been exposed to so many diseases. But, I have a very strong constitution, obviously. And good genes. . . . I'm gonna die probably very quietly, instead of in battle. [laughs] Or be blown into the middle of next week by a Nazi bomb, or whatever. Because any of those things could have happened to me, and they didn't.*

Here, she was referring to having dodged risky situations in her young and middle adult years. She had been a volunteer in the Spanish Civil War in the 1930s, survived more than one potentially life-threatening illness as a young adult, and suffered nearly disabling back problems in middle age. It is as if surviving these close calls were as only a reprieve granted by extraordinary luck and "good genes." She therefore saw no cause for complaint today because she "used [her] body so badly" as a young woman. What she felt she could accomplish at the time of the interviews was what the situation offered her—no more and no less. This is not the self-understanding of a radically free, rational agent striving toward mastery and control. On the contrary, much of her life had been shaped by the things beyond her control, and her self-understanding made room for this. She did not experience her body as an adversary, an object of disgust for having failed her. She accepted it, foibles and all, as if it were an old friend. Acknowledging and working within its constraints, she knew full well that challenging its limits would make her more uncomfortable by exacerbating symptoms.

> *"My creative unconscious serves me well."*

Ann's ability to see possibilities rather than obstacles in most situations seemed to have characterized her from an early age. Growing up in the rural Midwest, she turned numerous disappointments into exciting opportunities. When she and her family had to leave their beloved homestead and move into town when she was eight, she took up naturalistic studies of the frogs and snakes in the local drainage ditch. As she approached the end of high school, she was expecting to go on to college and medical school, but this dream was squelched by her family's financial losses in the Great Depression. Instead, she became a social worker, and eventually earned two master's degrees and a Ph.D. in middle adulthood. Through employment, commitment to social causes, and self-directed learning, she found outlets for her earliest passionate interests in science and nature, social justice, and creative writing.

In the second interview, Ann talked about her "creative unconscious," a term she explained is drawn from Jungian psychology. Soon after her husband died and before she herself became ill, Ann considered the possibility of her own eventual physical decline and the potential inaccessibility of her upstairs bedrooms. Realizing that this might someday prohibit her remaining in her own home, she added a bedroom and a large, well-equipped bathroom to the main level of the house. She explained how she came to do this:

> *My creative unconscious serves me well. And it can come up with a whole project. I mean, look at the addition to this. It's a project entirely out of my creative unconscious. I came upstairs one day for the unpty-umph time, and I said to myself, "I've got to do something about this." Now I didn't design the project, I didn't build the project, but I knew immediately who to ask, and what to do on the business end. And that's what your creative unconscious can do for you.*

Unfortunately, her foresight became reality two years later when she had a serious heart attack. Overnight, her remodeled house became an invaluable resource, affording her a degree of independence she would otherwise not have been able to enjoy. Knowing that her financial resources couldn't last indefinitely, she refinanced her house and took out a loan to have more cash to live on. As a result, she could afford the in-home services of a nutritionist to ensure that she maintain adequate nutrition given her scant appetite, and an acupressurist to treat her arthritis pain. She hired people to do her housecleaning and had her groceries delivered. Her prescience in these matters worked to shore up the embodied capacities she still had.

Ann said she is good at "seizing opportunities," which she described and demonstrated as a stance of engagement with her world and openness to what her circumstances could offer. "Listening to [her] creative unconscious" was an existential skill for her. Through her familiar habits, skills, and practices, she was solicited by the saliencies of the situation and its possibilities. Ann's story is an excellent example of "situated possibility" (Benner & Wrubel, 1989; Taylor, 1985b; Wrubel, 1985). She saw many aspects of her day-to-day life—things that might seem problematic to others—as holding meaningful possibilities. For example, Ann brought up her sleep patterns as "very bad," suggesting that they were at odds with what had previously been her pattern. But she had come to interpret her sleep disruption—tossing and turning in bed—as having some paradoxical advantage, a "form of exercise." In fact, it became a *new* habit for her, a routine happening that she made room for, and even endorsed, despite its annoyance. She did not fight her wakefulness, but instead worked with it and came to understand it as serving her rather than defeating or disabling her.

Through her lifelong habits, routines, and practices, Ann exemplified *involvement, not detachment* from concerns and desires. By way of her involvement, she was able to recognize that which is possible in her situation, in contrast to being committed to seeking idealized, and therefore unattainable versions of her desires or ways in which her life was deficient (Benner & Wrubel, 1989). As she said, "I would rather live. I would rather be strong. I would rather be young . . . but there are no choices here." She had a realistic appreciation of her limits, while at the same time being open to whatever her situation could offer.

We see this illustrated by Ann in numerous ways: Whereas her debility might have disrupted a long history of hostessing parties and holiday meals in her home, this was not the case. Although she was no longer capable of the planning, shopping, and food preparation it involved, she continued to entertain albeit on more modest terms. Shortly before our interviews began she invited eight family members and friends over for a dinner party. She explained, "I can't cook, so I ordered up an ever such a nice Chinese dinner, and everybody sat around, and I opened up two bottles of wine."

Despite being substantially debilitated and in nearly continuous pain, Ann did not "moan and groan" about it because "Who would come and visit an old *kvetch*?" She draws sustenance from a lifelong tradition of scholarship, appreciation of music and the arts, and an ongoing engagement with people. Her resourcefulness and personal attributes must not be construed as the sole explanation for her situated possibility, however. Her community of friends and family played a substantial part in preserving the web of familiar practices and habits that constituted her self-understanding. They continued their involvement with her as in previous years, but at her home. They sought her counsel. They were responsive to the hospitality she extended through spontaneous dinner parties. They complemented and filled in for her waning physical capacities.

Rather than change the rituals of the holidays, gatherings continued to take place at *her* home even though she was assisted by all the guests sharing in the tasks of preparing the meals and carrying out the usual traditions. She recognized that she was fortunate in having many supportive people around her. She entertained the notion of reciprocity in her relationships, but the relationships were not framed in terms of mere exchange. Instead, she accepted help without the burden of guilt or indebtedness, acknowledging goodness in the relationships in and of themselves:

> *I have loads and loads of visitors. I have a very large circle of friends. It's sort of a network. And I see them often and they do things for me. I don't exactly know what I do for them, but we have a high old time.*

Whereas she could no longer be the bustling "do-gooder" she was in younger years, her interviews suggested that she continued to artfully tend and nurture her social environment as if tending a garden. She attempted to be socially welcoming instead of sour or self-pitying:

> *I'm not depressed and I'm—most of the time—I'm quite happy. And I try to keep the people around me happy. You know there is a great deal to be said for creating a therapeutic environment because you're the one that lives in it. So that I'm absolutely reliable as far as mood swings are concerned. I don't say bad things or treat people badly or anything like that ever, ever. What happens then is that the house has an ambience, everybody is happy and comfortable. If you create it, you live in it and you're the luckiest one of all. [laughs] I dare say I shall live courted and die lamented because of the way I behave and the consistency of my temperament.*

Although Ann was dependent upon others for many things, she made it clear that she contributed to the effort and didn't need a "hoverer." She explained how she and the students who lived with her worked *together* to prepare a simple but elegant meal:

> *I can do very simple things. Last night, I pan-broiled some steaks, and the nurse who's with me now made the salad and the mashed potatoes, and we had steak and mashed potatoes and salad and then she made a fruit cup. It was a very elegant dinner.*

Ann's engagement with her community mutually constituted and created possibility for them both. In this sense, neither Ann nor her community invented or chose meaning for themselves individually. Meaningful life was not located in Ann as an individual—nor was it solely a matter of her personal traits, knowledge, or skills—but, rather, was made possible in this relational context. Ann's friends and family knew her history and what had always been significant to her. Their ability to respond to her in familiar ways in spite of her deteriorating physical capacities preserved her personhood and allowed her life to be so vibrant. It was as if there were a dance going on between Ann and the people and circumstances surrounding her life. The traditions and practices they participated in together were so ritualized that they *knew*—not necessarily consciously, but through embodiment—how to respond to each other in a very skilled way. As her body failed, the community filled in. As circumstances changed, their zones of participation shifted to preserve the familiar, constituting context.

When I asked Ann how she envisioned her future, she replied

> *I don't think I have much future except doing what I'm doing now. I'll probably stay home and read and knit and sort of supervise the house. . . . I have a lot of visitors.*

The social contact and engagement she had, both over the phone and with visitors, was clearly her lifeline because it provided a familiar, sustaining context within which her traditional ways of being constituted shifted and changed in response to the exigencies of her situation. Ann's existential ability to dwell in her relationships and world had been challenged by the increasing limitations imposed by her declining health and functional abilities. The meanings associated with the things Ann was doing in her early and middle adulthood—raising children, teaching in the university, helping friends in time of need, working for social causes, being hostess to visitors and social gatherings—were not identical to the meanings inherent in her activities at the time of the interviews, given her substantially reduced level of functioning and shrinking future. However, these earlier meanings had shifted and been reinterpreted: She "entertained" with take-out food, "hostessed" holiday meals cooked by her guests, read about historical figures in science for the pure enjoyment of it, and allowed herself to be cared for in the way she had previously cared for others. In this sense, she and her world embodied a living tradition that shifted in relation to her shifting concerns and abilities. These shifts in meaning were facilitated by the relational nature of her world, in that the people and things in her world skillfully knew how to be with each other, albeit changed and changing.

This idea runs counter to the assumption in much of gerontology that elders are autonomous agents, logically selecting and acting on adaptive choices in order to maintain continuity (Atchley, 1989; Becker, 1993; Luborsky, 1993). Some authors have noted that the notion of continuity itself—a construct that underlies geronotological theories of aging and life course development (Kiefer, 1974; Neugarten, 1979)—needs to be rethought because it overlooks and even pathologizes the impact of many of the changes, disruptions, and losses common in late life (Becker, 1993; O'Connor, 1994). Atchley's notion of "dynamic" continuity, involving strategies of adaptive management to "preserve and maintain existing internal and external structures" in the face of change (1989, p. 183) is a normative construct in that it applies only to those without disabling conditions or disease: those aging "normally." The experience of chronic illness, for example, is viewed as "pathological aging" in Atchley's conception despite it being common in old age (Becker, 1993). This understanding of continuity posits control/mastery as a primary, normative objective:

> *Individuals have strong motives for wanting to preserve internal continuity. To begin with, individuals perceive that internal continuity acts as a foundation for effective day-to-day decision making because internal continuity is an important part of individual mastery and competence. For example, continuity of cognitive knowledge is a major element of the individual's capacity to interpret and anticipate events. Without persistent cognitive knowledge, there is no predictability to the world.*

> *Without predictability, mastery (or even competence) is not possible. (Atchley, 1989, p. 185)*

However, as the end of life approaches, when the possibility of becoming disabled or chronically ill increases, the cultural paradigm of control/mastery is often our undoing. It absolutely fails us when we are hit in the face with our vulnerability and growing sense of finitude. At the individual level, the failure to regain continuity after a disruptive event can trigger a sense of defeat and despair. More fundamentally, the notion of continuity disregards the mutually constituting nature of the relation between person and world, and how one's experience of being-in-the-world prior to disruptive life events is often never fully restored. Several authors argued that continuity, wholeness, or coherence of the self is, in fact, an illusory phenomenon (Becker, 1993; Ewing, 1990; Luborsky, 1993). Ann's paradigm exemplifies openness to new possibilities for existential dwelling that is facilitated by the shifts in self-understanding taking place between Ann and her world. Giving absolute priority to the maintenance of continuity could undermine this process. Unfortunately, contemporary Western culture has no coherent vision for transition in aging that isn't seen as a problem to manage or control. What is needed is a cultural discourse on aging that accounts for our inherent vulnerability and supports flexibility and shifting of meanings as we proceed through the transitions and sometimes pivotal disruptions that may accompany old age without normalizing, pathologizing, or technologizing them.

I would assert that Ann's openness to the possibilities in her changing situation and her involvement with family and community was central to her skillful dwelling. Ann was constituted by her situation and responsive to the meanings inherent in it, rather than having *assigned* meaning to it from among an infinite number of possible meanings as a rationally calculating and radically free view of human agency would posit.

PARADIGM CASE #2: DAVID

David—an 81-year-old, married, former academic physician and researcher—suffered a severe stroke four years before participating in this research. The stroke resulted in his having the use of only one side of his body, making him reliant on a wheelchair and on other people for many basic activities of daily living. David struggled to once again experience an involvement in the world that made life meaningful prior to his stroke. When I interviewed him, he was disconnected from many habits, skills, and social practices that had previously constituted his self-understanding and given meaning to his work life and later to his retirement.

Before his stroke, David had spent more than ten years in a vibrant retirement, passionately pursuing the study of art and painting. He led an active and independent life, frequently attending galleries and museums where he lived on the East Coast, and working with a challenging painting teacher. His life dramatically narrowed after his stroke. He experienced his post-stroke life as discontinuous with his life before the stroke, as if he were "living a completely different life." This expression concisely captured the impoverished notion of possibility he experienced. David was struggling to experience himself in a way that could allow for a synthesis between his capable, vital past and his life as a physically disabled person. His self-understanding was informed, in part, by a world that didn't sufficiently understand who and what he was before the stroke, and was therefore limited in its ability to respond to him in ways that might have allowed him to experience himself as the same person he was before the stroke.

In our first interview, David told me that he considered himself to be in "pretty good health," yet he was in a state of great existential suffering as a result of his dependency and disconnection from the world that had been tremendously satisfying and meaningful. Although he had come a very long way since his stroke, the limitations in his functioning constantly reminded him of how he had changed and his dependency on others:

> *Well, it really was an earthquake-like—sudden. Everything changed. There was no preparation for this. Before this I was independent, I did what I wanted myself. And I enjoyed being by myself. In fact, I didn't want to go to a museum with anybody. I just wanted to look at things myself. And that was very satisfying to me: my painting and my life. And then suddenly the stroke. I couldn't drive—I, I had to be dependent. I never was dependent on people. They had to take care of my bladder. It was very, very difficult for me. And I was stuck in bed. And stuck in the wheelchair. So it really was the most revolutionary event in my life: completely changed me. I felt helpless and useless. Instead of being in charge of things, I couldn't anymore. And everything was like in the past, it was far away. It wasn't my world anymore.*

He continued, recounting a dream he frequently had that juxtaposed his pre-and post-stroke experience and expressed the helplessness and invisibility he felt as a disabled person:

> *I dream a great deal about the past. Not specifically, but symbolically. I'm usually in the suburban train going to the city to visit art galleries. But I find I'm very frightened because I'm through and I want to go home. I say, how am I gonna get home? I'm not in a wheelchair, or I am in a wheelchair? How am I getting to the train and back to my house? A taxi cab will take me. I can't drive my car. That's one*

problem. Another problem is I have no money. I have no change. How will I pay for the ticket? What will the conductor say to me? And the third problem in my dream, always, is getting food. I go to a restaurant or a hotel dining room, they don't serve me. They act like I'm not there. And it frightens and angers me. And sometimes I go in the kitchen and make myself eggs and toast and coffee. And I bring them back, and I lie down. And I put them here, and then I'll say I mustn't put the coffee here. It'll spill. So I reach for it, and there's no coffee there. There's no eggs there. And I say, wait a minute. This is all a dream. And I wake up as I feel the bed for the coffee. And I say, "Where is—is there any toast?" And [my wife] says, "There's no toast. I haven't made any toast. You're dreaming.

On recalling the grave state he was in immediately following the stroke and the progress that he'd made, David said the following ("I" represents the interviewer):

D: *They told me I was very sick. They didn't know if I would pull through. But I did with this residual paraplegia. I couldn't talk. I couldn't swallow. My breathing was difficult. They did a good job. . . . They did a trach on me . . . and he did a gastrostomy . . . and a cystoscopy. Oh boy, I was really full of tubes and everything . . . and doctors. I had a whole staff of doctors.*

I: *How do you feel about having been that sick?*

D: *Well, I'm depressed and I sometimes wish they hadn't pulled me through. What kind of a life is this? But people say, "Oh you look wonderful. You have a wonderful house. And the trees. And your daughters—your children live here. So what are you—you're lucky." And when I go to the rehab, I see I'm luckier than most people. I have enough money to buy anything I want. My wife takes good care of me. And people like you help me. I should be very grateful. But [I get] very, very lonely. And very, very depressed and frustrated. . . . I was always independent. I used to go to New York to the galleries and the museums all by myself. I still paint a little bit, but I don't enjoy it as much. My teacher says, "You know something. You're very good. You're active and your work is exciting." I don't find it exciting . . . at all.*

After David's stroke, he and his wife decided to move to the West Coast to be closer to their children and grandchildren, whom they saw frequently. He got out of the house most every day, made possible by the van his wife drove, which was specially equipped with a lift for his motorized wheelchair. Although he was accustomed to gallery and museum-hopping before his stroke, he rarely visited art exhibits after his stroke because getting around in a large, unfamiliar metropolitan area with his special needs posed a substantial obstacle for them.

He did participate in a number of organized activities, including swimming, painting classes, senior center groups, and psychotherapy sessions. Because his family and doctors believed they were important for him, he did these things, but they didn't answer his soul-felt need to be involved in life the way he was before the stroke. He felt that these activities, even the art class, were of limited value. Although he appreciated the kind acquaintances he made in classes and in senior activities, he yearned for stimulating discussion and intellectual banter with people he felt were his intellectual equals.

Never having been a man of small talk, David wanted to talk about "serious" things with people who enjoyed sophisticated discussions of ideas and issues. He wanted to continue to be challenged to demonstrate the capacities of his intellect, which were still intact in contrast to the inertia of his body. His self-understanding prior to the stroke was constituted by engaging with the world through challenging ideas and the prospects of what he could discover through his mind. His weekly attendance at a Senior Center discussion group after the stroke had occasionally provided him with the possibility of this experience.

> *And they welcomed me, and we talked around a circle a little bit and we got involved in child abuse and whether you can believe—fabrication that sort of . . . or the whole problem. And the two psychologists got into an argument. I was very amused, but I enjoyed this kind of adult discussion.*

It tended to be the group facilitators with whom David had the most satisfying interactions. Over the course of our interviews, he attended these discussion groups regularly, but it was inconsistently gratifying because he had a hard time relating to many of the participants who didn't have the same interests or demonstrate the intellectual sophistication David had:

> *So I go there every week. And they discuss around a circle the various feelings that people have during the week. Sometimes I find it very boring. Sometimes it's interesting. Some of the people are not very imaginative. I find myself a little bit exhibitionist, you know—showing off a little.*

He was referring to having talked about being familiar with and missing famous art collections in the East, a subject to which no one else in the group could relate. In contrast, others in the group spent time talking about subjects he considered petty or inconsequential. David had been confronted in the group about being "arrogant," which he accepted as a legitimate criticism, acknowledging that at times throughout his past he has been "impatient" with people. He admitted that this aspect of his personality sometimes worked against him in his career leadership roles. David's repertoire of conversational subjects was broad in the sense of being culturally and intellectually sophisticated. However, the emotional distance he kept from most of his peers in the group prevented him from experiencing his situation as part of the human condition in some way. To experience this would have required that he be able to relate to his senior center peers on a more "equal" level, but he had trouble seeing them as such.

Most of the people outside David's family with whom he had contact never knew him as he had been before his stroke, and they didn't *recognize* his distress, much less *understand why* he was distressed. He talked about how much energy he spent putting on a good social face, communicating that he was enjoying himself in the day-to-day when he really wasn't, so as to spare both his family and his acquaintances the despair he felt much of the time. By protecting them from his pain in this way, he further walled himself off.

Being so aware of his functional deficits, David's feelings of alienation from his present world were exacerbated when others around him remarked about his improvement. He mentioned on numerous occasions how "resentful" he was when people remarked about the substantial progress he had made since the stroke. When people congratulated him on how good he looked and how far he'd come, he felt patronized. It increased his sense of impotence and the painful feeling that a core part of the person he was did not show up to people, or at least was not being acknowledged. This came up in a conversation about his doctor and his medical care:

> **D:** *He says I'm doing very well. . . . I resent that when everybody [says] I look so well. . . . And I'm really not so well.*
>
> **I:** *What are they not seeing? What are they not acknowledging?*
>
> **D:** *Not seeing how difficult it is for me to be dependent and to be limited like this. They don't understand that. All they say to me is, "You look so well." Everybody says that to me.*

David's disability was particularly alien and unbearable to him. The fact that he was dependent was an enormous obstacle to showing the world who he really was, beyond being a man in a wheelchair:

> *Now I'm watching myself going through the day, am I really living it. And there's a separation there . . . of everything. Not what I am, but who I am. What I am is in this wheelchair. Who I am is inside of me. I find that very few activities or people who communicate this relate to me. They relate to the chair mostly.*

This passage repeats the theme of his invisibility. After having known what it was to be ascribed social status and power by virtue of his being well-educated and a physician, he was acutely aware of that loss of social recognition and power as a result of being an aged, disabled person. David's invisibility was constituted by both the stigma of being an aged, wheelchair-bound person as well as by his own self-understanding of what it is to be a person and have a social identity. The Cartesian dualism underlying Western notions of the hierarchical relationship between mind and body contributed to his sense of despair over being unable to project the authority of his autonomous subject self over his recalcitrant object body. This is a central ontological dilemma pervading our contemporary Western views of the aged, the infirm, and the dispossessed.

David's typical mode of engagement with his social environment prior to the stroke was animated and evocative. He took great pleasure in controversial discussions and intellectual and political debate. Before his retirement, he had run an academic department in a large medical center. He described himself as having been a leader with strong opinions and an authoritative style of management. In recounting stories from his entire life, from medical school to painting classes in retirement to stroke rehabilitation, David repeated the theme of having been faced with some challenge, doubting his capacity to succeed, being prodded by others who believed in him, and then struggling with it and discovering he could accomplish more than he'd expected. This "I can't/I can?/I did!" stance provided the context for a meaningful way of understanding himself in the world.

As he approached the apex of his successful and demanding career in midlife, the ground dropped out from under him. His first wife died suddenly, leaving him with four dependent children: "It destroyed me. It just took all the life out of—life of me." This was a devastating tragedy for him. However, he was determined to find a new life partner and mother for his children, and he succeeded in this. Within a year and a half, he married a woman who was able to gracefully and capably reconstitute his home and family life. As he explained, "I was in good shape then. I had a good mother for my children, and a good wife for me."

In retirement, as friends and colleagues moved away or died, he channeled his energy into learning about painting in a studied, intellectual way, not just as a fanciful form of entertainment. The familiar skills, habits, and practices that had constituted David's self-understanding in his career—involving challenge, intellectual stimulation, and the solitary experience of discovery that came after staring for hours into a microscope until he found something—readily found expression when he shifted in retirement to the serious study of painting in the exciting New York world of art. In painting, he studiously explored form and color, attempting new techniques and visiting galleries and museums to discover the techniques famous painters had used. His teacher at that time offered him the kind of challenge that his teacher after the stroke was unable to provide:

> *I find it rather hard to get good teachers. I need an aggressive, courageous critic. I don't need somebody to say, "Oh, isn't that nice. Isn't that interesting? You keep going. I like that. I like that." Every week, she says the same thing. "David, you go ahead. Look at what David's doing. It's wonderful." It's not wonderful. In New York, I had a teacher who would say to me, "Don't you ever do that again in my class." He'd say, "What's the matter with you? Are you afraid of corners? You better work on corners." And I did, and that really helped me. And then he said to me, "You never use grey. Everything you do is dark grey. What's the matter with you? Can't you handle grey?" I said, "I can't make grey." He said, "I'll show you how to make grey." And from then I always used grey in my colors. And then one time he said to me, "What's bothering you today?" And I said, "My work is coming out flat. How do you get depth?" He said, "I'll teach you a little trick." And I said, "Go ahead and teach me." He said, "Take a brush and a dark color and a lot of paint and go right across the whole canvas in a straight line. Just slash across it and see what happens." And you know what happened? Everything in the canvas was behind the line. And it suddenly became deep. I need that kind of a teacher with imagination, who's not afraid of me.*

> **"So you do something else, and you look at it, and then little by little over a day, it begins to talk to you. And then you do what we call "pinwheel." You take it and move it around right angles and another right angle, another right angle. So while I was doing that, I began to see the circus come out again out of my unconscious."**

In this kind of interchange, David was accompanied in confronting his fears and hesitancies and propelled toward mastering new challenges. In his retirement, the day-to-day activities David was involved in were different from those of his career life. However, through his solitary study of painting and art, his self-understanding as an independent, persevering person capable of aesthetic discovery and expression was reinforced. This was a context not unlike earlier experiences in his life when he was challenged to "show off" the intellectual stuff he was made of. Through these kinds of experiences, he discovered new capacities and new possibilities. He went on to describe his serendipitous discovery in painting and the pleasure it used to give him before his stroke:

> *What you do is put a color—it's instinctive or serendipitous, it's a happening. It just comes out of the canvas. For example, you pick up that. And then now you have a blue. You put a blue on the white canvas. Then you decide, "Today, I'm gonna try blue and red. Not red, because red's very hard. So I'm gonna try blue and green." So you put a little green next to it. Or a big dash of green (voice speeding up excitedly) and then you look at it and you say, "What's happening?" "Nothing." So you do something else, and you look at it, and then little by little over a day, it begins to talk to you. And then you do what we call "pinwheel." You take it and move it around right angles and another right angle, another right angle. So while I was doing that, I began to see the circus come out again out of my unconscious. Do you see what I mean? Just whatever you feel comes out on it. Then I say, "Oh my God, here comes the circus again." And I start playing with it. And little by little, it becomes real.*

In contrast, his ability to paint in a soul-felt way after his stroke was vastly diminished. Most of his painting was mechanical, uninspired, and with limited emotional content. He spoke about this difficulty:

> *Well, the point is that during my depression, which was a couple of years—I think I'm just coming out of it now—I no longer had any images in my head. My head was black. So when I painted, I just mechanically painted. Nothing happened.*

David's depression would be expected to have a substantial dampening effect on his affect and on his emotional access to art. On this basis, his difficulty experiencing the "images" in his head that engaged his creative imagination and nourished his soul might have improved as his depression improved. However, it is conceivable that the neurological effects of the stroke itself were also partially responsible for this difficulty. Because a stroke can have broad-reaching effects on sensation, movement, cognition, and emotions, it is possible that his physiological capacity to experience art may have been irretrievably altered from what it had once been. Neurological damage affecting any one of these areas of functioning could, by itself, interfere with painting as he had previously known it.

David explained that the technical aspects of painting with oils and large canvasses and "pinwheeling" the canvas to discover an image and feeling that "talks" to him was essentially impossible for him without his former strength and the use of the left side of his body:

> *But I wish I could paint in oil and paint standing up. And paint like that again. . . . And now I gotta paint these little things, which frustrate me.*

He entertained a glimmer of hope that he could paint as he had formerly when he referred to a photo he'd seen showing a severely disabled artist using a mechanical easel to allow the pinwheeling method he'd been accustomed to.

David kept returning to a description of the kind of social engagement he had found meaningful in the past and how frustrating it was finding this around the time of our interviews:

> *I like this [teacher] because she says, "I'll help you." So she helps me mechanically, but she has no image in her head. She likes conventional painting. And that puts me to sleep. She said all my things are "very nice." I'd like to find a man who'd get angry with me. That's what I need: a man.*

It is not, in fact, a person of a particular gender with whom David has throughout his life needed to engage, but with the work itself of struggling and wrestling with seemingly insurmountable challenges and mastering them. Although the stroke violently disrupted his satisfying retirement life, it did present another challenge for David to take up. Many people didn't expect him to recover nearly as well as he did. As with many challenges of his earlier adulthood, he needed to be persuaded that he could go farther in rehabilitation. He spoke of his physical therapist as someone with whom he struggled, finally being convinced he had capacities he hadn't imagined:

> *She used to say, "Don't be so passive. Get up and walk." And I did. And she said, "Let's go upstairs." I said, "I can't climb stairs." She said, "I'll show you how." And she did, holding on the banister, holding on. And she said, "Come on, let's take a shower." I said, "I can't." And she said, "Yes, you can." She was very aggressive. Very good. Very tough.*

Confronting the limits of his powers of physical rehabilitation, however, ushered in the period of despair and disconnection, which continued to the time of our interviews. He recalled his reaction when he first realized the implications of these limits:

> *I remember one day I was in the outpatient department of the hospital. I was having a conversation with the director of rehab. And I heard him say something. I never forget. He said, "You're not gonna make any more progress. You better just settle for this. You're gonna make a little, but you'll never walk." And so I realized it was over, and it was a very important lesson for me. It was destructive. It was just completely demoralizing.*

Up to the time of David's stroke, his self-understanding was constituted through experiences that confirmed for him the belief that he had the individual strength and capacity to surmount any challenge, but not without struggle or sacrifice. Progress and the promise of a pay-off for hard work provided him the horizons for a meaningful life and work. By applying himself with single-minded determination to overcome his fears and doubts and tackle the hard work, study, or practice that his goals required, he was usually successful.

This was the way he excelled in college, medical school, research, and throughout his professional life. It was also reflected in the way he was able to mobilize himself from a position of intense grief when his first wife died. Taking stock of his situation and realizing that he already knew the woman who could turn his life around, he doggedly courted her until they were married. As a means to a satisfying retirement, he deliberately immersed himself in painting in much the same way, voraciously studying the techniques used by the masters and with which his teacher challenged him. David's successes in his career and in painting were a measure of how well his stance—embodied in daily habits, routines, practices, and ways of relating to others—worked for him throughout most of his adult life.

> **"I can't go out into the world. It's out there, but it's somebody else's world. It isn't mine anymore. I feel strange. You lose all your self-confidence and your ambition to go out and do things. You want to pull back in and be protected like a child with his mother."**

This way of being, or ontology, based on both the notion of continuous progress and hard work paying off and a stance of autonomy, objectification, and control, is consistent with the Protestant work ethic and a technological self-understanding (Benner, 1984b; Benner & Wrubel, 1989). It also happens to be the preeminent cultural paradigm of the Western world.

This paradigm is very effective in contemporary life until the limits of control become apparent. When David's doctor told him not to expect continued improvement, at least not to the point of walking, he was confronted—perhaps on a gut level for the first time—with the possibility that there would be limits to his body's capacity to recover from the stroke. David experienced his doctor's words as a condemnation, an instantaneous dismissing of the autonomous, competent, and enterprising man he had been. It was "over," and the open horizon for "progress" that structured meaningfulness for him was also over. The physical world in which he lived, while made up of equipment (wheelchair, ramps, poles, and bars)—which were, ironically, intended to enable him to be as independent as possible—contradicted this self-understanding.

On our fourth and final meeting, after having shown me the fleeting glimmers of possibility he'd experienced over the previous months in senior center discussion groups and in his painting, he made a very poignant, moving statement that seemed to sum up his absolute loss of an existential place in which to dwell. He described his experience of himself at that time in relation to the past:

> *When I was in pediatrics, I used to teach that the fetus was inside the mother, and then with birth, the baby came out, but really still, psychologically and emotionally part of the mother. And then when he began to walk, the world became a little bit more interesting other than the mother, but still frightening and the baby would come back to the mother. And then when the baby began to socialize with the world, the world got bigger and bigger. And then in school, the child finally left the mother. And a world was outside for him to explore. That was his life, the exploration outside the mother. And I feel that, myself, I used to be [inside] my mother, and I held on. And I gradually got my world outside. It was a big world. I explored medicine, parenthood, marriage, and the war. All the things about life were outside in the big world. And then as I grew older it began to come back inside again. Enough so like now, I'm back inside again. I can't go out into the world. It's out there, but it's somebody else's world. It isn't mine anymore. I feel strange. You lose all your self-confidence and your ambition to go out and do things. You want to pull back in and be protected like a child with his mother.*

David's words speak truth to all of us. He captured the universal human predicament of the finitude of our being. The body is our universal existential dwelling place. Following its lead, we are opened out to the world, but in disability, our access to the world may be compromised. This predicament is heightened when a stance of hyper-independence, mastery, and control—which David had previously embodied with physical capacities under girded by willpower—is contradicted through one's confrontation with the realistic limits of control over the body.

Winnicott (1953/1986, p. 256) talked about the "intermediate area of experiencing": the part of the human being where the ability to recognize self and others and to accept reality develops. In infants, it is an area of illusory experience, where transitional objects and transitional phenomena facilitate beginning object relationships. Winnicott asserted that this domain of illusion prevails in adulthood because the tension between inner and outer reality can never be completely reconciled. It is in this region, outside the authority of any kind of reality testing, where artistic experience, religious feeling, dreaming, and creativity exist and provide a bridge between inner self and world. David's access to the world was once through his will and imagination, and later through his art, but without these channels of access, he can find no other meaningful way to dwell in the world.

The feeling of impotence in David's words parallels Arthur Frank's (1991) poignant testimony to the existential authority of the "will of the body" in illness. In contrast, an infirm body, in the modern technological self-understanding, is evidence of the failure of the autonomous mind to harness the potential resource of the body (Benner, Janson-Bjerklie, Ferketich, & Becker, 1994). This is a cultural-level background meaning implicit in the modern Western self-understanding that explains, in part, why the loss of self-reliance is experienced with such ambivalence and even shame in our culture. In light of David's self-understanding, perhaps his "arrogance" and detachment in his senior center discussion group worked to preserve a semblance of the autonomous, self-reliant agency he so desperately needed to shoulder the moral burden of his dependency.

Having taken up this technological self-understanding as his *primary* way of being, David was left without sustainable meanings for dwelling in the world because his body was no longer an instrument of autonomy and control. Without the opportunities to comport himself through the embodied skills and practices that constituted his autonomous, control-oriented self-understanding—including the somewhat confrontational style of social interaction that mobilized him so well—he felt cut off from his sense of personhood. He said, "I have nothing useful to do. I'm finished. It's somebody else's world. It's not mine anymore." In some ways, his despair became his only project: It was the realm within which his fears laid. Those who were willing to confront his terror with him, rather than avoid or deny it, offered him some sense of possibility. However, constituted by this ontological self-understanding, the possibilities that could show up for him were limited.

COMMENTARY

These two narratives were presented because they are strong examples of how cultural level paradigms can be interpreted and taken up by aged participants in early–21st century American culture. They are meant to show how different self-understandings "work" to allow various possibilities for meaning in the context of some of the disruptions occurring in late life. These self-understandings are not chosen, but are given by the personal events and social circumstances that shape people's lives. In late life, personal and social meanings change, but not to the extent that we end up with a whole new set of meanings.

Although Ann's physical capacities were severely compromised, she continued to experience a sense of possibility because her habits, rituals, and practices allowed for dwelling in family and community relationships. At the same time, her community supported her and filled in for her, preserving what was meaningful. Ann's relational self-understanding shifted to make a place for being cared for as well as being the giver of care. In contrast, David's way of understanding himself made no allowance for being a recipient of care without it also diminishing his sense of self. With the loss of his autonomous body and the radical changes in his life circumstances, his self-understanding as a capable, self-reliant subject was called into question. Dependency and infirmity, then, represented assaults on his identity and self-understanding, as well as exacting a heavy moral burden on him for failing to live up to the expectations of an autonomous self of possession (Benner et al., 1994; Leonard, 1994; Sandel, 1982).

Gender could be posited as a factor distinguishing between Ann's and David's self-understandings. Since Gilligan's (1982) work on women's psychological and moral development, there has been prolific and heated discussion about the influence of history, biology, and culture in shaping notions of gender, identity, relationship, and morality (Benhabib, 1992; Benjamin, 1988; Gilligan, 1982, 1993; Keller, 1985; Vetlesen, 1994; Whitbeck, 1984). I am referring to the controversial proposition that women and girls are either intrinsically or developmentally situated in a relationally oriented ontology of care, responsibility, and interdependence *in contrast to* a justice- and rights-orientation attributed to men and boys in which autonomy, rationality, and deference to universal roles and principles are highly valued. That the latter stance has been privileged throughout the history of patriarchal society—including its centrality in scientific epistemology since the Enlightenment—is not in dispute (Benhabib, 1992; Benjamin, 1988; Gilligan, 1982, 1993; Keller, 1985; Vetlesen, 1994; Whitbeck, 1984). However, controversy persists over the ways gender has become socially and historically constituted as well as whether such an ontological dichotomy between men and women can be asserted, particularly as the basis of moral reasoning (Benhabib, 1992). Regardless of the answer to this question, Benhabib pointed out that moral theory in the Kantian tradition, which has privileged the autonomous individual, has overlooked the "nurture, care and responsibility" that is essential to the development of the mature, self-sufficient adult individual (p. 188):

> *Not only as children, but also as concrete embodied beings with needs and vulnerabilities, emotions and desires we spend our lives caught in the "web of human affairs," in Hannah Arendt's words, or in networks of "care and dependence" in Carol Gilligan's words. Modern moral philosophy, and particularly universalist moralities of justice, has emphasized our dignity and worth as moral subjects at the cost of forgetting and repressing our vulnerability and dependency as bodily selves. Such networks of dependence and the web of human affairs in which we are immersed are not simply like clothes which we outgrow or like shoes which we leave behind. They are ties that bind; ties that shape our moral identities, our needs, and our visions of the good life. The autonomous self is not the disembodied self; universalist moral theory must acknowledge the deep experiences in the formation of the human being to which care and justice correspond.* (ibid., p. 189)

The research I am presenting is not intended to respond to questions concerning oppositional ontologies between men and women, but rather to lay out how one's ontological basis for being-in-the-world, whatever it may be, holds up and offers various possibilities in aging, given some of the difficult circumstances that may arise in late life—circumstances that tax or exceed the limits of our embodied capabilities and challenge our assumed autonomy and self-reliance. Although the two paradigm cases highlighted in this chapter show strong contrasts that may suggest a gendered dichotomy, they are not being presented to support the argument of a distinct dichotomy or to hold up one self-understanding as superior to another. On the contrary, we do not usually take up our self-understandings in an absolute way, nor are our self-understandings completely fixed and unchangeable. As the circumstances of our lives change, the personal and social meanings associated with the activities of our existential habitus are reshaped; new experiences challenge our previous self-understandings while simultaneously illuminating possibilities not evident previously.

If our life circumstances dramatically change without this concomitant shift in the way we understand ourselves, without a means of connecting with the possibilities associated with transformed meanings and new saliencies—as David's story illustrates—we are likely to experience a crisis of meaning. Following David's stroke, his life was up-ended. He was dependent, and he felt invisible. His embodied self-understanding became incoherent when he could no longer project himself into the world in the same way he had previously. The channels that had been his access and connection—art and intellectual repartee—became impeded by his neurological losses, physical limitations, and psychic pain. His experience of dependency was so alien and untenable given his previous social stature and self-understanding that he had trouble revealing his inner despair to many people. This further closed off new involvements that might have illuminated new ways of being and a shift in self-understanding. By relocating across the country, he was closer to most of his family, yet far removed from the places, patterns, and practices that had been central in constituting much of his life. His existential suffering reflected the loss of much that had been meaningful to him in the past as well as the relative incoherence of his way of knowing himself in the present because of the limited access he had to the world.

EXISTENTIAL SKILLS OF "DWELLING"

It appears, therefore, that dwelling in the world requires particular existential skills: ways of bridging personal experience and social reality. The research data suggest that the following existential skills promote and sustain dwelling in the world:

- **Physical and cognitive capacities,** including memory and access to emotions, which facilitate embodied participation in meaningful habits, rituals, and practices

- **Ways of being with people,** characterized by a self-in-relation-to-others based on practices of mutual recognition

- **Caring or having current concerns or structures of meaning** such that people and things matter; what is salient shows up in light of these concerns

Depending upon one's existential skills of dwelling, self-understandings can work to facilitate meaning or to limit possibilities for meaningful existence. Assaults on meaning can occur when any of these skills or aspects of dwelling become eroded. However, the optimal configuration and relative importance of these existential skills varies among people. The breakdown of any one particular skill will be more devastating to one person than to another based on the ways that they are constituted and understand themselves. David was hit particularly hard given his pre-stroke technological self-understanding—one that is shared to some extent by everyone in contemporary Western society—and the impact his stroke and resulting life changes had on his existential dwelling skills. To a great extent, Ann's self-understanding was constituted via a way of being in relationships that more readily allowed for alternation between providing for others and being vulnerable and requiring care for oneself. While her physical and cognitive capacities were diminished, her ability to experience a meaningful world was not closed off because of this self-understanding; it allowed her to be open to new ways and new possibilities of being a person in her situation. Dwelling in the world is thus the existential manifestation of the paradox of the self both constituting and being constituted by personal social meanings.

CONCLUSION

This chapter presents paradigm cases and exemplars to illustrate ways in which "dwelling-in-the-world" can be compromised in late life. Basic to this ability to understand ourselves as connected to the possibilities for meaning that our changing circumstances bring forth are particular "existential skills." The erosion of these skills—through illness; impairments in physical, cognitive, or social functioning; losses of loved ones; or environmental disruptions, for example—challenges one's self-understandings such that familiar meanings may no longer be available. The challenge requires finding new ways of understanding oneself that account for one's history, one's embodiment, and the saliencies of the new situation. However, as we saw in David, irretrievable neurological deficits can work against one's best efforts to regain access to the meaningful world, leaving one "without a place to dwell."

References

Becker, G. (1993). Continuity after a stroke: Implications of life-course disruption in old age. *Gerontologist, 33*(2), 148-158.

Benhabib, S. (1992). *Situating the self: Gender, community and postmodernism in contemporary ethics*. New York: Routledge.

Benjamin, J. (1988). *The bonds of love: Psychoanalysis, feminism, and the problem of domination*. New York: Pantheon Books.

Benner, P. (1984a). *From novice to expert: Excellence and power in clinical nursing practice*. Menlo Park, CA: Addison-Wesley.

Benner, P. (1984b). *Stress and satisfaction on the job: Work meanings and coping of mid-career men*. New York: Praeger Scientific.

Benner, P. (Ed.). (1994a). *Interpretive phenomenology: Embodiment, caring, and ethics in health and illness*. Thousand Oaks, CA: Sage Publications.

Benner, P. (1994b). The tradition and skill of interpretive phenomenology in studying health, illness, and caring practices. In P. Benner (Ed.), *Interpretive phenomenology: Embodiment, caring, and ethics in health and illness*. (pp. 99-128). Thousand Oaks, CA: Sage Publications.

Benner, P., Janson-Bjerklie, S., Ferketich, S., & Becker, B. (1994). Moral dimensions of living with a chronic illness: Autonomy, responsibility, and the limits of control. In P. Benner (Ed.), *Interpretive phenomenology: Embodiment, caring, and ethics in health and illness* (pp. 225-254). Thousand Oaks, CA: Sage Publications.

Benner, P., & Wrubel, J. C. (1989). *The primacy of caring: Stress and coping in health and illness*. Menlo Park, CA: Addison-Wesley.

Dreyfus, H. L. (1991). *Being-in-the-world: A commentary on Heidegger's Being and Time, Division I*. Cambridge, MA: The MIT Press.

Dreyfus, H. L. (1992). *What computers still can't do: A critique of artificial reason*. Cambridge, MA: The MIT Press.

Ewing, K. P. (1990). The illusion of whole: Culture, self, and the experience of inconsistency. *Ethos, 18*, 251-278.

Frank, A. W. (1991). *At the will of the body*. Boston: Houghton Mifflin.

Gilligan, C. (1982). *In a different voice: Psychological theory and women's development*. Cambridge, MA: Harvard University Press.

Gilligan, C. (1993). *In a different voice: Psychological theory and women's development*. (2nd ed.) Cambridge, MA: Harvard University Press.

Heidegger, M. (1962). *Being and time*. (John Macquarrie and Edward Robinson, Trans.). New York: Harper & Row. (Original work published 1927).

Keller, E. F. (1985). *Reflections on gender and science*. New Haven: Yale University Press.

Kiefer, C. (1974). *Changing cultures, changing lives*. San Francisco: Jossey-Bass.

Leonard, V. W. (1994). A Heideggerian phenomenological perspective on the concept of person. In P. Benner (Ed.), *Interpretive phenomenology: Embodiment, caring, and ethics in health and illness* (pp. 434-464). Thousand Oaks, CA: Sage Publications.

Luborsky, M. R. (1993). The romance with personal meaning in gerontology: Cultural aspects of life themes. *Gerontologist, 33*(4), 445-452.

Neugarten, B. L. (1979). Time, age, and the life cycle. *American Journal of Psychiatry, 136*, 887-893.

O'Connor, P. (1994). Salient themes in the life review of a sample of frail elderly respondents in London. *Gerontologist 34*(2), 224-230.

Polanyi, M. (1962). *Personal knowledge: Towards a post-critical philosophy*. Chicago: University of Chicago Press.

Sandel, M. J. (1982). *Liberalism and the limits of justice*. Cambridge, UK: Cambridge University Press.

Taylor, C. (1985a). *Human agency and language: Philosophical papers I*. Cambridge, UK: Cambridge University Press.

Taylor, C. (1985b). *Philosophy and the human sciences: Philosophical papers 2*. Cambridge, UK: Cambridge University Press.

Taylor, C. (1989). *Sources of the self: The making of the modern identity*. Cambridge, MA: Harvard University Press.

Taylor, C. (1991a). The dialogical self. In D. R. Hiley, J. F. Bohman, & R. Shusterman (Eds.), *The interpretive turn: Philosophy, science, culture* (pp. 304-314). Ithaca, NY: Cornell University Press.

Taylor, C. (1991b). *The ethics of authenticity*. Cambridge, MA: Harvard University Press.

Vetlesen, A. J. (1994). *Perception, empathy, and judgment: An inquiry into the preconditions of moral performance*. University Park, PA: Pennsylvania State University Press.

Whitbeck, C. (1984). A different reality: Feminist ontology. In C. C. Gould (Ed.), *Beyond domination: New perspectives on women and philosophy* (pp. 64-88). Totown, NJ: Rowman and Allanheld.

Winnicott, D. W. (1986). Transitional objects and transitional phenomena: A study of the first not-me possession. In P. Buckley (Ed.), *Essential papers on object relations* (pp. 254-271). New York: New York University Press. (Original work published 1953).

Wrubel, J. C. (1985). *Personal meanings and coping processes: A hermeneutic study of personal background meanings and interpersonal concerns and their relation to stress appraisals and coping*. Unpublished doctoral dissertation, University of California, San Francisco.

CHAPTER 15

Patients' and Family Members' Experiences of Hospital End-of-Life Care

ELISABETH SPICHIGER

INTRODUCTION

For professional health care providers, the hospital is the everyday workplace with which they are very familiar. People who enter the hospital as patients or family members, however, are confronted with an unfamiliar situation. Given the context of health care providers working in their taken-for-granted world of the hospital, and of patients and their families who are thrown into a more or less unfamiliar situation where they may face the patient's death, in this chapter, I explored the question: What are adult patients' with a terminal illness and their family members' lived experiences of hospital end-of-life care?

The chapter is based on a study that was conducted in a tertiary care hospital in Switzerland, where I worked as a nurse for many years. A review of the literature showed that publications on experiences of hospital end-of-life care were rather scarce and frequently focused on specific aspects. With my study, I thus aimed at providing a necessarily local but comprehensive description of patients' with a terminal illness and their family members' experiences of hospital end-of-life care.

Interpretive phenomenology (IP) was chosen as methodological approach (Benner, 1994b). This method is most suitable for exploring questions about human issues and concerns (Plager, 1994). It allows researchers to uncover common meanings and everyday experiences, habits, skills, and practices in a specific context, which often get overlooked because they are aspects of human beings' taken-for-granted background (Leonhard, 1994). IP was, therefore, well suited to researching terminally ill patients' and their families' experiences of end-of-life care in a particular hospital.

BACKGROUND AND SIGNIFICANCE

In the United States and several European countries, more than 50% of patients die in hospitals (World Health Organization [WHO], 2004). In Switzerland, approximately 37% of patients died in hospitals in 2001 (Fischer, Bosshard, Zellweger, & Faisst, 2004). Most hospital units provide end-of-life care but do not specialize in palliative care even though this approach is widely acknowledged as state of the art for patients with a terminal illness and their families (Sepulveda, Marlin, Yoshida, & Ullrich, 2002). End-of-life care means all the diagnostic and therapeutic interventions initiated and provided by the interdisciplinary team of health care professionals in the hospital within the context of their relationships to patients and family members with the goal to improve the patients' situation.

Palliative care, according to WHO (2003), is an approach that improves the quality of life (QoL) of patients and their families facing problems associated with life-threatening illness, through the prevention and relief of suffering by means of early identification and impeccable assessment and treatment of pain and other problems, whether physical, psychosocial, or spiritual. Furthermore, in palliative care, life is affirmed, and dying is considered as normal process; subsequently, death is neither hastened nor postponed. Patients are supported in living as actively as possible until death, and families are helped to cope during illness and bereavement. An interdisciplinary team addresses patients' and families' needs (WHO, 2003). It is also recognized that palliative care should be applied early in the course of an ultimately fatal illness. Disease-modifying therapies decline when the illness progresses, but palliative care measures increase toward the end of life (WHO, 2002). Symptom control in cancer patients, however, may be best achieved through the control of neoplastic growth, or through the alteration of tumor biology or metabolic activity; thus, disease-modifying interventions such as chemotherapy or radiotherapy are included as components of palliative care provided that adverse effects do not outweigh potential symptom improvement and that the patient's comfort may be enhanced (Doyle, Hanks, Cherny, & Calman, 2005). Standards of palliative care are often not achieved in hospitals, however, because of insufficiently educated care providers and structural aspects of the health care system (Bruera, 2006; Meier, Morrison, & Cassel, 1997; McGrath, 2001).

Research on care experiences of patients with a terminal illness is scarce; the literature on families' experiences is more extensive but still limited (Heyland et al., 2006). Regarding symptom control, substantial groups of patients with life-threatening diagnoses experienced severe symptoms in the second week of a hospitalization during the last six months of their life (Levenson et al., 2000; Lynn et al., 2000; McCarthy, Phillips, Zhong, Drews, & Lynn,

2000; Roth et al., 2000; The SUPPORT Principal Investigators, 1995). In contrast, Grond et al. (1991) demonstrated that with a rigorous application of the WHO guidelines for cancer pain relief (1986), good pain control could be achieved for a majority of patients at the end of life. Family members remembered patients as exhibiting many symptoms, and that symptoms were often unsatisfactorily controlled (Bucher, Trostle, & Moore, 1999; Lynn et al., 1997; McCarthy, Lay, & Addington-Hall, 1996; Miettinen, Tilvis, Karppi, & Arve, 1998; Teno et al., 2004; Tolle, Tilden, Hickman, & Rosenfeld, 2000; Tolle, Tilden, Rosenfeld, & Hickman, 2000). Family members expected health care providers to attend rapidly to the patients' symptoms and to ensure comfort as much as possible (Czerwiec, 1996; Hanson, Danis, & Garrett, 1997).

Studies investigating communication showed that patients considered good communication skills as relevant for care providers (McCormick & Conley, 1995; Wenrich et al., 2001). Family members valued communication with staff that gave them honest and appropriate information, was timed to their needs, respected their standpoints, and allowed them to ask questions and make contributions. Often, however, they experienced problems with communication (e. g., with lack of information, or with the way bad news was given) that overshadowed the whole experience of care (Andershed & Ternestedt, 1998, 1999; Berns & Colvin, 1998; Dunne & Sullivan, 2000; Keegan et al., 2001; McGrath, 2001; Rogers, Karlsen, & Addington-Hall, 2000; Teno et al., 2004).

In these studies, family members also highly praised caring health care providers, and uncaring staff members were experienced negatively. Family members considered the patient's dignity compromised when personal needs were disregarded and stated that the maintenance of patients' personal hygiene facilitated their being present at the bedside (Andershed & Ternestedt, 1998; Czerwiec, 1996; Hawker et al., 2006; Keegan et al., 2001; McGrath, 2001; Pierce, 1999; Rogers et al., 2000). A common finding of several surveys was that a majority of the families reported great overall satisfaction with care even though they raised problems: for example, unavailability of care providers (Baker et al., 2000; McCarthy et al., 1996; Tolle et al., 2000).

In summary, publications show that what patients and families value in end-of-life care corresponds well with the goals of palliative care. However, study findings provide only fragments of patients' and families' experiences, not a full picture. Lacking in the literature are comprehensive descriptions of hospital end-of-life care from the patients' and family members' perspectives. With this study, I aimed at exploring care in a Swiss university hospital, and at providing a necessarily local but broader account of patients' with a terminal illness and their family members' experiences of hospital end-of-life care (Spichiger, 2004).

METHOD

Interpretive phenomenology (IP), as described and used by Benner and her colleagues for nursing research (Benner, 1984, 1994b; Benner, Hooper-Kyriakidis, & Stannard, 1999; Benner, Tanner, & Chesla, 1996) was chosen to explore patients' with a terminal illness and their family members' experiences of hospital end-of-life care. The method assumes that results are embedded in the context of a study, that researchers are part of this context, and that their pre-understandings shape the project. Thus, this study's context and my position are briefly outlined.

Context

This study was conducted in Switzerland in a public university hospital during 2002 and 2003 to document patients' with a terminal illness and their family members' experiences of hospital end-of-life care. The study was approved by the university hospital, the clinic management team, and the Institutional Review Board of the University of California San Francisco, where I was a student.

Switzerland has a well-developed healthcare system, with compulsory health insurance for basic care, ambulatory healthcare mostly delivered by physicians in office-based, independent practices, fairly comprehensive home health care coverage, and a well-developed hospital infrastructure for the delivery of acute care, with 6.3 beds per 1,000 inhabitants (Undritz, 2004). In Switzerland, palliative care is increasingly recognized as the required standard for end-of-life care, but currently, only a minority of patients and families in need of palliative care can receive care from expert palliative care practitioners in Switzerland (Raemy-Bass, Lugon, & Eggimann, 2000; Spichiger, 2003).

The hospital where the study took place had about 1,000 beds, providing specialized as well as basic care. Data were collected in the clinic for general internal medicine, which is the clinic where most patients died from terminal diseases. The clinic had 140 beds, with two departments for acute care and one department for rehabilitation. Mean duration of hospitalization was about 12 days for acute care and 42 days for rehabilitation. The clinic had 11 units, with one or two resident physicians per unit; senior physicians as supervisors; and three senior consultants, each in charge of one department.

A charge nurse was responsible for each unit, and a nurse manager and an assistant nurse manager supervised each department. Nurse staffing levels were approximately 0.9 nursing and 0.2 nursing assistant positions per bed (calculated on a yearly basis, with 5 weeks of holidays for staff members). Team nursing or primary nursing were used, and nurses worked in three shifts.

The clinic offered practical training to nursing and medical students. Services of social workers, dieticians, physiotherapists, occupational therapists, and chaplains were available. Even though good end-of-life care was an agreed-upon goal as stated in the clinic guidelines, palliative care was not an explicit approach, and thus no specialized palliative care services were available.

I worked as a staff nurse, charge nurse, and clinical nurse specialist for many years at this clinic and was always very interested in end-of-life care. After studies in the United States, I returned to the clinic for data collection but was not involved in direct patient care during the time of study.

Sample

Study participants were 10 adult patients and 10 close family members. The patients comprised 3 women and 7 men, with a mean age of 62.7 years (range = 38–85); all suffered from an advanced cancer, were no longer treated curatively, and were expected to die during their current hospital stay or within a few months. The family members were 7 women and 3 men (4 spouses, 3 partners, 1 mother, 1 brother, and 1 sister-in-law), with a mean age of 64.6 years (range = 41–82). All patients and family members were Caucasian, and all but one were Swiss. One patient was an immigrant from Eastern Europe. The former or current occupation of patients and family members varied widely (e.g., housewife, public employee, scientist). The patients were hospitalized on average for 33 days (range = 5–72).

For recruitment, patients who met the inclusion criteria were first approached by a nurse manager. She briefly explained that a nurse researcher was conducting a study that explored patients' and their families' experiences of care in this hospital. I contacted only those patients who wanted to hear more about the project. The closest family member was approached in a next step. All participants provided written informed consent.

Data Collection and Analysis

Interpretive phenomenology aims at articulating everyday taken-for-granted meanings and practices as well as how participants experience breakdowns in this taken-for-grantedness (Benner, 1994a; Leonard, 1994). Accordingly, a data collection method was chosen that allows as good an approach to the participants' world as is feasible. For this study, data collection included repeated participant observations, conversations with patients, interviews with the closest family members, and reviewing medical and nursing records. Conversations with patients were rather informal; length and content were adapted to the patients' health status. Conversations and interviews were tape-recorded and transcribed in German. Quotes were later translated into English. Data from 22 observational sessions as well as 36 conversations with patients and interviews with family members provided the text for analysis.

Data analysis—that is, interpretation—began as soon as text was available, paralleled further data collection and extended beyond data collection to the final interpretation and articulation (Benner, 1994a; Leonard, 1994). The interpretive process involved three parallel strategies:

- Paradigm cases illustrate strong patterns of meanings and were fully interpreted.

- Exemplars were searched and used to discover qualitative distinctions.

- Thematic analysis, finally, meant reading the whole text across cases for common themes.

From the thematic analysis, an interpretive plan emerged and major themes were then developed further (Benner, 1994a; Leonard, 1994).

To improve the rigor of the research, I discussed interpretations with other researchers. This was in accordance with participants' informed consent. Validation of results through participants (Benner, 1994c) was limited to offering reflections of my understanding of their stories to participants during conversations and interviews as often as possible, asking them to comment on my interpretation.

RESULTS

Some patients who participated in this study were admitted to the hospital with severe symptoms and then diagnosed with a terminal illness; for others, the diagnosis was known, and they were admitted because of a serious deterioration in their health status. Some patients died in the hospital, one was transferred to a palliative care unit, and others recovered enough to return home once again.

Results describe how these patients and their families experienced the care providers' efforts to achieve the best possible QoL for them as well as how the professionals balanced advantages and disadvantages of medical procedures, managed symptoms, provided information and anticipatory guidance, attuned care activities to patient and family needs, and prevented—or, at times, provoked—difficulties for patients and families. Consequences for professionals are discussed within the result section as far as this seems adequate.

Achieving the Best Possible QoL

According to patients and family members, the professional care providers tried hard to achieve the best possible QoL for them; that is, they tried to alleviate symptoms; ameliorate patients' health status if feasible; respect the patients' autonomy; and take patients' and families' psychological, social, and spiritual needs into consideration. The care providers also acted as patients' advocates, and were willing to do more than just the requested tasks. The following examples illustrate this: A patient who suffered from severe constipation was offered rosemary compresses in addition to laxatives and enemas. Patient and family member were very pleased with this complementary measure. The following interview (where the patient is identified as P and the interviewer as I) is illustrative:

> **P:** *I actually only have a bowel movement with an enema, not otherwise. And with laxatives; this certainly also helps, in order not to get hard stool, but laxatives are not sufficient, and they are unpleasant, these laxatives! And rosemary compresses, which aid, which stimulate the peristalsis, this is very pleasant.*
>
> **I:** *They are doing this as well?*
>
> **P:** *They are doing it here. The nurses buy it themselves or let the family bring it, and that is incredibly pleasant, these rosemary compresses. It stimulates, it frees a bit, and it smells wonderfully.*

The nurses in this situation took the initiative and extra effort to provide a very welcomed treatment that improved the patient's well-being as well as the patient's and the family member's satisfaction with care.

During observation, another nurse gave the patient's need priority over the work flow in the X-ray department, when she refused to send the patient there without pain medication.

> *The patient tells me (observer) that the X-ray department wanted her to get there earlier this morning, but that this would not have been possible. The nurse says that they had asked if she could come earlier, but she denied, because she had agreed with the patient to give her an injection against pain prior to transportation. She did not want to deviate from this.*

Thanks to this injection, the patient was then pain-free during transportation to the X-ray department and the computer tomography she had to undergo.

These examples show the care providers' successful efforts to improve the situation for patients and family members, to achieve a better QoL for them. Achievement of the best possible QoL is a major goal of palliative care. Thus, the professionals acted in accordance with this goal. Although "the best possible QoL" has a positive connotation, the other side should not be overlooked. The word "possible" points it out; only the possible can be achieved, not the impossible. The constipated patient, for instance, enjoyed the rosemary compresses, but she still suffered from her condition and had to swallow horribly tasting laxatives. Hence, the care providers could do their best to improve patients' and family members' situations; however, the terminal illness still robbed the patients of their physical and sometimes of their cognitive abilities, provoked symptoms, and rendered them dependent upon the care and support of others. The existential suffering that accompanies a terminal illness cannot be remedied; patients and families must somehow endure it and live through it.

Balancing Positive and Adverse Effects of Medical Procedures

All patients in this study suffered from far advanced cancer. According to palliative care, thus, the ultimate goal of medical procedures should have been to improve these patients' QoL. The approach calls for balancing potential positive and adverse effects of any intervention and for suggesting measures that would most likely contribute to a patient's well-being. Although a palliative-care approach was not explicitly adopted in the study clinic, patients and families nevertheless experienced this balancing of potential effects of medical procedures and reported differing situations. For instance, for a patient diagnosed with vertebral metastases causing severe pain and paralysis, a disease-modifying intervention—radiation therapy—was suggested. The patient agreed and later stated that his pain completely disappeared after the first treatment even though he never mentioned any problems with side effects from radiotherapy. When another patient got diagnosed with severely advanced esophageal cancer, surgery, radiotherapy, chemotherapy, or the insertion of a stent was not suggested because, according to the specialists' judgment, none of these treatments would contribute anything to the patient's QoL. This explanation was acceptable for the patient and his wife.

The decision for or against diagnostic tests and medical treatments or the choice between available therapies, however, was not always easily made as the following example shows. This patient suffered from shortness of breath attributable to aspiration pneumonia and pleural effusions. Shortly after his admission, a tube was inserted to drain pleural effusions. This first drainage worked quite well, and the patient's breathlessness was relieved to some extent but only for a rather short time. Two weeks later, the physicians suggested a second drainage. At this time, the patient left decisions to his wife (W), and she only reluctantly agreed.

> **W:** *And they inserted the tube once more. Well, at this moment, I did not fully agree anymore first. I said: "Well, does it have do be done?" "Yes, in order for him to breathe more easily." Then I had to say, yes, because suffocating, that must be horrible.*
>
> **I:** *And did you get the impression that the tube had some effect?*
>
> **W:** *Not at all. Well, I don't know how it would be, if they had not inserted it. But what the effect was. . . . The physician just told me one could not say that it had been useless, but what effect it had?*

The second drainage was problematic and hardly effective because the effusions were encapsulated. The pain from the tube was well controlled; the patient did not suffer from the treatment. However, it did not alleviate his shortness of breath. The patient died a few days later. In retrospect, any positive effect of this second drainage seems questionable from a professional perspective, and this was clearly also the view of the family member. It can be speculated that without the drainage, breathlessness would have increased. But given this patient's clearly stated wish to die as soon as possible, symptom control might as well have been possible with opioids. According to the wife, this was not suggested as an alternative way for proceeding.

The example sheds some light on the difficulties involved in balancing advantages and disadvantages of interventions. A clear judgment is not always possible: The consequences of procedures cannot always be predicted. In addition, it is (of course) easier to judge the adequacy of any intervention in retrospect, but tremendously more difficult to do so prospectively because it is impossible to fully know an individual patient's reactions and illness trajectory in advance. But even though the situation outlined earlier is recognized as problematic and the difficulty in making the best decision is acknowledged, questions arise: When the second drainage was suggested, was the patient's wish to die taken into account? Was symptom control with opioids as an alternative option considered?

> **"Care providers must be aware of their own sense of helplessness when confronted with suffering and death, and reflect on their coping strategies: on their reasons for acting.**

In similar situations, the care providers mostly seemed to suggest rather invasive procedures. One questions whether they did so, in part, to deal with their own need to act and their experience of helplessness in the face of death. Without doubt, witnessing patients' suffering is difficult for the professionals, and they may feel compelled to do something. Taking action may too often mean initiating medical procedures; conversely, other options may not be considered as "doing something." However, caring relationships, being with and talking to patients and families, recognizing them as persons, and providing excellent comfort care have been shown to be powerful measures to improve patients' and families' well-being in the hospital. In fact, although often overlooked, these aspects are challenging for professionals because of the courage needed to get emotionally involved and the skill to find an adequate level of engagement (Halpern, 2001). Reacting to problems by prescribing and carrying out medical procedures may be easier for some professionals.

The example also highlights that if the perceptions of patients, family members, and care providers differ, the care providers have the upper hand. They have the medical knowledge from which they can argue convincingly, but the lay persons depend upon the information provided to them for their decisions. Not astonishingly, patients and family members usually, albeit at times reluctantly, follow the professionals' advice. This fact leaves the care providers with the responsibility to fully consider and carefully balance advantages and disadvantages of any medical procedure they suggest, and to discuss alternative treatment options if available, thereby taking patients' and families' whole situation into account and keeping the goal in mind: the best possible QoL for patients and family members. To do this fully, the care providers must be aware of their own sense of helplessness when confronted with suffering and death, and reflect on their coping strategies: on their reasons for acting.

Managing Symptoms

The patients experienced a variety of symptoms, with pain as the most frequent. According to patients and family members, care providers were eager to alleviate symptoms although their success varied; and, even though effective treatment was readily available for some symptoms, there was none for others.

Some patients experienced effective symptom management within a short period of time. For instance, a patient related how her pain regimen was effectively adjusted in the hospital. Prior to admission, her excruciating back pain from a not-yet-diagnosed metastatic cancer was treated with nonsteroid anti-inflammatory drugs, which were ineffective and caused side effects. In the hospital, she got Fentanyl patches as an around-the-clock medication, supplemented with morphine as needed. Subsequently, this patient's pain was satisfactorily controlled, and she could enjoy meals again.

> *Yeah, before I had very, very bad pain everywhere. Only had weak pills, they didn't help at all; and it also ruined the stomach, when I swallowed many pills. But now I get the right ones, and not so incredibly many, but they are effective. Before I couldn't eat; because of the many pills, I had stomachaches. But now I can eat again, not an awful lot, but always a bit, every day. Sometimes I also feel hungry again. I think that's nice.*

Unfortunately for several patients, satisfying symptom control was not always achieved. Some symptoms proved to be intractable: for instance, a patient's dizziness and tendency to fall to the right side from brain metastases. Neither radiotherapy nor cortisone brought about any positive effect. The world kept turning around the patient: an endless ride on the merry-go-round that confined him to the hospital and nursing home.

Another patient suffered from severe pain from vertebral metastases. In addition, she was nauseated, vomited repeatedly, and was constipated. Although her pain was fairly well controlled through radiotherapy and medication, the other symptoms were not. Throughout the four weeks of her hospital stay, the patient's experiences alternated between good and bad times. She was nauseated, unable to eat, and vomited frequently for one or two days; then she felt much better for a couple of days before she started vomiting again. Constipation was an ongoing problem; the patient never achieved good bowel function.

> **P:** *I again vomited, vomited, vomited. Yesterday it eased, but I didn't really have a bowel movement. Now I believe, that we will finally gain control over it. When I am not nauseated, I am a completely different person. When it is like that for two days, then I don't have much resistance anymore. Sorry . . . then I tell my husband: "Oh, I would like to die, then everything would be over." Well, then I recovered during the day yesterday, and this morning I could eat half a muesli and some bread and coffee. It goes upwards like that.*
>
> **I:** *And as soon as you feel better, you don't want to die anymore. . . .*
>
> **P:** *No, no. [laughs]*

The care providers and the patient identified multiple potential reasons for the symptoms: the patient's proneness for constipation before her illness, her immobilization from pain, opioids interfering with bowel movement, fecal impaction, radiotherapy affecting the gastrointestinal tract, psychological problems, and even a basiliaris syndrome. A variety of interventions were tried—for instance, antiemetics, laxatives, enemas, black olives and plums, a tranquilizer, and a collar to stabilize her neck. However, all these endeavors did not bring about the hoped for symptom relief. In fact, shortly before the patient's discharge, the medical record stated optimistically that bowel functioning had finally been achieved even though the patient vomited again the next day, and an X-ray revealed fecal impaction.

The patient's accounts and the medical and nursing record provided a somewhat confusing and fractured picture of a repeated trial-and-error approach to symptom control. The interrelatedness and the multiple potential causes of the symptoms made effective management very difficult. What seemed to be missing was a comprehensive consideration of the patient's situation and a rigorous, stepwise approach to symptom management as suggested in palliative care (Twycross, 2003).

The experience of this patient who suffered from common symptoms—nausea, vomiting, pain—highlights the importance of optimal symptom control. With untreated or untreatable symptoms, suffering can become overpowering and take up the patient's whole life. The horizon of the patient's world closes down; going on with life means suffering on. Life becomes pointless, and death—the end of suffering—is welcomed. With effective symptom management, suffering is forced back; with symptom relief, the patient's world opens up again, her horizon widens, life regains meaning and becomes worthwhile once more.

Providing Information and Anticipatory Guidance

For patients and family members in limbo, with tormenting thoughts floating about their mind and tremendous insecurity, adequate information and anticipatory guidance were extremely helpful. A family member related that the patient had talked a lot about death with a specialist. He had reassured him not to be afraid: that he would likely sleep more and more, and die in his sleep. Thinking about death as falling asleep forever was very comforting for the patient: He hoped for this development, and in fact, did die in his sleep.

A couple, facing the recurrence of the woman's lung cancer and several diagnostic tests to decide upon a palliative chemotherapy, experienced the counselling of a specialist as very supportive and clarifying, as the wife stated: "The dreadful unknown that floats one's mind is bad. So he explained to us why each time when a new diagnostic test was done." However, because of the unknown illness trajectory, clear information was not always available. Further treatment decisions often depended upon effects and side effects of the current therapy and were, therefore, postponed until these effects became apparent, leaving patients and families in great uncertainty: "It is a constant back and forth and unclear, how it will go on."

Eventually, not all consultations were experienced as supportive. One family member, when asked whether she felt supported by repeated conversations with the patient's physicians, explained that these meetings brought along an agreement on the best care for the patient, but nothing for her: "I would like to say that the physicians were not relevant for me, and they did not give me what I would have needed." She experienced the information regarding the patient's prognosis as unsatisfactory, and stated that the advice to have her own life besides caring for the patient was misguided. For the family member, living her life at this moment meant accompanying the patient through his terminal illness. Being distant and attempting to live a separate life temporarily was untenable.

Attuning Care Activities Individually

All the patients needed nursing care, and for some, additional professionals were involved. The professionals aimed at individual care for patients and families. With the wide range of situations they encountered, the frequent and at times rapid changes in patients' health status, the care providers were constantly challenged to adapt their activities in order to fine-tune them to the shifting needs of patients and families. According to patients' and family members' accounts, the care providers' abilities to live up to this challenge varied.

Patients and family members repeatedly related satisfying interventions, which brought about positive outcomes. For instance, the massage of the physiotherapist helped a bedridden and spastic patient relax. Patients and family members valued the good coordination among nurses. Their observance of details was also welcomed, for instance, the timely changing of sweaty bed linen.

At times, however, professionals' interventions did not match the needs of patients and families. This could have different reasons, such as lack of experience, poor attention to details, or adherence to routines. For instance, a mother was dissatisfied with how her deceased son was dressed. She did not like to see him in a shroud with a bow tie.

> *I don't know, why they do this, but they dressed him with a bow tie or so, completely unnaturally. And I think, in death one should remain as natural as possible. From the beginning, I said: "Could you dress him in a polo shirt?" And they said that it was difficult.*

The mother stated that the inadequate dress was a hassle at the time, but it became irrelevant later. The issue can be seen as a drop of bitterness in what the family otherwise experienced as a peaceful death—an avoidable drop of bitterness because the hospital guidelines allowed personal clothes for the deceased. Unfortunately, the nurses seemed not to be aware of this possibility.

The following observed care episodes further illustrate nurses' successes or break downs in attuning activities to a patient's needs. The patient was a 40-year-old man with a glioma. He was wheelchair-bound because he was hemiplegic, and he suffered extremely from his dependency. He also suffered from some apraxia and from aphasia, but he could still answer questions with yes or no. During observation, his nurse asked him whether he would like to take a shower. The patient agreed. In the shower, she repeatedly asked whether the water temperature was alright. She also said that she would like to wash his hair, and the patient agreed. Thus, the nurse respected his wishes. She encouraged him to do as much as possible himself. As soon as he got stuck, she guided him or took over, passing silently over his disabilities. The patient, when asked whether he had enjoyed the shower, said yes. He could not utter his experiences more precisely, but the showering went by smoothly, and he never appeared unhappy. The approach of this very experienced nurse seemed appropriate, mainly because she focused on the patient's remaining abilities rather than on his disabilities. Through her respectful and attuned care, the nurse recognized the patient as an independent person.

I observed a less favorable approach when a nursing student was feeding breakfast to the same patient. She cut his roll in two halves and spread them with butter. She prepared a feeding cup with hot chocolate. She gave one half of the roll to the patient and told him: "Take a bite!" This was difficult for him; he repeatedly succeeded only after several demands. The nurse explained: "You don't have to open the mouth that much—like 'that' is sufficient." [She demonstrated it.] "And now bite. Doesn't it work?" She alternated with feeding roll and hot chocolate, feeding the hot chocolate to the patient with the feeding cup. In the beginning, the nurse asked questions, for instance, whether he had already had a shower. "Do you still remember? No? Or can't you say it?" She did not get any answer. Later, she asked less and looked out of the window at times. Then she prepared the gathering device of the napkin to protect the patient's clothes from food and hot chocolate. She mentioned to the patient that everything would fall into it, and in the end, one could eat dessert out of it. Finally, the patient had eaten the whole roll and almost finished the hot chocolate. The nurse left the cup within reaching distance and carried the tray away. The patient grasped the cup and drank.

Observation showed that this nursing student did not know the patient well; she was unaware of the extent and limits of his abilities. For weeks, his rolls had been cut into bite-sized pieces, but he was still able to drink himself although he needed some guidance at times. He was unable to answer her questions. It seemed likely that she was not always focusing her attention on the patient and the task at hand because she was either talking about unrelated issues or staring out the window. Her demanding way of talking to the patient and her repeated requests to do things he was no longer able to do had the potential of bringing his deficits fully to his attention, and may have caused unnecessary distress. Finally, her remark about eating dessert out of the napkin highlighted his spillage and was simply tactless. This nursing student lacked the knowledge, empathy, and experience required to feed this patient in an adequate way. She was unable to attune her care to his needs. Feeding someone is often thought of as simple and doable by anybody. The episode illustrates that this seemingly simple task becomes a complex and challenging nursing intervention in the context of physical and mental disability and suffering from dependency.

These observations highlight that the care providers' expertise and their knowledge of the patient heavily influence the attuning of care activities to a patient's needs. Fine-tuning is a much bigger challenge for a nursing student than an experienced nurse. The latter—the expert—can intuitively rely upon her extensive theoretical knowledge, practical know-how, and comparisons with prior similar cases; the former—the novice—may rely upon textbook knowledge about brain tumors as well as hemiplegia, aphasia, and apraxia, but has never met a patient with a specific and frequently changing pattern of symptoms from these conditions (Benner, 1984).

Removing Stumbling Blocks

At times, the care providers intervened skillfully on behalf of patients and family members to prevent difficulties or the escalation of a problematic situation. The following story of a patient illustrates this. The woman shared a room with a second patient who had been admitted during the night. According to her health insurance, this patient was entitled to a private room; however, none had been available at night. When her husband arrived in the early morning, he insisted on his right to be present around the clock as in a private room, without considering the needs of the other patient. The latter said:

> *One morning, I almost freaked out. There was another patient, and her husband arrived at seven in the morning. Put up the divider, and then he just was in the*

room. I was waking up, had not yet been on the toilet, nothing, and he was just walking around the room. And the nurses could not get rid of him. He said that he was a private payer and had the right to be in the room. And I almost freaked out. I could not go to the toilet, I could not do anything. And when they had brought him out, after five minutes, he was back again. I would have freaked out as a nurse. But they ushered him out again and again with a saintly patience. And there, I realized that after all, I lacked any vigor, I just said: "He has to leave."

Within two hours, the nurses organized a private room for the second patient and moved her out. In both the patient's and the family member's view, the nurses showed great social competencies in dealing with this awkward situation. The patient was very relieved that they acted on her behalf and saved her from the additional distress of an escalating conflict.

Care providers, and especially nurses, often act preventively, usually in relation to physical problems like pressure sores. The preceding story told highlights that care providers also act preventively in other realms. They use their social competency to deal with upcoming interpersonal problems and ensure the smooth running of the units; stumbling blocks are removed. Disputes with patients, family members, other visitors, or among care providers can be disruptive and cause considerable distress. However, the brewing storm in the air whose breakout was competently prevented is easily overlooked. In other words, the competent social interactions of the care providers remain almost invisible to other care providers, the hospital management, or the public. Yet in the context of the distress of terminal illness and an enforced hospital stay, such social competence is essential for patients and families, thereby making their life easier.

Putting Stumbling Blocks in the Way

Although patients and family members mostly felt well cared for in the hospital, they also related some negative experiences, which were more or less tolerable. Usually, patients and family members found a way to cope with these negative aspects; for instance, time might remedy the issue, they considered it as a minor aspect in the context of their overall positive experiences, or they found an acceptable explanation or excuse such as a staffing shortage. However, patients and family members also related a few care episodes that affected them very negatively. These situations hurt them deeply and were neither easily forgotten nor forgiven. They stuck in peoples' memories and came up again and again in conversations as stumbling blocks put in their way by care providers, as the next example illustrates.

A patient and his family were told that the patient had to apply for a place in several nursing homes because he could not stay in the hospital. The patient had been admitted with a recurrence of brain metastases. His health status was quite stable; an unlimited hospital stay, therefore, was not justifiable. Because the patient had been living alone, was now wheelchair-bound, and was in need of nursing care, returning home was also not an option. The patient was very satisfied with his care in the hospital and wished to stay on the unit. It was hard for him to accept that this was not possible, but he finally came to terms with this fact and looked forward to the transfer to the nursing home. What he could not cope with was the physician's message. He remembered the conversation with the physician:

> **P:** *Well, I just have to leave. Cost-and-effect calculation, that's it. The physician told my brother. He explained the disease, and that radiotherapy did not respond, and that chemotherapy would be useless, ineffective, and well, that I cannot stay here when there are no tests, treatments, therapies. Cost-and-effect. That shocked my brother. That is impudent, cost-and-effect: exactly like in a butcher's shop.*
>
> **I:** *Well, and how was it for you to hear that?*
>
> **P:** *In any case, I did not forget it so far!*

For the patient's brother and sister-in-law, this conversation was also a disturbing experience. The brother mentioned that it would be okay to let him know, but it seemed brutal that such things were said in the patient's presence. The sister-in-law said that the physician mentioned the cost-and-effect relation several times. And she added: "That seemed rather disturbing to me. That one just says this so frankly, you know, cost-and-effect for a human being . . . the relation of cost and effect isn't right anymore."

For the patient, when talking about cost-and-effect, the physician seemed to make a comparison with, for instance, a butcher calculating which goods might be profitable for his shop, with the patient as a good. Stated otherwise, the patient extended the cost-and-effect appraisal to his own worthiness: He felt objectified and dehumanized. The family members experienced the message as inadequate and reacted angrily but coped by rationalizing: Health care costs had to be taken into account. They were mainly concerned about the negative consequences of the message for the patient. As they mentioned, the degrading message remained a sting in the flesh for the patient.

Regardless to whom it is given, patient or family, a message with such a nonbeneficial outcome seems unjustifiable to me from an ethical perspective. The sister-in-law is right:

Talking about cost-and-effect in relation to a human being is harmful. The discussion of costs in relation to the effectiveness of interventions for specific groups of people is necessary for health care policy. This discussion must not be taken, however, to the level of individual patients. The message, as perceived by patient and family, heavily damaged the relationship between the patient and his physician. In ethical terms, it can be seen as an offense against the rule of nonmaleficence. The slippage into economic language leaves behind the care provider's concern for the patient's well-being. The physician neither takes fully into consideration the patient's vulnerability and dependency nor the responsibility, which acting from the more powerful position comprises.

Although the physician was obliged to inform his patient about the impossibility of an unlimited hospital stay and the necessity of a nursing home move, it was up to him to formulate this message in an acceptable way—to choose the right words, which he did not. The patient felt kicked out by the care providers for financial reasons rather than learning what the consequences of insurance and hospital guidelines were in his case, how the care providers could support him in finding an acceptable solution, and that he would still be cared for in the hospital until the transfer to the nursing home.

The example shows how blatant failures of care providers are experienced extremely negatively by patients and families. Such situations are problematic because they add avoidable burden to the already distressed patients and families: stumbling blocks put in their way by awkwardly acting care providers. Furthermore, the care providers may not learn how badly their actions affected patients and family members because the latter remain silent. Thus, putting stumbling blocks in patients' and family members' way may occur with the same invisibility as the removing.

DISCUSSION

A comparison of findings in the literature to results of this study reveals correspondence in some areas. Publications on patients' and families' experiences pointed out communication among patients, families, and care providers as an important aspect of hospital end-of-life care (Andershed & Ternestedt, 1998, 1999; Berns & Colvin, 1998; Dunne & Sullivan, 2000; Keegan et al., 2001; McCormick & Conley, 1995; McGrath, 2001; Rogers et al., 2000; Teno et al., 2004; Wenrich et al., 2001). Similarly, patients and family members in this study experienced understandable, honest, and timely information provided by knowledgeable professionals as very helpful. The couple who faced the recurrence of the woman's lung cancer serves as an example. However, the same couple was left in limbo regarding the next steps because further treatment decisions depended upon the effect of the current radiotherapy. This highlights that the trajectory of the terminal illness is often unpredictable and, therefore, the much desired information is not always available. Thus, even with excellent interactions, professionals may be limited to explaining which factors will influence future decisions and that questions cannot be answered at the moment because of the ever-variable and unpredictable illness trajectory. With the aspect of limited available information that may hamper conversations, this study adds a perspective which has hardly been addressed so far in the literature.

> *"Even with excellent interactions, professionals may be limited to explaining which factors will influence future decisions and that questions cannot be answered at the moment because of the ever-variable and unpredictable illness trajectory.*

Across studies, the patients' well-being had priority for family members, and in several publications the relevance of support in activities of daily living was mentioned (Hawker et al., 2006, Pierce, 1999; Rogers et al., 2000). For the participants in this study, adequate support in activities of daily living for patients was also essential. In addition to other publications, the concrete narratives in this study highlight that mundane care activities, such as feeding or bathing, become challenging and complex in the presence of illness, suffering, and disability. The results illustrate that patients may well accept such interventions from care providers who act as experts (Benner, 1984), but may experience interventions as degrading, when provided by inexperienced or uncaring nurses.

The discrepancy between insufficient symptom control and high satisfaction with care described in the literature (Lynn et al., 1997; McCarthy et al., 1996; Rogers et al., 2000; Teno et al., 2004; Tolle, Tilden, Hickman et al., 2000; Tolle, Tilden, Rosenfeld et al., 2000) also appears in the current study. For instance, the patient with unrelieved vomiting and constipation still highly praised the professionals for their caring and concern. The study provides an explanation for this contradiction and points to a conclusion: Patients and family members who do not know what they can expect regarding symptom management, but who feel that the professionals try hard, will likely be satisfied with their care and assume that a better symptom control is impossible. Thus, the professionals are responsible to provide optimal treatments according to palliative care standards.

In summary, this analysis shows that what patients and family members experienced as good end-of-life care corresponds well with the standards of excellence in palliative care. In many situations, the care providers' endeavors yielded positive results for patients and families. However, the professionals were not always able to actualize palliative care standards.

Their great compassion was at times jeopardized by a lack of scientific knowledge and expertise in palliative care.

Limitations

This study explores experiences of ten terminally ill patients and their family members in one university hospital in Switzerland. Thus, the results provide a particular and local account of patients' and family members' experiences. Taking the study context into account, readers must decide whether and which particular aspects of the findings described in this study are transferable to other settings.

Methodologically, there is no clear end-point to interpretations in phenomenology. The option of a deeper, more comprehensive or more convincing interpretation always remains available (Leonard, 1994). Thus, these findings represent one account of patients' and families' experiences that is neither exhaustive nor the only possible interpretation.

CONCLUSION

The fact that no cure is available, never means that "nothing can be done" for patients with a terminal illness and their families. The professional health care providers in the hospital can decisively influence patients' and families' experiences. Care providers, who lack a caring stance toward patients and families, are inattentive, or do not have the needed skills and expertise are unable to recognize patients and family members as persons, to act adequately and attune care interventions to particular patients. Inappropriate actions, such as the use of cost-and-effect language, are painful for patients and family members, and they experience being disregarded and devalued as dehumanizing. Inadequate care adds avoidable suffering to patients' and families' burden of living with a terminal illness and being in the hospital.

However, the results also show the power of adequate and finely tuned care interventions to improve patients' and their families' well-being. Committed and caring providers who give individualized care enable patients and families to accept this care and feel well cared for; the hospital stay becomes more bearable.

Patients with a terminal illness and their family members value expert professionals who can carry out requested tasks and achieve excellent results without unduly burdening patients; stated otherwise, Aristotle's productive knowledge or *techne* is welcomed (Dunne, 1997). The responsibility to acquire the needed scientific knowledge and technical skills and to transfer them appropriately into practice rests with the care providers because patients and families are not always aware of the best possible outcomes.

However, *techne* is not sufficient; patients' and families' good or bad experiences with hospital care do not depend upon outcomes only. Rather, their lived experiences are strongly related to the process of caregiving, to their relationships with professionals, to the latter's way of acting. *Phronesis*, embodied practical knowledge about how to act well, is also required (Dunne, 1997). Phronesis calls for care providers, who engage in their actions and with patients and families, to apply universal knowledge in a particular context to individual patients and families and to strive for excellence while continually learning from their experiences. The complex area of end-of-life care, with unspecific situations, rapid changes, and often undetermined illness trajectories calls for phronesis in order to respond to patients' and families' particular needs over time and to achieve the best possible QoL for them.

ACKNOWLEDGMENTS

My great thanks go to the patients and family members who participated in the study, to the care providers in the hospital, to the members of my dissertation committee: Patricia Benner, Ph.D., R.N., FAAN (chair); Annemarie Kesselring, Ph.D., R.N.; Margaret Wallhagen, Ph.D., G.N.P., R.N.; and Jeanie Kayser-Jones, Ph.D., R.N., FAAN. I also thank Rebecca Spirig, Ph.D., R.N. and Heleen Prakke, Ph.D., R.N. for her review of an early draft of the manuscript. Funding of the author's studies from the following sources is gratefully acknowledged: Regents Fellowship and Non-Resident Tuition Scholarship, University of California San Francisco; Bernese Cancer League's Grant; Inselspital Bern University Hospital; and Lindenhof, Bern, Switzerland.

References

Andershed, B., & Ternestedt, B. M. (1998). Involvement of relatives in the care of the dying in different care cultures: Involvement in the dark or in the light? *Cancer Nursing, 21*, 106-116.

Andershed, B., & Ternestedt, B. M. (1999). Involvement of relatives in care of the dying in different care cultures: Development of a theoretical understanding. *Nursing Science Quarterly, 12*(1), 45-51.

Baker, R., Wu, A. W., Teno, J. M., Kreling, B., Damiano, A. M., Rubin, H. R., et al. (2000). Family satisfaction with end-of-life care in seriously ill hospitalized adults. *Journal of the American Geriatrics Society, 48*, S61-S69.

Benner, P. (1984). *From novice to expert: Excellence and power in clinical nursing practice*. Menlo Park, CA: Addison-Wesley.

Benner, P. (1994a). The tradition and skill of interpretive phenomenology in studying health, illness, and caring practices. In P. Benner (Ed.), *Interpretive phenomenology: Embodiment, caring, and ethics in health and illness* (pp. 99-127). Thousand Oaks, CA: Sage.

Benner, P. (Ed.). (1994b). *Interpretive phenomenology: Embodiment, caring, and ethics in health and illness.* Thousand Oaks, CA: Sage.

Benner, P. (1994c). Introduction. In P. Benner (Ed.), *Interpretive phenomenology: Embodiment, caring, and ethics in health and illness* (pp. xiii-xxvii). Thousand Oaks, CA: Sage.

Benner, P., Hooper-Kyriakidis, P., & Stannard, D. (1999). *Clinical wisdom and interventions in critical care: A thinking-in-action approach.* Philadelphia: Saunders.

Benner, P., Tanner, C. A., & Chesla, C. A. (1996). *Expertise in nursing practice: Caring, clinical judgement, and ethics.* New York: Springer.

Berns, R., & Colvin, E. R. (1998). The final story: Events at the bedside of dying patients as told by survivors. *American Nephrology Nurses' Association Journal, 25,* 583-587.

Bruera, E. (2006). Foreword. In H. Neuenschwander, R. Baumann, E. Bergsträsser, S. Eberhard, S. Eichmüller, H. Gudat, et al., *Palliativmedizin* [Palliative medicine] (p. 11). Bern, Switzerland: Krebsliga Schweiz.

Bucher, J. A., Trostle, G. B., & Moore, M. (1999). Family reports of cancer pain, pain relief, and prescription access. *Cancer Practice, 7,* 71-77.

Czerwiec, M. (1996). When a loved one is dying: Families talk about nursing care. *American Journal of Nursing, 96*(5), 32-36.

Doyle, D., Hanks, G. W. C., Cherny, N., & Calman, K. (Eds.). (2005). *Oxford textbook of palliative medicine* (3rd ed.). Oxford, UK: Oxford University Press.

Dunne, J. (1997). *Back to the rough ground: Practical judgment and the lure of technique.* Notre Dame: University of Notre Dame Press.

Dunne, K., & Sullivan, K. (2000). Family experiences of palliative care in the acute hospital setting. *International Journal of Palliative Nursing, 6,* 170-178.

Fischer, S., Bosshard, G., Zellweger, U., & Faisst, K. (2004). Der Sterbeort: 'Wo sterben die Menschen heute in der Schweiz?' [The place of death: Where do people in Switzerland die today?] *Zeitschrift für Gerontologie und Geriatrie, 37,* 467-474.

Grond, S., Zech, D., Schug, S. A., Lynch, J., & Lehmann, K. A. (1991). Validation of World Health Organization guidelines for cancer pain relief during the last days and hours of life. *Journal of Pain and Symptom Management, 6,* 411-422.

Halpern, J. (2001). *From detached concern to empathy: Humanizing medical practice.* New York: Oxford University Press.

Hanson, L. C., Danis, M., & Garrett, J. (1997). What is wrong with end-of-life care? Opinions of bereaved family members. *Journal of the American Geriatrics Society, 45,* 1339-1344.

Hawker, S., Kerr, C., Payne, S., Seamark, D., Davis, C., Roberts, H., et al. (2006). End-of-life care in community hospitals: The perceptions of bereaved family members. *Palliative Medicine, 20,* 541-547.

Heyland, D. K., Dodek, P., Rocker, G., Groll, D., Gafni, A., Pichora, D., et al. (2006). What matters most in end-of-life care: Perceptions of seriously ill patients and their family members. *Canadian Medical Association Journal, 174,* 627-633.

Keegan, O., McGee, H., Hogan, M., Kunin, H., O'Brien, S., & O'Siorain, L. (2001). Relatives' views of health care in the last year of life. *International Journal of Palliative Nursing, 7,* 449-456.

Leonard, V. W. (1994). A Heideggerian phenomenological perspective on the concept of person. In P. Benner (Ed.), *Interpretive phenomenology: Embodiment, caring, and ethics in health and illness* (pp. 43-63). Thousand Oaks, CA: Sage.

Levenson, J. W., McCarthy, E. P., Lynn, J., Davis, R. B., & Phillips, R. S. (2000). The last six months of life for patients with congestive heart failure. *Journal of the American Geriatrics Society, 48,* S101-S109.

Lynn, J., Ely, E. W., Zhong, Z., McNiff, K. L., Dawson, N. V., Connors, L., et al. (2000). Living and dying with chronic obstructive pulmonary disease. *Journal of the American Geriatrics Society, 48*, S91-S100.

Lynn, J., Teno, J. M., Phillips, R. S., Wu, A. W., Desbiens, N., Harrold, J., et al. (1997). Perceptions by family members of the dying experience of older and seriously ill patients. *Annals of Internal Medicine, 126*, 97-106.

McCarthy, E. P., Phillips, R. S., Zhong, Z., Drews, R. E., & Lynn, J. (2000). Dying with cancer: Patients' function, symptoms, and care preferences as death approaches. *Journal of the American Geriatrics Society, 48*, S110-S121.

McCarthy, M., Lay, M., & Addington-Hall, J. (1996). Dying from heart disease. *Journal of the Royal College of Physicians of London, 30*, 325-328.

McCormick, T. R., & Conley, B. J. (1995). Patients' perspectives on dying and on the care of dying patients. *Western Journal of Medicine, 163*, 236-243.

McGrath, P. (2001). Caregivers' insights on the dying trajectory in hematology oncology. *Cancer Nursing, 24*, 413-421.

Meier, D. E., Morrison, R. S., & Cassel, C. K. (1997). Improving palliative care. *Annals of Internal Medicine, 127*, 225-230.

Miettinen, T. T., Tilvis, R. S., Karppi, P., & Arve, S. (1998). Why is the pain relief of dying patients often unsuccessful? The relatives' perspectives. *Palliative Medicine, 12*, 429-435.

Plager, K. A. (1994). Hermeneutic phenomenology: A methodology for family health and health promotion study in nursing. In P. Benner (Ed.), *Interpretive phenomenology: Embodiment, caring, and ethics in health and illness* (pp. 65-83). Thousand Oaks, CA: Sage.

Pierce, S. F. (1999). Improving end-of-life care: Gathering suggestions from family members. *Nursing Forum, 34*(2), 5-14.

Raemy-Bass, C., Lugon, J.-P., & Eggimann, J.-C. (2000). *Palliative Care in der Schweiz: Bestandesaufnahme 1999-2000*. Geneva, Switzerland: Association François-Xavier Bagnoud.

Rogers, A., Karlsen, S., & Addington-Hall, J. (2000). 'All the services were excellent. It is when the human element comes in that things go wrong': Dissatisfaction with hospital care in the last year of life. *Journal of Advanced Nursing, 31*, 768-774.

Roth, K., Lynn, J., Zhong, Z., Borum, M., & Dawson, N. V. (2000). Dying with end stage liver disease with cirrhosis: Insights from SUPPORT. *Journal of the American Geriatrics Society, 48*, S122-S130.

Sepulveda, C., Marlin, A., Yoshida, T., & Ullrich, A. (2002). Palliative care: The World Health Organization's global perspective. *Journal of Pain and Symptom Management, 24*, 91-96.

Spichiger, E. (2003). Palliative care in Switzerland: Look back, current endeavors, and outlook. *Journal of Hospice and Palliative Nursing, 5*, 161-167.

Spichiger, E. (2004). *Leading a life with a terminal illness: An interpretive phenomenological study of patients' and family members' experiences of hospital end-of-life care*. Unpublished doctoral dissertation, University of California San Francisco, San Francisco.

The SUPPORT Principal Investigators. (1995). A controlled trial to improve care for seriously ill hospitalized patients: The study to understand prognoses and preferences for outcomes and risks of treatments (SUPPORT). *Journal of the American Medical Association, 274*, 1591-1598.

Teno, J. M., Clarridge, B. R., Casey, V., Welch, L. C., Wetle, T., Shield, R. et al. (2004). Family perspectives on end-of-life care at the last place of care. *Journal of the American Medical Association, 291*, 88-93.

Tolle, S. W., Tilden, V. P., Hickman, S. E., & Rosenfeld, A. G. (2000). Family reports of pain in dying hospitalized patients: A structured telephone survey. *Western Journal of Medicine, 172*, 374-377.

Tolle, S. W., Tilden, V. P., Rosenfeld, A. G., & Hickman, S. E. (2000). Family reports of barriers to optimal care of the dying. *Nursing Research, 49*, 310-317.

Twycross, R. (2003). *Introducing palliative care*. Oxon, UK: Radcliffe Medical Press.

Undritz, N. (2004). Krankenhaus [Hospital]. In G. Kocher & W. Oggier (Eds.), *Gesundheitswesen Schweiz 2004-2006: Ein aktueller Ueberblick [Health care in Switzerland 2004-2006: An actual overview]* (pp. 130-143). Bern, Switzerland: Hans Huber.

Wenrich, M. D., Curtis, J. R., Shannon, S. E., Carline, J. D., Ambrozy, D. M., & Ramsey, P. G. (2001). Communicating with dying patients within the spectrum of medical care from terminal diagnosis to death. *Archives of Internal Medicine, 161*, 868-874.

World Health Organization (1986). Cancer pain relief. Geneva: World Health Organization.

World Health Organization. (2002). National cancer control programmes: Policies and managerial guidelines (2nd ed.). Geneva: World Health Organization.

World Health Organization. (2003). *WHO Definition of palliative care*. Retrieved 02/28, 2009, from http://www.who.int/cancer/palliative/definition/en

World Health Organization (2004). *Palliative care: The solid facts*. Retrieved 02/28, 2009, from http://www.euro.who.int/InformationSources/Publications/Catalogue/20050118_2

CHAPTER 16

End of Living: Maintaining a Lifeworld During Terminal Illness

JUDITH WRUBEL, MICHAEL ACREE, STEFFANIE GOODMAN, SUSAN FOLKMAN

CORRESPONDING AUTHOR: JUDITH WRUBEL

INTRODUCTION

The focus in recent decades on the provision of palliative care for terminally ill people has been a welcome shift in support offered to people who are nearing death. However, the label of end-of-life care reflects an ongoing bias toward viewing people's lives in terms of their static end point instead of in terms of the possibilities for living meaningfully while they are still alive. This study focuses on the phenomenological concept of lifeworld. The *lifeworld* is the dynamic horizon in which people live and by which all things and experiences have meaning. The study examines how 32 people, judged to have 6 months to a year to live, were characterized by either the maintenance of or the interruption in the way they maintained connections to aspects of their lives that defined who they were as a person (i.e., their lifeworld).

Social science research about the final phase of life for seriously ill individuals diagnosed as having one year or less to live[1] tends to focus on depression (e.g., Block, 2001); the success of pain management (e.g., Lo, Woo, et al., 2002; Roth et al., 2000; Steinhauser et al., 2000; Stewart, Teno, Patrick, & Lynn, 1999); and existential concerns such as hope (e.g., Chochinov, 2006) and spirituality (e.g., Lo, Ruston, et al., 2002; Nakashima & Canda, 2005). This research focus has provided an important impetus to discover the best ways to support dying patients and alleviate their suffering.

Some research on people nearing death proceeds from the assumption that we are culturally disposed to deny death (Becker, 1973). This research emphasizes ways of helping people come to terms with their mortality in order to facilitate acceptance, which a prerequisite for a "good death" according to Friel (1982). The importance of "accepting" death became widely popularized with the publication of Kubler-Ross' (1973) work about the stages of grief.

Another line of research questioned the assumption that we are a death-denying society (Zimmermann, 2004, 2007), argued for the importance of distinguishing between illness and disease, and recommended the subordination of the outsider perspective (e.g., observing the individual in terms of sick role or illness behaviors) in favor of an insider perspective that speaks to how illness is experienced by the people affected by it (Benner & Wrubel, 1989; Conrad, 1990; Kleinman, Eisenberg, & Good, 1978). Examples of research taking this direction include Cohen, Mount, Tomas, and Mount (1996), who pointed out that the physical domain is usually over-emphasized in quality of life (QoL) measures and that other life aspects that reflect what matters to people (e.g., relationships, spirituality, meaning) are neglected. This view coincides with findings of Chochinov et al. (2005) from their study of 189 persons with end-stage cancer in which they observed strong relationships between existential and social variables and the will to live. Physical distress was correlated less strongly with the will to live than were the existential and social variables. These authors noted that, "No one wants to be viewed merely as the embodiment of a disease process" (Chochinov, Hack, et al., 2005 p. 9).

In a similar vein, Clark (2002) criticized the "medicalization of dying," noting that the focus on death and dying obscures how people live until they die. This point has been vividly illustrated by recent research on people with amyotrophic lateral sclerosis (ALS; Lou Gehrig's disease), which is a progressively debilitating, fatal disease with a survival prognosis of 2 to 5 years. Rabkin et al. (2005) reported in their study of 80 people with late-stage ALS that only a small percentage of the participants were depressed and that no one became more depressed as he or she neared death. The absence of depression—an expected outcome from an outsider perspective in a disease that destroys the nerves that innervates muscles so the person gradually becomes unable to move, to speak, to swallow or breathe—has been anecdotally illustrated in the life of Dr. Richard Olney. Dr. Olney founded the ALS clinic at the University of California, San Francisco and ironically developed the disease himself at age 55. He is wheelchair-bound and communicates using a word/phrase board and a laser pointer attached to his glasses, but he is not depressed: He interacts meaningfully with his family and continues to keep up with the literature in his field and to publish articles (Russell, 2008).

We propose that living a life that is meaningful and coherent with respect to the things that matter to the person with a terminal illness may be as important for well-being or even more important than accepting death. Exploring how people with terminal illnesses stay open to positive experiences while dealing with the physical challenges of managing their illness could lead to a better understanding of this phase of human life. One way of exploring these positive aspects is to examine the lifeworlds of people with terminal illnesses. The term *lifeworld* has been defined by Agre and Horswill (1997) as referring to

> The familiar world of everyday life, and specifically to that world as described in the terms that make a difference for a given way of life. Cats and people, for example, can be understood as inhabiting the same physical environment but different lifeworlds. Kitchen cupboards, window sills, and the spaces underneath chairs have different significances for cats and people, as do balls of yarn, upholstery, television sets, and other cats. (p. 114)

In their 35 case studies of doctor-patient interviews, Barry et al. (2001) found that the best patient outcomes occurred when the doctors recognized their patients' lifeworlds and allowed them to give voice to lifeworld concerns in the interview. Hyden (1997), in a review of 10 years' worth of studies on illness narratives, concluded that "a central aspect of being ill in modern society [is] the difficulty of giving voice both to suffering and to the lifeworld context of illness" (p. 64).

In examining individuals' lifeworlds, we do not try to capture the larger existential issues of the meaning of life, but, following Frankl (1963), the meaning *in* life. As Frankl noted: "What matters is not the meaning of life in general, but rather the specific meaning of a person's life at a given moment" (p.171).

This study explores how people with a terminal illness live out their lives. Through analysis of monthly interviews with people judged by their physicians to have 6 months to 1 year to live, we came to see the challenge that people face at this juncture as living rather than facing death. Our goals are to articulate the ways how people nearing the end of their life maintain their lifeworld and engage with life, and to examine the associations between different kinds of engagement and potential constraints attributable to their illness and their psychological states of mind.

METHODS

Study Sample and Procedures

Data for this study were collected as part of The Care Preferences Study of 88 people diagnosed with a terminal illness (cancer or AIDS) and their primary family caregiver. The study was conducted in San Francisco and New York City between January 2003 and September 2005. Qualitative data were gathered only at the San Francisco site.

Potential participants were referred by their physicians. Participants were adult, nondemented cancer or AIDS patients who, according to their physicians

- Had a survival prognosis of 6 months to one year
- Were receiving their care at home at study entry
- Had an identified family member, significant other, or close friend who was primarily responsible for care.

Interviewers received informed consent at the time of the first interview. The Institutional Review Boards at the recruitment sites approved the study's consent procedures.

The present analysis is based upon the narrative accounts of ill participants from the San Francisco site who completed two or more qualitative interviews (32). Ill participants were interviewed separately from their caregivers every month until death or until the study ended. If their health stabilized or improved, they were interviewed bimonthly. By the end of the study, 20 of the 32 were deceased. Demographics for the sample are summarized in Table 16-1.

Table 16-1 Demographics of Study Participants

	AIDS	Cancer
Race		
Black	11	0
Caucasian	4	16
Other	0	1
Disposition		
Deceased at end of study	4	16
Not deceased	9	3
Other		
Age range	39–61	27–73
Income range	<$15K to $50–$75K	$15–$25K to >$200K
Educational range (years)	11–16	14–20

Study Qualitative Analysis

The participants were asked the following semistructured interview questions:

- Tell me a little about your life before you got sick. (First interview)
- Can you tell me a little about your illness? (First interview)
- Tell me, how do you spend your day?
- Have you noticed any problems with memory or concentration?
- How would you describe your current health status?
- What do you expect in the coming year regarding your health?
- Has your doctor said anything about what to expect in the future, and if so, what has he/she said?
- Is there anything that you would have liked to tell us that we didn't ask about?
- What are some of the things that keep you going or help you get through the day?

Responses were recorded by audio tape and transcribed. For this thematic analysis, we used three approaches: coding, case study, and cross-case analysis. A case comprised all the interviews that a participant completed. We used a team-based analytic approach (MacQueen, McLellan, Kay, & Milstein, 1998; Ryan & Bernard, 2003) for identifying and coding themes in the narratives that were responsive to the question of interest for this study: Namely, how do people with a terminal illness live their lives until they die? Two analysts developed the coding protocol based upon 10 cases. The remaining cases were divided between two coders, with each analyst coding half and verifying the codes of the other half. Disagreements were resolved through discussion. Case studies were written by the first author, who then performed a cross-case analysis to identify similarities and differences between cases. The qualitative analyst was blind to the quantitative outcomes until the completion of the qualitative work.

Study Quantitative Measures

Depression: Beck Depression Inventory: BDI-II and BDI-PC. The 21-item self-report BDI-II (Beck, Steer, Ball, & Ranieri, 1996) was administered to participants at baseline, and the briefer BDI-PC (primary care) version (Steer, Cavalieri, Leonard, & Beck, 1999) was given thereafter. The seven-item BDI-PC is intended for medically ill patients, and has the advantages of brevity and exclusion of somatic symptoms. Scores and their significance are

- <10: Absence of depression
- 10–16: Mild symptoms
- 17–29: Moderate symptoms
- 30+: Severe symptoms

The Patient Health Questionnaire (PHQ) (Spitzer, Kroenke, & Williams, 1999). This self-administered form of the earlier PRIME-MD (Spitzer, Williams, Kroenke, & Linzer, 1994) was developed for primary care patients. It inquires about symptoms and also their functional significance. It provides information about threshold mood disorders (DSM-IV diagnoses) and subthreshold disorders, and also yields a measure of depressive severity that can be used to track changes.

Visual Analog Scales (VAS). The VAS comprised 22 items that asked the participant to assess on a 10-point scale positive and negative aspects of well-being (e.g., "How depressed have you been feeling?"; "How much pleasure have you been experiencing?"). As recommended by Cohen and Mount (1992), we used a 3-day time frame to maximize recall and to avoid very transient fluctuations often observed in very sick patients. With respect to the validity of single item measures for the seriously ill, Chochinov, Wilson, Enns, and Lander (1997) compared a standard interview and three brief screens for depression in 197 advanced cancer patients receiving palliative care. The most accurate screen was the single item asking, "Are you depressed most of the day nearly every day?" It correctly identified all cases, with no false positives.

Lawton Instrumental Activities of Daily Living (Lawton & Brody, 1969). This assesses performance on eight everyday tasks instrumental to independent functioning.

Katz Index of Activities of Daily Living (Katz ADL) (Katz, Ford, Moskowitz, Jackson, & Jaffe, 1963). This assesses six self-care functions among patients with chronic disease and disability. It was administered only to patients who could not perform one or more activities on the Lawton IADL.

Symptom checklist. This checklist was used to record 15 symptoms reported by at least 10% of patients (Field & Cassel, 1997). The instrument asks for two ratings during the past 3 days for each checked symptom: severity and functional impairment.

RESULTS

Study Qualitative Analysis

Narrative data were collected only at the San Francisco site. The present analysis is based on ill participants who completed two or more qualitative interviews. In this section, we first describe how these participants understood their lives given their terminal diagnoses. Then we discuss the two groups that emerged from the analysis that were characterized by either the maintenance of or the interruption in the way they maintained connections to aspects of their lives that defined who they were as a person (i.e., their lifeworld).

END OF LIVING VERSUS END OF LIFE

Instead of "end-of-life," which bears connotations of a biomedical approach to death (Lock, 1996; Oakes-Greenspan, 2007), we use the phrase "end of living" as reflecting the insider perspective of the people with terminal diagnoses who are not in a static state but still living their lives. As Ira Byock, a leader in palliative care has noted: "There is a tendency within contemporary culture and reflected in medical practice to assume that on receipt of a terminal diagnosis meaningful life has ended" (1996, p. 245).

The participants in our study were aware that they had a disease that was going to be the cause of their death. For two reasons, most of the time participants did not see their lives in terms of approaching death. They had received their initial diagnosis an average of 7.2 years prior to the study. Most of them had lived with a terminal illness for years longer than predicted, and many had been adjudged near death one or more times previous to their enrollment in the study. As one participant (P: a man with AIDS for 16 years, now deceased) voiced to the interviewer (I)

> **P:** *You know, nobody feels like obsessing about it [death]. I've been living with it for years and years. It's been bad a few times, faced that, lived through it; it really <u>does</u> make it easier. You know there's no point in getting upset because it doesn't do anything–it just adds a layer you don't need (laughs). I think that once you live through a period where you <u>have</u> experienced the anxiety, you realize that it doesn't make a damn bit of difference (laughs), so what's the point? You get real philosophical about it.*

I: *What do you expect in the coming year regarding your health?*

P: *Not sure. I suppose if you look at the statistics, the chances are that it's going to get worse, but it hasn't. It's gotten worse and gotten better several times now, so I don't want to look at it that way. [woman with cancer for 8.4 years, nondeceased]*

Participants also frequently experienced a disjunction between clinical indicators and how they felt. Sometimes patients reported feeling worse although the doctor told them their laboratory test results were good. Other times, they reported feeling fairly well physically despite ominous clinical findings. Consequently, although participants had treatments, doctor appointments, and other health care activities, there were times that they had the time and energy to attend to other interests and life concerns.

LIFEWORLD: MAINTAINED VERSUS INTERRUPTED

Two groups emerged from the narrative analysis: Maintained Lifeworld and Lifeworld Interrupted. The groups were characterized either by

- The way they preserved connections to aspects of their lives that defined who they were as a person (i.e., their lifeworld)

- What interrupted that connection or made the connection weaker

The participants who maintained their lifeworld did so in the face of their declining health and the limitations their illnesses placed on them.

Maintained Lifeworld

Nineteen participants described living daily lives that embraced centrally self-defining concerns despite the spatial and temporal constrictions imposed by their illness. Of the 19, 12 died before the end of the study. Three types of central concerns embodied the participants' core values and personhood:

- Relational

- Spiritual

- Goal-oriented

These were not mutually exclusive categories. Most participants' narratives reflected more than one concern. Maintaining engagement with one or more of these central concerns was a source of positive feelings in the midst of the ups and downs of the illness as well as recurring or ongoing pain and suffering.

Relational concerns. Participants recounted a range of relational concerns, from close relationships with family and friends, to a connection to a wider community. Although these relational concerns differed among participants, they shared a common focus that was outward toward others.

Those whose relational concerns were more focused on family and friends emphasized the affective dimension of their connectedness and articulated how the connection affected them emotionally. Here are two responses:

> *I can't say that I've felt depressed. I don't know if there are parts that we haven't touched yet, but I haven't really felt depressed. Because again, I feel like I'm in such a cocoon of love. [woman with cancer, deceased]*

> *An interesting comment here is that my daughter was up to visit and how happy I am to see her and my dad together. He loves her. She loves him. I mean, it's just good to see the two of them together. That has an effect on me and my mood and the responses I'm giving to you in this survey. [man with cancer, deceased]*

In his first interview, one participant described being treated for lymphoma 4 years earlier and said that the birth of his nephew at that time was a major motivation for him to fight the cancer and survive. The nephew continued to be extremely important in this participant's daily life.

> *You know, because of all the medication I take, I don't have the luxury of forgetting that I've <u>got</u> this disease. And it really is a luxury. I've got the reminder every day of the drug regimen and the injections and everything, so at some point, you just want to have other things occupy your time and your mind. And that's why the boy upstairs [his 4-year-old nephew] is a great gift, you know? He'll <u>immediately</u> pull you out of whatever your situation is. You're always outside of yourself when you're around him. [man with AIDS, deceased]*

Some participants focused their relational concerns on a wider group than their immediate family. The following participant had a long-standing role in supporting the local high school swim team.

> **I:** *Tell me, how do you spend your day?*
>
> **P:** *I get up and watch some TV in the morning, and I leave here around 2:30 and go to the swimming pool every day. We have a local swim team, and I have been the grandmother for all the swimmers for about 12 years now. So I go down and take them cookies and spend about 3 to 4 hours every day down there at the swimming pool. Some I pick up and take to the pool and some I take home, and make sure that none of them sneak out and do something bad. I just love kids. [woman with cancer, nondeceased]*

At the beginning of the study, her health had declined, she was on portable oxygen, and she limited her driving to local destinations only and no longer drove to out-of-town meets. However, she continued going to the pool every afternoon for swim practice.

Relational concerns also included more formal community service. The following participant described his involvement in a number of AIDS organizations:

> *This is my day [takes out paper, chuckles]. Normally I get up and go to Oakland to meet with support groups. And I also go to AIDS Project of the East Bay, do client referrals. I also sit on the planning council of Alameda County. I stop by the planning council's office, turn in reports like demographics on clients that are positive, people who are trying to get into health care. I'm basically a volunteer. I do it because I—I care. And generally, every Thursday I go to doctor appointments. Then do some departmental meetings, it depends on what day of the week it is. When I'm in downtown Oakland, then I do Medicine Tray. I'm one of the advocates for that. I help clients with set-up. I give them a call and let them know how many clients I'm at that need some medicine and service and get them to deliver it to them. [man with AIDS, deceased]*

In his first interview, this participant recounted a conversation with his physician, who tried to convince him to do less and put his health first. She attempted to impress on him that he had advanced AIDS and told him he was "in denial" when he refused to heed her warning. In her concern to give him as long a life as possible, she couldn't hear how important it was to him to maintain the meaningful connections to his lifeworld.

Spiritual concerns. The participants who expressed a strong spiritual concern understood their lives and the world in spiritual terms.

> *I've always believed in God and tried to be a good Christian, and I can tell you, every time something happens, it just draws me closer, so my faith becomes stronger. [woman with cancer, deceased]*

That is, their everyday lives and actions were imbued with their spiritual understanding. They were active in being spiritual in that they had regular daily practices. For example, one participant was very committed to her spiritual practice, which involved nearly daily visits to her dojo.

> **I:** *Tell me, how do you spend your day?*
>
> **P:** *Four or 5 days a week, I go to the dojo for about 6 hours. The dojo is like a temple or a church, and that is where I do my spiritual practice. By the time I get home, I'll have something to eat. It takes me about an hour for my spiritual work, to pray, and do things like that. I always do my spiritual stuff before I go to bed. [woman with cancer, deceased]*

It should be noted that maintaining their lifeworld did not depend upon the participants being physically active. One spiritually oriented participant's world horizon was very constricted. He had AIDS, hepatitis-C, and kidney failure. He needed help managing daily activities. He required a walker and walked with difficulty. He had to go to dialysis three times per week, which was an exhausting process. He very often felt weak and fatigued—not well enough to do things. Those were his internal limits. His external limits came from living in a building with a broken elevator, so he was often confined to his apartment. Even with these limitations, he inhabited a meaningful lifeworld. He was a very spiritually oriented Christian, who daily watched ministers preaching on TV and listened to gospel music. These experiences made him feel good and reflect positively on his life.

> **I:** *What are some of the things that help you get through the day?*
>
> **P:** *My television, of course. And I love my gospel music. It's what keeps my spirituality, it's what I believe is keeping me going, my love for the Lord (enthusiastically). It keeps me going. I told the Lord that I never wanted to do anything [other than] his will. [man with AIDS, deceased]*

Goal-oriented concerns. By goals, we refer to setting specific objectives and working toward them. In order to have a goal-oriented perspective that helped them maintain their lifeworld, participants had to have goals that were possible to attain. For some, this required a re-orientation to the limitations imposed by their illness.

> *It's just a big change for me to be so sedentary. I was an <u>extreme</u> traveler. I was traveling <u>all the time</u> to a lot of very interesting and exotic places. So It's been a shift for me to kind of learn how to enjoy being in one spot. [woman with cancer, nondeceased]*

When she could no longer go to far-off places, this participant "traveled" through the cyberworld and connected with people over the Internet and by phone. She stayed abreast of new cancer treatments, belonged to online support groups, and constantly e-mailed friends. She took on the goal of learning as much as she could about treatments for her disease and of maintaining a wide network of friends and fellow cancer patients. In this way, her lifeworld constricted geographically, but it expanded relationally.

> *I am on the Internet a huge amount, looking at new drugs, looking at programs that might be useful to me. I get lots of calls from people who want to be cheered up who have cancer. People will say, "Call J because she is upbeat, she is on top of things." So I get a lot of calls from people who need a cheerleader or need suggestions of what to do next. And then all of my friends calling to see how I am doing.*

Another participant had written a nonfiction book and had it accepted for publication just prior to starting the study. During the study, when it was physically possible for him, he continued to be involved in promoting his book and in writing another.

> **I:** *What are some of the things that keep you going or help you get through the day?*
>
> **P:** *Being involved with projects and that would include writing and the PR end of it. Yeah, I'm involved with a lot of exciting things that have great possibility. [man with AIDS, nondeceased]*

One participant articulated the importance to him of planning and anticipating doing something. His interviews were punctuated by events that he was happily looking forward to or happily remembering how much fun he had. He recognized the emotional benefit to him of having something planned and anticipated.

As long as someone has something to look forward to, they have great medicine. [man with cancer, deceased]

Lifeworld Interrupted

Thirteen participants (8 deceased, 5 nondeceased) did not share any of the central concerns held by the Maintained Lifeworld group. One or more of the following life aspects or disease conditions among these participants appeared to prevent the maintenance of a lifeworld:

- Relocation just before or during the study
- Disease-caused cognitive impairment or pre-existing psychiatric condition
- Commitment to pre-illness goals that were no longer tenable
- Ongoing substance abuse

Relocation. A surprising number of participants (6) in this group moved during or just prior to the study. These were all relocations to another house or apartment. None of the participants moved into a nursing home or hospice. Moving is stressful, even for people in good health. A change in residence for the study participants disrupted life at many levels. The act of moving, if the participant had to be involved in the physical aspect of it, was exhausting. Leaving a familiar household setting, neighborhood, and neighbors was a loss. And even when the move was initially appraised as positive, as the requirements of adjustment to a new setting were encountered, the move came to be viewed as negative.

> **I:** *Tell me a little about your life before you got sick.*
>
> **P:** *I was working at a company down at Orange County. We had a big house [chuckles], a pool, had a lot of friends down there, had a good job. And of course, then we moved up here, because of the hospital situation.*
>
> **I:** *Was it difficult to have to move?*
>
> **P:** *I don't see my friends and that's the difficult thing, not having my friends. I mean, they were really close, close friendships. [woman with cancer, deceased]*

The participant and her husband in the preceding narrative chose to relocate to San Francisco for her medical care. And although they were very happy with her care and liked the city, the rupture in her social fabric was too severe to be repaired.

In one case, the participant did not initiate the move, and the move was emotionally catastrophic. The participant had to move in with his brother following a hospitalization because his elderly mother could no longer care for him in their third-story walk-up apartment. The move was planned and carried out while he was hospitalized and cognitively challenged.

I: *Have you had to make any difficult decisions recently?*

P: *Yeah, difficult decisions about having to move sooner than expected, and I feel that I have been stripped of my decisions of what I want to do. I can't make decisions like I want to or used to or supposed to. I feel like I've just been stripped of everything–stripped of my life. [man with AIDS, deceased]*

Cognitive impairment. One of the unfortunate and not uncommon sequela of cancer and of AIDS is cognitive impairment. Although participants were screened for severe cognitive impairment and dementia, some participants suffered mild cognitive impairment, which affected their ability to understand issues involved with their treatment, to maintain social networks, or do necessary self care. Here are two interview excerpts:

I: *Have you noticed any (more) problems with memory or concentration?*

P: *Some. Like I can't find things, my camera, my watch, can't find . . . my DiscMan. I can't remember things like with medication, my mom and K are helping me with meds. I won't remember when to take it or where it is. [man with AIDS, deceased]*

I: *Have you noticed any problems with memory or concentration?*

P: *I have short-term memory loss.*

I: *And you have trouble finding words, too?*

P: *Yes, I know what I want to say: I just can't get the word out. [woman with cancer, deceased]*

This participant had turned all medical decision-making over to her caregiving husband. She reported that at doctor appointments, she just smiled and nodded and let the words go by her. She knew her husband would follow up as necessary.

Commitment to untenable goals. While pursuing desired goals was a way for some participants to maintain their lifeworld, having untenable goals was a source of unhappiness and inability to find pleasure in the world.

> **I:** *Tell me a little about your life before you got sick.*
>
> **P:** *Overall, I had a life. This makes you feel like you don't have a life.*
>
> **I:** *Tell me, how do you spend your day?*
>
> **P:** *Moping, depressed, trying to get as close to the life I had before I got sick.*
>
> **I:** *What are some of the things that keep you going or help you get through the day?*
>
> **P:** *I have goals I want to complete, things I want to do.*
>
> **I:** *What do you expect in the coming year regarding your health?*
>
> **P:** *A great deal. Self-sufficiency. Get off this payment crap. A healthier body, healthier living. A new life. Not even a new life, but a new life without health problems. [man with AIDS, nondeceased]*

Ongoing substance abuse. Even in physically healthy people, addiction to drugs or alcohol can unravel people's engagement with their lifeworld. The lifeworld of an addict is severely restricted in that the person's primary relationship eventually becomes to the addiction itself. In the case of the participants with addictions, their lifeworlds had been interrupted prior to their diagnoses. Researchers on addiction have proposed that 12-step programs are effective in recovery because they provide clear goals, social interdependence, and spiritual engagement (Miller, 1998; Peteet, 1993). These three aspects match the concerns that we found in the participants who maintained their lifeworld.

LIVING WITH THE WAY IT IS

There is a tendency to view people who live admirable lives in the face of adversity as heroic and courageous. This can lead to a distorted view of what their lives are actually like day to day. It is important to recognize that participants who maintained their lifeworld did so in the face of their declining health and the limitations their illnesses placed upon them, and that they had their ups and downs, just as the rest of the population does. They were not unremittingly cheerful and upbeat, but at times gave vent to anger, frustration, and emotional weariness.

> **I:** *What would make things easier or better for you?*
>
> **P:** *Yes, answer the fatigue problem, get rid of the pain. Well, you know what I'm saying, it's the <u>shits</u>. And on top of that, there's room to get old-fashioned pissed-off every now and then. 'Cause, like a dog howling at the moon, whatever, you just got to let it out, get it out. [man with cancer, deceased]*

Participants also made clear that no matter how positive an attitude one has, or how much one embraces the moment, there remains the daily reality of illness, symptoms, and suffering. There is no "good" way to cope that will make those things go away.

> **I:** *What kinds of problems with regard to your health have you had in the past month? I know you mentioned backaches?*
>
> **P:** *Well, all that stuff is kind of small. It's more the mental emotional stuff that comes with being ill. It's a sense of, "When is this ever going to be done? And am I ever going to get to where it's not the biggest part of my life?" I think I have an incredible attitude, and even <u>I</u> have times when it's just—<u>enough is enough</u>. And I think probably more than physical symptoms—'cause I have kind of learned to just let them come and go 'cause they do. But emotional stuff—it's like you question everything you ever thought was true about life, and you do that on a daily basis. And that can wear on a person (softly). But sometimes it's <u>really</u> positive when you do that, and sometimes it's <u>really</u> exhausting—and you wish you could be ignorant and go back to life before. [woman with cancer, deceased]*

QUANTITATIVE ANALYSIS

The quantitative analysis used measures of symptoms, physical functioning, and assessment of impact of illness on various aspects of life to provide further description of the groups. We compared the Maintained Lifeworld and Lifeworld Interrupted groups on the averaged scores of each participant's responses to the quantitative measures over the course of the study. The number of completed interviews among this sample range from 2 to 15, with a mean of 6.7.

The Maintained Lifeworld and Lifeworld Interrupted groups did not differ by type of disease (AIDS, cancer) or by demographics (see Table 16-2).

Table 16-2 Demographics of Study Participants by Group

	Maintained Lifeworld	Lifeworld Interrupted
Sex		
Male	9	7
Female	10	6
Race		
Black	4	7
Caucasian	15	6
Other	1	0
Disease		
AIDS	8	7
Cancer	11	6
Disposition		
Deceased at end of study	12	8
Not deceased	7	5
Other		
Age	27–73	38–65
Income range	<$15K to >$200K	<$15K to >$200K
Education range (years)	12–20	11–18

The groups also did not differ when compared by disease (AIDS, cancer) or by status (deceased, not deceased before the end of the study) on the following outcomes:

- Somatic Symptoms Checklist
- Activities of Daily Living

- Physical limitations or depressive symptoms (BDI)

They also did not differ on items from the Visual Analog Scale (VAS) asking about energy, pleasure, weariness, will to live, and overall quality of life.

However, the two groups differed significantly on other VAS items. Compared with participants in the Maintained Lifeworld Group, the participants in the Interrupted Lifeworld group were

- More bothered by symptoms [$F(1, 31) = 5.50; p\ .0264$; adjusted $\eta^2 = .13$]
- Had more pain [$F(1, 31) = 13.23, p\ .0011; \eta^2 = .33$]
- Suffered more [$F(1, 31) = 4.38; p\ .0456; \eta^2 = .11$]
- Felt more anxiety [$F(1, 31) = 6.51, p\ .0165; \eta^2 = .17$]
- Felt more worry [$F(1, 31) = 9.45, p\ .0047; \eta^2 = .25$]
- Felt more sadness [$F(1, 31) = 4.65, p\ .0399; \eta^2 = .11$]

We did not correct the alpha level to take into account the number of tests. Our approach is to interpret results only when they exhibit a theoretically meaningful pattern. In the present case, the variables on which the two groups did and did not differ constitute clearly coherent clusters.

DISCUSSION

This study provides important support for the idea that many people in the final phase of life continue to focus on living and remain engaged in the contexts of their lives rather than focusing on life's terminus. One key to this engagement with life is the capacity to maintain a lifeworld. It is notable that a lifeworld orientation was maintained by 19 of 33 (57%) participants in this study. A lifeworld orientation was not a rare exception, but rather the orientation of a majority of participants. Maintenance of lifeworld included continued engagement with family, friends and community; the ability to relinquish untenable goals if necessary, and substitute new, realistic ones; and, for many, engagement in spirituality and a spiritual practice. Those who maintained their lifeworld reported lower scores on how much their symptoms bothered them; the experience of pain, suffering, depressed mood; and illness-related worry and anxiety. Surprisingly, this engagement was not related to physical symptoms, activities of daily living, or physical activity levels. In short, those who maintained their lifeworld were physically compromised by their illness in much the same way as those whose lifeworld was interrupted; but, nonetheless, they still maintained an active engagement in living.

The picture we see of these people who have maintained their lifeworlds, most of whom have been living with terminal illness for years, differs starkly from the picture in which individuals are focused on death, either struggling with the preparation for death or working towards acceptance of death. People who maintain their lifeworlds are not denying the imminence of their deaths: They are simply more focused on the commitments that define their day-to-day living.

The outcome of a positive quality of life in the period just preceding death has been documented elsewhere. In a study of the last months of life for 539 people with congestive heart failure, Levenson, McCarthy, Lynn, Davis, and Phillips (2000) found that while functional status decreased and symptoms increased, the majority of patients reported good to excellent quality of life even in the last month of their lives. (The sample for the study was drawn from the larger Study to Understand Prognoses and Preferences for Outcomes and Risks of Treatments, or SUPPORT.) However, our study demonstrates not only that it is possible to have a good quality of life even in the last days or weeks of life, but we also describe how such positive experiences occur through relational, spiritual, and goal-oriented processes.

Furthermore, the current study illustrates what can interfere with the possibility of positive experiences and the maintenance of lifeworld in the last stage of life. Another study drawn from SUPPORT that examined a sample of 575 people with end-stage liver disease with cirrhosis (Roth et al., 2000) found that in contrast to the Levenson et al. study (2000), most participants rated their quality of life as fair or poor in the last year of life. However, the authors noted that many participants had a prior history of alcohol abuse, and the majority of them also experienced mental confusion in their last months of life. We identified both cognitive impairment and substance abuse as lifeworld interrupters.

There is thoughtful discussion in the literature about dignity and end of life (Chochinov, 2006). One aspect of dignity is to respect people's choices to maintain their lifeworlds by supporting their commitments and their engagement. Our findings could serve to guide formal care providers in their interactions with patients to assist in the continuation—or in the repair, when possible—of the patients' lifeworld. For example, an interesting finding of this study is the association of moving one's residence and having an interrupted lifeworld. Moving is obviously disruptive, and in many cases, it is confounded with cognitive impairment. When individuals with terminal illnesses must move, attention could be given, to the extent possible, to addressing the concerns the move disrupts.

LIMITATIONS

Limitations of the study include small sample size and restricted disease conditions. In addition, because the parent study recruited both patients and their family/friend caregivers for interviews, all the participants in this study had a family or friend caregiver throughout the study. We were not able to assess the effect of having such a caregiver on the participants' maintenance or interruption of their lifeworld.

ACKNOWLEDGEMENTS

We wish to express our gratitude to the participants who so generously shared their life experiences with us. Our goal is to honor their lives and their words. This study was supported by National Institutes of Health grant NR008293.

CONCLUSION

This study supports the notion that our ethical requirement to care for people with terminal illnesses includes a commitment to help them maintain or repair engagement with their lifeworld. Nurses are uniquely positioned to address this need because of their contact with people receiving treatment for serious illnesses, either inpatient or outpatient, and because of their role in hospice care. Nursing education should recognize the importance of the nursing role in assisting terminally ill people to maintain a continuing engagement with their lifeworld.

References

Agre, P., & Horswill, I. (1997). Lifeworld analysis. *Journal of Artificial Intelligence Research*, 6(1), 111-145.

Barry, C. A., Stevenson, F. A., Britten, N., Barber, N., & Bradley, C. P. (2001). Giving voice to the lifeworld. More humane, more effective medical care? A qualitative study of doctor-patient communication in general practice. *Social Science & Medicine*, 53(4), 487.

Beck, A. T., Steer, R. A., Ball, R., & Ranieri, W. (1996). Comparison of Beck Depression Inventories -IA and -II in psychiatric outpatients. *Journal of Personality Assessment*, 67(3), 588-597.

Becker, E. (1973). *The Denial of Death*. New York: Free Press

Benner, P., & Wrubel, J. (1989). *The primacy of caring: Stress and coping in health and illness*. Reading, MA: Addison-Wesley.

Block, S. D. (2001). Psychological considerations, growth, and transcendence at the end of life: The art of the possible. *Journal of the American Medical Association*, 285(22), 2898-2905.

Byock, I. R. (1996). The nature of suffering and the nature of opportunity at the end of life. *Clinics in Geriatric Medicine, 12*(2), 237-252.

Chochinov, H. M. (2006). Dying, dignity, and new horizons in palliative end-of-life care. *CA: A Cancer Journal for Clinicians, 56*(2), 84-103.

Chochinov, H. M., Hack, T., Hassard, T., Kristjanson, L. J., McClement, S., & Harlos, M. (2005). Understanding the will to live in patients nearing death. *Psychosomatics, 46*(1), 7-10.

Chochinov, H. M., Wilson, K. G., Enns, M., & Lander, S. (1997). "Are you depressed?" Screening for depression in the terminally ill. *American Journal of Psychiatry, 154*(5), 674-676.

Clark, D. (2002). Between hope and acceptance: The medicalisation of dying. *BMJ, 324*(7342), 905-907.

Cohen, S. R., & Mount, B. M. (1992). Quality of life in terminal illness: defining and measuring subjective well-being in the dying. *Journal of Palliative Care, 8*(3), 40-45.

Cohen, S. R., Mount, B. M., Tomas, J. J. N., & Mount, L. F. (1996). Existential well-being is an important determinant of quality of life: Evidence from the McGill quality of life questionnaire. *Cancer, 77*(3), 576-586.

Conrad, P. (1990). Qualitative research on chronic illness: A commentary on method and conceptual development. *Social Science & Medicine, 30*(11), 1257-1263.

Field, M. J., & Cassel, C. K. (1997). *Approaching death: Improving care at the end of life.* Washington, DC: National Academies Press.

Frankl, V. E. (1963). *Man's search for meaning.* New York: Washington Square Press, Simon & Schuster.

Friel, P. B. (1982). Death and dying. *Annals of Internal Medicine, 97*(5), 767-771.

Hyden, L.-C. (1997). Illness and narrative. *Sociology of Health and Illness, 19*(1), 48-69.

Katz, S., Ford, A. B., Moskowitz, R. W., Jackson, B. A., & Jaffe, M. W. (1963). Studies of illness in the aged. The index of ADL: A standardized measure of biological and psychosocial function. *Journal of the American Medical Association, 185,* 914-919.

Kleinman, A., Eisenberg, L., & Good, B. (1978). Culture, illness, and care: Clinical lessons from anthropologic and cross-cultural research. *Annals of Internal Medicine, 88*(2), 251-258.

Kubler-Ross, E. (1973). *On death and dying.* New York: Routledge.

Lawton, M. P., & Brody, E. M. (1969). Assessment of older people: Self-maintaining and instrumental activities of daily living. *Gerontologist, 9,* 179-186.

Levenson, J., McCarthy, E., Lynn, J., Davis, R., & Phillips, R. (2000). The last six months of life for patients with congestive heart failure. *Journal of the American Geriatrics Society, 48*(5).

Lo, B., Ruston, D., Kates, L. W., Arnold, R. M., Cohen, C. B., Faber-Langendoen, K., et al. (2002). Discussing religious and spiritual issues at the end of life: A practical guide for physicians. *Journal of the American Medical Association, 287*(6), 749-754.

Lo, R. S. K., Woo, J., Zhoc, K. C. H., Li, C. Y. P., Yeo, W., Johnson, P., et al. (2002). Quality of life of palliative care patients in the last two weeks of life. *Journal of Pain and Symptom Management, 24*(4), 388-397.

Lock, M. (1996). Death in technological times: Locating the end of meaningful life. *Medical Anthropology Quarterly, 10*(4), 575-600.

MacQueen, K. M., McLellan, E., Kay, K., & Milstein, B. (1998). Codebook development for team-based qualitative analysis. *Cultural Anthropology Methods, 10*(2), 31-36.

Miller, W. R. (1998). Researching the spiritual dimensions of alcohol and other drug problems. *Addiction, 93*(7), 979-990.

Nakashima, M., & Canda, E. R. (2005). Positive dying and resiliency in later life: A qualitative study. *Journal of Aging Studies, 19*(1), 109-125.

NIH (2004). National Institutes of Health State-of-the-Science Conference Statement on Improving End-of-Life Care. http://consensus.nih.gov/2004/2004EndOfLifeCareSOS024html.htm

Oakes-Greenspan, M. (2007). Running toward: Reframing possibility and finitude through physician's stories at the end of life. Unpublished doctoral dissertation, University of California, San Francisco.

Peteet, J. R. (1993). A closer look at the role of a spiritual approach in addictions treatment. *Journal of Substance Abuse Treatment, 10*(3), 263.

Rabkin, J. G., Albert, S. M., Del Bene, M. L., O'Sullivan, I., Tider, T., Rowland, L. P., et al. (2005). Prevalence of depressive disorders and change over time in late-stage ALS. *Neurology, 65*(1), 62-67.

Roth, K., Lynn, J., Zhong, Z., Borum, M., & Dawson, N. (2000). Dying with end stage liver disease with cirrhosis: insights from SUPPORT. *Journal of the American Geriatrics Society, 48*(5).

Russell, S. (2008, March 22). Researcher with ALS finds solace with expertise. *San Francisco Chronicle*, p. 1A.

Ryan, G. W., & Bernard, H. R. (2003). Techniques to identify themes. *Field Methods, 15*(1), 85-109.

Spitzer, R. L., Kroenke, K., & Williams, J. B. (1999). Validation and utility of a self-report version of PRIME-MD: The PHQ primary care study. Primary care evaluation of mental disorders. Patient health questionnaire. *Journal of the American Medical Association, 282*(18), 1737-1744.

Spitzer, R. L., Williams, J. B. W., Kroenke, K., & Linzer, M. (1994). Utility of a new procedure for diagnosing mental disorders in primary care: The PRIME-MD 1000 study. *Journal of the American Medical Association, 272*(22), 1749-1756.

Steer, R. A., Cavalieri, T. A., Leonard, D. M., & Beck, A. T. (1999). Use of the Beck Depression Inventory for Primary Care to screen for major depression disorders. *General Hospital Psychiatry, 21*(2), 106-111.

Steinhauser, K. E., Christakis, N. A., Clipp, E. C., McNeilly, M., McIntyre, L., & Tulsky, J. A. (2000). Factors considered important at the end of life by patients, family, physicians, and other care providers. *Journal of the American Medical Association, 284*(19), 2476-2482.

Stewart, A. L., Teno, J., Patrick, D. L., & Lynn, J. (1999). The concept of quality of life of dying persons in the context of health care. *Journal of Pain and Symptom Management, 17*(2), 93-108.

Wuthow, R. (1998). *After heaven: Spirituality in America since the 1950's.* Berkeley, CA: University of California Press.

Zimmermann, C. (2004). Denial of impending death: A discourse analysis of the palliative care literature. *Social Science & Medicine, 59*(8), 1769.

Zimmermann, C. (2007). Death denial: obstacle or instrument for palliative care? An analysis of clinical literature. *Sociology of Health & Illness, 29*(2), 297-314.

Footnote

[1] The period of time known as end of life has become of increasing interest to both biomedical and social science researchers over past decades. Social scientists and some sectors of the biomedical world have to attempted an exploration of the best ways to support people at the end of life. An initial obstacle to achieving this goal has been differences about what constitutes end of life. A National Institutes of Health State-of-the-Science conference statement on improving end-of-life care (NIH, 2004, section 1, ¶1) issued the consensus that "the evidence does not support a precise definition of the interval referred to as end of life or its transitions."

INDEX

A

acceptors, 130
adolescents with spina bifida, 253–254
adversarial caregiving (teen mothers), 227–228
age of possibilities, 29
aging, humanity and, xxviii–xxix
aging experience, 288
    Ann, 289–296
        connection with others, 290
        creative unconscious, 292
        curiosity of, 291
        future, 294–295
        involvement, 293
        pleasurable activities, 290
        possibilities rather than obstacles, 291
        preparing for physical decline, 292
        relationships, 293–294, 308
        seizing opportunities, 292
        studies, 290
        wakefulness, 292
        youthful risk taking, 291
    being in the world and, 308–309
    David, 296
        desire for interconnectedness, 299
        entering the world, 306
        existential suffering, 297
        feelings of alienation, 300
        losses, 301
        others' recognition of distress, 300
        painting, 302–304
        participation after move, 299
        realization of limits, 305–306
        stroke effects, 297
        stroke's effects on painting, 303–304
    debility, 289
    elders as autonomous agents, 295
    existential suffering, 297
    experiences in youth, 291
    future, 294–295
    gender, 308–309
    involvement, 293
    limits, adapting to, 289
    physical decline, planning for, 292
    relationships, 293–294
    wakefulness, 292
agnostics in religious metaphor xxviii, 273–276
AIDS, xxviii
    caring and, 261
    co-factors, 283
    holistic approach, 282
    patients responses to, 261
alternative therapies, HIV-positive patients, 269

Alzheimer's, 17
American Academy of Pediatrics, 147
ANA (American Nurses Association), model definition of nursing practice, 147
APNs (advanced practice nurses), 148
Aristotelian tradition *versus* Platonic, 120
Aristotle, 93
   virtuous mean, 284–285
asymptomatic HIV infection, 273
atomistic individualism, xxi
attending to situation, 169
authentic care, 243
AZT in HIV treatment, 280–281

meanings of, 35
new students, xxii
Other and, 38
physical, xxi
social, xxi
Sri Lankan woman, 33–34
technology and, 34–36
bodily changes, world and, 59
bodily self, 245
body. *See also* lived body
   as universal existential dwelling place, 306
body schema (PD patients), 63
Bradyphrenia (PD), 65
British Empiricism, 128
burnout, stress an, 172

B

back rubs, 47
background
   cultural, 102
   emotions, 127
   general, 102
   individual, 102
   meanings, 25
balance within self, 172
basal ganglia, PD and, 66
Beck Depression Inventory, 341–342
bed bath, 47
bedside nursing, 25
Being-in-the-World, 28
Being-With, 28, 41
believers, xxviii
   religious metaphor, State Church, 269–272
Benner, Patricia, 3
biomedical industry, 262
biomedicine, metaphor of war, 262
birth
   Hispanic couple, 31–32

C

California AB 394 (nurse-patient ratios), 58
care
   ethics, 27
   partners, 47
   phenomenon of, 243–244
   relationship and, 170–171
care of others, interrelatedness with self-care, 170–171, 179–180
caring
   human beings, 4
   meaning and purpose and, 169
   practice and, 4, 169
   quiet knowing and, 182
   as things mattering, 28
caring practices
   how to study, 14–16
   possibility for health care and, xxi
   in postmodern, 38–39
   reasons to study, 13–14
   vulnerability in institutions, 9–11
Carnegie Foundation study, 147

Cartesian epistemology, IP overcoming, 116
Cartesian interpretation of human beings, xvii
Cartesian Medicine, xx
Cartesian science and epistemology, 114
categorization through generalization, xxxi
cerebral cortex, PD and, 66
chart notes
    historical forms, 48
    narrative proximity and, 48
    SOAP, 48
    structure, 48
Chassy, 123–124
chess in debate over AI and expert systems, 126
circadian rhythms, SAD and, 82
classification systems, 75
clearings, 30–34
    opening up to students, 37
clinical concrete cases, 25–26
clinical empathy, 106
clinical encounter components, 154
clinical forethought, 97
clinical grasp, 97
clinical imagination, forming, xxii
clinical judgment, xxix
clinical perception, 151
clinicians
    development of certainty, 94
    expert, abilities, 98
    moral distress, 107–108
CNSs (clinical nurse specialists), 146
    Consulting Role of the Nurse, 157
co-workers, connectedness with, 180–182
cognitive decline of PD patients, 65
cognitive impairment of terminally ill patients, 350–351
cognitivism *versus* Dreyfus Model of Skill Acquisition, 124
collaboration with patients, 149

coming to terms with illness, 130
communications
    families of terminally ill patients, 315
    relevance for care providers, 315
communities of practice, 27
community, 25
    spina bifida and, 254
community service of terminally ill patients, 346
comparative analysis of practice situations, 156–158
competence, 121–122
complementary therapies
    HIV-positive patients, 269
    language, 133
comportment, 96–97
connections
    to co-workers, 180–182
    nurses and, 87
    with others, 182
    postmodern human being, 29
    to self, 180–182
    shared humanity and, 88
consciousness, projection into physical world, 69
Consulting Role of the Nurse, 157
consumption of services, 52–53
context, 169
context-bound lifeworlds, xix
continuity of care, NPs, 156–159
coping as restoration of meaning, 81
cost-and-effect, 329
courage in terminally ill patients, 352
creative unconscious, 292
cultural background, 102
cultural epoch, 28–29
cultures
    as connection source, 88
    nature and, 82
    styles, 29
curing *versus* healing, 149
curiosity of humans, xvii

D

Dasein (human being), 288
death
    denial, 338
    in ED, 104
    ED patient's certainty of, 106
    as falling asleep forever, 324
    medicalization of dying, 338
    as part of life, 107
decade of the brain (1990s), 87
degrading interventions, 331
depression. *See also* SAD (Seasonal Affective Disorder)
    Beck Depression Inventory, 341–342
    as source of life's richness, 76
Descartes, xvii
details about patients, 50
device paradigm, 197
diagnoses
    deficit view of persons and, 75
    disconnection of individuals and, 75
    ordinary life becoming, 76, 82
dialogue between nurse and patient, back rub and, 47
dinnertime as family gathering practice, 200–201
    Brannon family, 202–207
    Brown family, 210–214
    description, 201
    dis-comforting, 211–212
    as disengaged activity, 210–214
    inclusiveness, 205–206
    invisible work involved, 202
    marginalization, 201
    occasional practice, 208
    restaurant eating, 208
    as source of conflict, 207
    Switzer family, 207–210
    teenagers and, 203
    TV during dinner, 203–204, 211
disability and self, 245
disabled students
    adolescence, 252
    dating rituals, 252
    mainstreaming of, 249–251
    wheelchair and isolation, 252
disaster survivors, 78
discharge, available beds and, 29
disease
    existential and biological terms, 59
    versus illness, 338
disorders, normality as, 80
distal nursing, xxii
    dangers, 49–52
    versus proximal, 51–52
distance from family, retreat and, 185–187
distractions, self-care and, 184–185
distrust of professional authority, 268
dividing practices, 53
doctor-priest, distrust of, 268
doctoring a drink, 148
Domains and Core Competencies of NP practice, 150
Domains of Skill and Practice of Nurse Practitioners, xxv
double standard between physicians and nurses, 148
Dreyfus Model of Skill Acquisition, 119
    versus cognitivism, 124
    expertise, embodiment, 120
drinks, doctoring *versus* nursing, 148
Dunne, Joseph, xxi
dwelling in the world, 288
    artistic creativity, 288
    body as dwelling place, 306
    existential skills of, 310–311
    scientific discovery, 288
    skills of, 288

E

eating practices, 6
ecumenists in religious metaphor, xxviii, 277–281
ED (emergency department), 91
   death in, 104
   end-of-life care and, 92
   family of patients, 105
   as microculture, 104
   patients
      backgrounds, 105
      certainty of death, 106
   physical proximity, 107
   as place of transition, 105
embedded thinking, engaged reasoning, 125
embodied habitus, 5
embodied intelligence, 120
   intuition, 121
embodied practices, 5
embodied sensations, self-care and, 188
embodiment, 94
   expertise (Dreyfus model), 120
emergency workers, stress and, 81
emotional attunement, 121
   RHP (reflective healing practice), 173
emotions
   background, 127
   perception and, 127
   primary, 127
   rationality and, 127
   self-care retreat, 190
empathy, 37
   clinical empathy, 106
empiricism, xviii, xxxi
   British Empiricism, 128
emplacement, 46
end-of-life care, xxiv, xxix
   as core value, 92
   ED and, 92
   as label, 337
   versus palliative care, 314
   philosophical approach, 92
end-of-life social science research, 337
end of living, 343
ending life of patient, 50
engaged care, 87
engaged reasoning as embedded thinking, 125
engagement, 37
English's critique of Benner, 122
environment, understanding through getting away, 183
environmental influences on motility, 67
epistemological approach to personhood, xvii
epoch, 28–29
ethical blindness, 10
ethics, 27
existential skills of dwelling, 310–311
experience-near narratives, 115
experiences
   assigning meaning, 69
   background meanings, 25
   history of person and, 94
   illness, 69
   intermediate area of, 307
   interpretation and, 95
   lived, xix
   perceptions that are open dialectical, 94
   phronesis and, 94–95, 96
   phronetic knowledge and, 94
experiential learning, 37
expert, situated, 119
expertise
   Dreyfus model of skill acquisition, 119
      embodiment, 120
   interpretations of *(FNE)*, 118–120
   Template Theory (TempT), 124
expressive individualism, xxi
external goods, 7–8, 26–27

F

failure discourse, teen motherhood, xxvii
families
    experience with dying, 108
    focal practices, 31–32
    focus change from patient to, 10
    of patients in ED, 105
    routines and rituals, 195
    treatments delegated to, 10
family
    identity, 196
    legacy, 195
    rituals, xxvi
        family's world, 196
    routines, 196–197
        teenagers and, 197, 203
    solidarity, 196
    as undifferentiated oneness, 196
family practices, 197
    dinnertime, 200–201
        Brannon family, 202–207
        Brown family, 210–214
        description, 201
        dis-comforting, 211–212
        as disengaged activity, 210–214
        inclusiveness, 205–206
        invisible work involved, 202
        marginalization, 201
        occasional practice, 208
        restaurant eating, 208
        as source of conflict, 207
        teenagers and, 203
        TV during dinner, 203–204, 211
    focal practice, 197
    health concerns, 198
    recognition practices, 197–198
    Switzer family, 207–210
family's world, rituals, 196
feelings, *POC* (Benner & Wrubel), 132
first-person experience accounts, 115
flexible response to significance of situation, 125

Flexner's report, 147
FNPs (family nurse practitioners), 158. *See also* NP (nurse practitioner)
focal practices, 4, 31
    birth, Other and, 38
    centering force, 37
    families, 197
    family, 31–32
    technology and, 37
focus, hearth and, 31
formulating problems, 13–14
FPs (family physicians), 158
freedom
    radical freedom, 99
    situated freedom, 99
From Novice to Expert (Benner), 114–115
    Cash's critique, 122
    competence, 121–122
    English's critique, 122
    expertise, 118–120
    intuition, 121
    reception by nursing community, 117–118
    skill and, 118–119
Frontier Nursing Service, 146
fusion of horizons, 23, 37
fuzzy resemblances, 172

G

gender, aging experience and, 308–309
gendered spatiality, 43
general background, 102
gestalt of situation, 121
goal-oriented concerns of terminally ill patients, 348–349
goals of terminally ill patients, 351
Gobet, 123–124
God's-eye view, 24
grasp of clinical situation, 125–126

grip of technology, 30
group retreat benefits, 183
gut feelings, 121

H

habits, participation in life and, 288
habitus, 60
    practice as, 5
healing begins with listening, 159
healing relationship, establishing, 160
healing *versus* curing, 149
health
    relationships and, 171
    stress and, 172
health care system, orientation to, 260
health-care *versus* person-care, 10
health professional education, 163
hearth, focus and, 31
heretics in religious metaphor, 263–269, xxviii
hermeneutics, 3
heroism in terminally ill patients, 352
HHP (Heideggerian hermeneutic phenomenology), 113–114
history of IP, xxiv–xxv
HIV (human immunodeficiency virus), 259
    asymptomatic HIV-positive gay men and competing therapies, 277
    asymptomatic infection, 273
        beliefs about, 283
    holistic attitudes, 266
    individual lives and, 262
    metaphors of war and religion, 262
    T cells, 265–266
HIV study, religious metaphor, 260
holism, HIV-positive patients, 269

holistic care, 149
    AIDS and, 282
    HIV-positive patients, 266
home, leaving and entering the unfamiliar, 42
hope, 160
Horrocks, 134
    Heidegger and, 135
hospital as archetypal institution, 262
hospital nurses, shortage, 53
hospital nursing, spatial-structural practices, 42
human, as habitus, 60
human beings
    caring, 4
    Dasein, 288
    dwelling in the world, 288
    inhabiting the world, 288
    meaning and, 25
    as placeholders, 29
    as resource, 29
    as self-interpreting, 288
    as standing reserve, 29
human experience, pathogenic paradigm and, 79
humanity, old age, xxviii–xxix

I

IDEA (Individuals with Disabilities Education Act), 249
identity, family, 196
illness
    coming to terms with, 130
    versus disease, 338
    experience of, 69
    Western meanings, 129
importance of place, 169–170
impressions
    from a place, 60

stored, 60
individual background, 102
individualism
    atomistic, xxi
    expressive, xxi
inhabiting the world, 288
insider perspective, 338
intelligence, embodied, 120
intentional arc, 91, 92, 99–100, 125
intentionality, 26, 133
intermediate area of experience, 307
internal goods, 8, 26–27
interpersonal relationship skills, 160
interpretations
    of expertise *(FNE)*, 118–120
    leaning and, 25
interpretive phenomenology. *See* IP (interpretive phenomenology)
interventions as degrading, 331
interviews
    medical, functions, 161
    practices, 18–19
    small group, 115
intuition, *FNE*, 121
invisibility of nursing, 8
IOM (Institute of Medicine), 92
IP (interpretive phenomenology), xvii
    evolution, 117
    introduction, 114
    narratives and, 114
    and NP practice, 145
    origins, 113
    philosophical discourses and debates, xx
    research development, 114–117
    studies, research practices, 115
    theoretical discourses and debates, xx

K

Katz ADL (Katz Index of Activities of Daily Living), 342
knowledge
    iterativeness, 95
    wisdom and, 97

L

Lawton Instrumental Activities of Daily Living, 342
legacy, family legacy. *See* family legacy
life
    death as part of, 107
    meaning in, 339
    participation in through habits, routines, and practices, 288
    understanding backward, 97
lifeworld, 337
    definition, 339
    terminally ill patients, 339
        interrupted, 349–351
        maintained, 344–349, 354
lived body
    as intertwining of intentionality and materiality, 59
    situation as an orientation in space, 64
living relationship with self, 69
logic, practice and, 11
Lord, Loretta, 148

M

mainstreaming of youth with disabilities, 249–251
    cruelty of other children, 251
    recess experience, 250

maintained lifeworld, 344–349
maximum grip, 91, 92, 100–104
mealtime rituals, 195
meaning
   caring and, 169
   humans and, 25
   of practice, 25–27
medical interview, functions of, 161
medical science humanistic approach to human problems, 267
medicalization of dying, 338
medicine
   boundaries between nursing, 147
   nursing overlap, 148
meditation, 171–172, 175
mental illness, xxiii
mentalism, 131
   definition, 132
   pure mentalism, 133
metaphysics, 28
midlife, disruptions, 287
mind-body-world relationships, 132
mobility of PD patients, improving, 66
model definition of nursing practice, 147
modesty, 27
monological observers, xxi
moral distress, 107–108
moral perception, 151
moral proximity, 44, 45
   disruption of, 49
mothers. *See* teen mothers
motility, environmental influences and, 67

N

narrative proximity, 44, 57
   chart notes and, 48
   physical proximity necessity, 48
narratives
   experience-near, 115
   IP approach and, 114
   Kierkegaard and, 115
National Organization of Nurse Practitioner Faculties (NONPF), 150
nature
   to be out of sync with, 82
   culture and, 82
nested proximities, 43
neurological determinism, 87
Nightingale, Florence, on observation and experience, 87–88
NIH (National Institutes of Health), 92
NONPF (National Organization of Nurse Practitioner Faculties), 150
normality as disordered, 80
normalizing discourses, xix
Norwegians
   darktime experience, 82–83
   respect for nature, 82
NP (nurse practitioner), xxv. *See also* FNPs (family nurse practitioners)
   agenda, 155
   collaboration, 155
   continuity of care, 156–159
   division of programs, 153
   Domains and Core Competencies of NP practice, 150
   Domains of Skill and Practice of Nurse Practitioners, xxv
   education, 162
   hope, 160
   interpersonal relationship skills, 160
   as junior doctor, 147, 162
   as junior doctors, 154
   partnering with patient, 155
   patient involvement, promotion, 161
   patients' life experiences and, 155–156
   personalized interventions, 156
   physical exam, 156
   practice, 145
      collaborative, 161–162
      historical practice, 146
      holistic, 161–162

nature of, 146–150
    patient-centered, 161–162
  as primary care provider, 150
  reclaiming nursing practice, 147
  as sounding boards, 155–156
  teachable moments, 156
nuns compared to nurses, 284
nurse practitioner. *See* NP (nurse practitioner)
nurses
  APNs (advanced practice nurses), 148
  as apologists, 284
  comparison to nuns, 284
  decline in, 57
  double standard with physicians, 148
  as evangelists, 284
  human connections and, 87
  meaning in practice, 8
  as overseers, 47
  philosophical issues, 135
  as role models, 178–179
  as technicians, 50
nursing
  boundaries between medicine, 147
  hospital, spatial-structural practices, 42
  as interdisciplinary, 149
  invisibility, 8
  medicine overlap, 148
  nature as timeless and enduring, 148
  paradigms of study and practice, 77
  spatial aspects, 42
nursing a drink, 148
nursing advocacy, 149
nursing community, *FNE* and, 117–118
nursing education, taken-for-granted skills, 25
Nursing Philosophy, 135
nursing practice
  central aspects, 153
  limiting of scope, 147
  model definition by ANA, 147
  RHP (reflective healing practices) similarities, 172–173
  structure's undermining of self-care opportunities, 171

O

observing, practices, 16–17
ontological questions of understanding human, xvii
optimal grasp, xxiv
ordinary life becoming a diagnosis (depression), 76, 82
organistic technology, 30
orientation in space, 67
  lived body and, 64
Other, 28
  authentic care of, 243
  focal practice of birth, 38
  moral proximity, 45
outsider perspective, 338

P

Paley, John, 128
  psycho-somatic illness, 128–129
palliative care
  disease-modifying therapies and, 314
  versus end-of-life care, 314
  Switzerland, 316
paradigms of study and practice of nursing, 77. *See also* pathogenic paradigm; salutogenic paradigm
Parkinson's disease. *See* PD (Parkinson's disease)
particularistic attitude, 58
particularity, 57
pathogenesis, 77
pathogenic paradigm
  human experience and, 79
  objective data, 77

pathologizing of facts of life, 86
patient involvement, promotion, 161
patients
    disengagement from, 51
    distinctions among, 51
    ED, backgrounds, 105
    experience with dying, 108
    focus change to families, 10
    as instances of a category, 50
    nurses ending life, 50
    orientation to powerful structures in society, 262
    remembering details about, 50
    terminally ill (*See* terminally ill patients)
PD (Parkinson's disease), 59, xxiii
    body schema, 63
    cognitive decline, 65
    experience because of changing capabilities, 61–70
    external sensory information to initiate movement, 66
    focus, changing, 62
    gait, 65
    immobility situations, 62
    intentional being, 63
    living and experiencing, 68
    mobility, improving, 66
    movements, requirements, 61
    objective signs of, 68
    physical symptoms, 65
    rhythm and, 62
    space, 63–64
    unpredictable motility, 64
perceiving and orienting to situations, 27
perceptions
    emotions and, 127
    schizophrenia, 84
person as thrown into the world, 219
person-care *versus* health-care, 10
personhood, epistemological approach to, xvii
perspective, gaining, 183–184

PHN (public health nursing), begin with people as they are..., 219
PHQ (Patient Health Questionnaire), 342
phronesis, xxix, 9, 91, 93
    end-of-life care, 92
    experiences and, 94–95, 96
    perceptiveness (nous) and, 96
    self-correcting experience, 95
    ultimate particulars (eschaton) and, 96
    virtue and, 95
phronetic knowledge
    experience and, 94
    refinement of, 106–107
phronimoi, 96
physical birth, xxi
physical contact, time available, 47
physical proximity, 44
    ED and, 107
    as livable relation with body, 44
    necessity for narrative proximity, 48
physical world, consciousness, 69
physician assistants, xxv
physicians
    double standard with nurses, 148
    false belief of superiority of care, 148
place
    grasping, 43
    importance of, 169–170
    impressions from, 60
    ontological meaning of, 60
    ontological primacy of, 43
    relationship to lived experience, 60
    space and, 43
    as thirdspace, 60
    world as, 60
placeholders, persons as, 29
Platonic tradition, *versus* Aristotelian, 120
possibility, trust and, 170
power, 43
    dynamics, 52–53
practical belief as state of the body, 5

practical knowledge, theoretical knowledge and, 152
practical reasoning, nature of situation and, 125
practice
  caring and, 4, 169
    as cluster of patterned and interrelated ways of being, 25
  communities of, 27
  connections, 6
  definition, 4
  eating practices, 6
  embodied practices, 5
  excluding attention to itself, 12
  external goods, 7–8
  focal practices, 4, 31
  generations and, 5
  as habitus, 5
  internal goods, 8
  logic and, 11
  as mechanical reaction, 5
  nurses' meaning in, 8
  purpose of, 4
  teleological nature of, 4
practice of nursing *versus* accomplishing tasks, 27
practice professions, beginners in, 7
practices. *See also* family practices
  being and, 26
  development of, 26
  dividing, 53
  interviews, 18–19
  learned, 7
  meanings of, 25–27
  observing, 16–17
  participation in life and, 288
  as social embedded human actions, 26
  text interpretation, 19–21
praxis, 91, 93
  end-of-life care, 92
  unreflectiveness, 93
presencing, 87
primary care provider, NP as, 150

primary emotions, 127
primordial familiarity with world, 28
problem formulation, 13–14
protocols, 9
proximal nursing, spatial resistance, 53
proximal nursing *versus* distal, 51–52
proximities, 42
  among nurses, 47
  back rubs, 47
  moral, 44, 45
  narrative, 44, 57
  nested, 42, 43
  physical, 44
  structural spatial changes affecting, 46–49
proximity
  reduction, 47
  temporal nearness, 47
  temporary staff and, 47
  and time, 46
psychiatric labels, effects of, 84
psychiatry as drive-through practice, 87
psycho-somatic illness, 128–129
psychologizing culture, xxiv
PTSD (Post-Traumatic Stress Disorder), 75, xxiii
  comparing self against checklist, 81
  debut, 80
  emergency workers, 81
  trauma as outside objective agent, 81
purpose, caring and, 169

Q

quadriplegic African-American man, 45–46
quality of life
  palliative care and, 314
  physical domain over emphasis, 338
  terminally ill patients, 319–320

R

radical freedom, 99
rationalist inquiry, xviii
rationality, emotions and, 127
reasoning, snapshot, 116
reasoning from particulars rather than abstract principles, 57
recognition, lack of, 10
recognition practices, families, 197–198
reductionistic science, 77
reflection, darktime for, 83
Reiki, 171–172, 174
relational concerns of terminally ill patients, 345–346
relationship, xxi
    aging experience, 293–294
    burnout cure, 171
    care and, 170–171
    health and, 171
    with self, 170–171
    spatial aspects, 42
religious metaphors, 260
    agnostics, 263, 273–276
    believers, 262
    State Church and, 269–272
    ecumenists, 277–281
    heretics, 263–269
reordering, 30
representational spaces, 53
representations of space, 53
rescuers, xxiii
research practices, 115
RHP (reflective healing practices), 170
    attunement, 173
    enhancing coping, 173
    as self-care, 171–172
    similarities to nursing practice, 172–173
role models, nurses as, 178–179
routines, participation in life and, 288
routines and rituals. *See* families' routines and rituals

S

SAD (Seasonal Affective Disorder), xxiii, 75
    circadian rhythms, 82
    dangers of diagnosis, 83–84
    definition, 82
    drivers of treatment, 83
    Norway's changes, 83
    reflection time, 83
    symptoms, 82
salutogenesis, 77
    positivity, 78
salutogenic paradigm, 77–78
sameness, xxi
schizophrenia, 75
    other people's interference with life of sufferer, 85
    perceptions and, 84
    psychiatric labels and their effects, 84
    psychiatric paradigm and, 76
    reconnection, importance of, 85
    separation from self and world, 85
scientific pluralism, xxiv
Seasonal Affective Disorder. *See* SAD (Seasonal Affective Disorder)
self, 60
    bodily self, 245
    connectedness with, 180–182
    disability and, 245
    living relationship with, 69
    relationship with, 170–171
    understanding of, xviii
self-care, xxv
    balance, 172
    decision to incorporate, 188–190
    distractions and, 184–185
    embodied sensations, 188

interrelatedness with other-care, 170–171, 179–180
nurses as role models, 178–179
quiet knowing, 182
retreat
   distance from family, 185–187
   emotions, 190
   journal keeping, 175–177
   options, 174–175
   perspective, gaining, 183–184
   results, 178
   setting, 185–187
RHP (reflective healing practices) as, 171–172
selfishness, 169
undermining of opportunities for, 171
self-focus, 182
self-reflection, 12
self-understanding, 182
   possibilities for meaning, 308
service partners, 47
SES (socioeconomic status), 221
setting of retreat, importance of, 185–187
shared disclosive spaces, 116
shortage of nurses, hospital, 53
situated freedom, 99
situated lifeworlds, xix
situated possibility, 246
situatedness, 245
situation, attending to, 169
skill
   Dreyfus Model of Skill Acquisition, 119, 127
   embodied, intuition, 121
   FNE and, 118–119
   iterativeness, 95
skill acquisition, 97
skilled know-how, 96–97
skillful coping, 102
skills, improving, 102
small group interviews, 115
snap-shot reasoning, 116

SOAP (subjective, objective, assessment, plan), 48
social birth, xxi
social discontinuities, xxviii
social situation, 116
socioeconomic status (SES), 221
solicitation, 125
solicitude, 28
solidarity, family, 196
space
   neutrality, 43
   orientation in, 67
      lived body in, 64
   passivity, 43
   PD patients, 63–64
   representations of, 53
   shared disclosive spaces, 116
space and place in philosophy, 42–43
spaces, representational, 53
spatial aspects of human relationships, 42
spatial aspects of nursing, 42
spatial resistance, proximal nursing as, 53
spatial-structural change in NP practice, 154
spatial-structural power dynamics, 52–53
spatial-structural practices of hospital nursing, 42
spatial vulnerabilities, 43
spatiality, gendered, 43
spina bifida, xxvii
   adolescents, 253–254
   biopsychosocial possibility and, 244–245
   bullying of youth, 254
   community, 254
   dating rituals among youth, 252
   description, 244
   interpretive approach to study, 246
   mainstreaming of youth, 249–251
      cruelty of other children, 251
      recess experience, 250
   relationships, 253–254

social interactions of students, 253–254
social marginalization, 249
    isolation, 253
socialization of youth, 249
stigma, 253
study
    analysis, 247–248
    data collection, 247
    findings, 249–253
    interview categories, 248
    sample, 246–247
victimization of youth, 254
wheelchair and isolation, 252
spiritual concerns of terminally ill
    patients, 347
standing reserve, 29
stress
    burnout and, 172
    definition, 81
    emergency workers, 81
    health and, 172
    work as, 81
stress-distancing techniques, 81
structural spatial changes affecting
    proximities, 46–49
studies, research practices, 115
style, personal, history and psychological
    structure, 98
styles of a culture, 29
substance abuse among terminally ill
    patients, 351
substantia nigra, PD and, 66
subthalamic nucleus, PD and, 66
suffering, Western meanings, 129
superiority of physician care, false belief
    of, 148
Swiss healthcare system, 316
symptoms
    insufficient control, 331
    managing in terminally ill patients,
        322–324
    reduction or elimination, 87

T

T cells, HIV and, 265–266
tai chi, 171–172, 175
taken-for-granted skills, 25
teachable moments (NPs), 156
technological paradigm, 197
technological understanding of being, 29
technology
    birth and, 34–36
    focal things and, 37
    grip of, 30
    organistic, 30
teen mothering
    contributing to despair, 225
    Coping Interview, 221
    as critical turning point, 235
    Family Routines Interview, 221
    future, creating, 234
    insistence of no change, 230
    moral compass and, 224
    physical violence, 230–231
    risks of, family's concerns about, 219
    rite of passage to adulthood, 218–219
    as social-technical problem, 218
    as syndrome, 218
    withdrawal of grandparents, 234
teen mothers, xxvi–xxvii
    13-year-old, 236
    children's paths, 234–235
    as diamonds in the rough, 236
    emotional responsiveness to baby, 226
    emulation of parents, 229
    family caregiving legacies, 229–233
    family relationships, 227–228
    future stops dead at adolescence, 225
    grandparents
        adversarial caregiving, 227–228
        over-involvement by grandparents,
            228
        responsive caregiving, 228

inheriting a diminished future, 225–227
Jenna, 229–230
LaKeisha, 224
    aunts' impact, 232–233
    cookie baking, 232
Maya, 230
Meg, 230–231
memories of female kin, 232
new aspirations, 224
new standards, 224
opinions of child's attitude, 231
passivity, 226
repeating the past, 231
risking future, 218, 226
Tamika, 225–226
therapists and, 233
third group, 227
welfare, 224
teen pregnancy as syndrome, xxvii
teenage childbearing, increase in focus on, 218
teenagers, family routines and, 197, 203
Template Theory (TempT) of expertise, 124
temporal determinateness, 38
temporary staff, 47
terminally ill patients
  admittance to nursing home, 329
  assumption that life has ended, 343
  care activities, positive/negative interventions, 325–327
  cognitive impairment, 350–351
  community service, 346
  courage, 352
  death as falling asleep forever, 324
  depression, Beck Depression Inventory, 341–342
  family
    dignity of patient, 315
    expectations, 315
    unsatisfactory interactions with care givers, 325
  goal-oriented concerns, 348–349
  heroism, 352
  interventions as degrading, 331
  Katz ADL (Katz Index of Activities of Daily Living), 342
  Lawton Instrumental Activities of Daily Living, 342
  lifeworld and, 339
    interrupted, 349–351
    maintained, 344–349, 354
  medical procedures, positive and adverse, 320–322
  nurse's help with shower, 326
  PHQ (Patient Health Questionnaire), 342
  positive experiences, staying open to, 339
  priorities, 319–320
  quality of life, 319–320
  reasons for admittance to hospital, 318
  relational concerns, 345–346
  relationships, 345–346
  relocation, 349–350
  research on care, 314
  spiritual concerns, 347
  substance abuse, 351
  symptom checklist, 342
  symptom management, 322–324
  techne, 332
  unfavorable experience with student, 326–327
  untenable goals, 351
  VAS (Visual Analog Scales), 342
thalamus, PD and, 66
The Other America (Harrington), 218
The Primacy of Caring (Benner & Wrubel)
  feelings, 132
  mind-body-world relationships, 132
theoretical knowledge, practical knowledge and, 152
things mattering, care as, 28
thinking-in-action, 97
thirdspace, place, 60
time, proximity and, 46
trauma, psychological, xxiii

treatments, delegation fo families, 10
trust and possibility, 170

U

uncertainty, 158
understanding
   background meanings, 25
   living, 25
understanding of self, xviii
undifferentiated oneness, family as, 196
unpredictable motility of PD patients, 64

V

VAS (Visual Analog Scales), 342
Vietnam War veterans, 80
view from nowhere, 24
virtue
   iterativeness, 95
      phronesis and, 95
virtuous mean (Aristotle), 284–285

W

war metaphors, 262, 263
war veterans, 80
will to mastery, 30
wisdom, description, 97
work, as stress, 81
world as giant medical institution, 262
world as place, 60
world-defining commitments, 274
world-transforming identity, 27

X–Y–Z

yoga, 171–172, 175